Medical Informatics

Medical Informatics

Medical Informatics

Editor: Isabel Madison

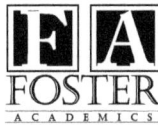

FA
FOSTER
ACADEMICS

www.fosteracademics.com

www.fosteracademics.com

FA
FOSTER
ACADEMICS

Cataloging-in-Publication Data

Medical informatics / edited by Isabel Madison.
    p. cm.
Includes bibliographical references and index.
ISBN 978-1-63242-671-0
1. Medical informatics. 2. Medicine--Data processing.
3. Medical care--Technological innovations. 4. Medical technology. I. Madison, Isabel.
R858 .M43 2019
610.285--dc23

Foster Academics,
118-35 Queens Blvd., Suite 400,
Forest Hills, NY 11375, USA

ISBN 978-1-63242-671-0 (Hardback)

Contents

Permissions

List of Contributors

Index

Preface

Medical informatics, also known as health care informatics, is a branch of health care involving the application of information engineering to the field of health care. It is a field which uses health information technology for improving health care. It generally revolves around the study of the IT-based innovations in planning, delivery and management of healthcare services. This includes the methods and devices required for the storage and use of information in health and biomedicine. Some of the common sub-fields of medical informatics include imaging informatics, pathology informatics, clinical bioinformatics, community health informatics, consumer health informatics, etc. This book provides significant information of this discipline to help develop a good understanding of medical informatics and related fields. It strives to provide a fair idea about this area and to help develop a better understanding of the latest advances within this field. The extensive content of this book provides the readers with a thorough understanding of the subject.

All of the data presented henceforth, was collaborated in the wake of recent advancements in the field. The aim of this book is to present the diversified developments from across the globe in a comprehensible manner. The opinions expressed in each chapter belong solely to the contributing authors. Their interpretations of the topics are the integral part of this book, which I have carefully compiled for a better understanding of the readers.

At the end, I would like to thank all those who dedicated their time and efforts for the successful completion of this book. I also wish to convey my gratitude towards my friends and family who supported me at every step.

Editor

Real-Time Tele-Auscultation Consultation Services over the Internet: Effects of the Internet Quality of Service

Sinchai Kamolphiwong, Thossapon Kamolphiwong,
Soontorn Saechow and Verapol Chandeeying

Abstract

A real-time tele-auscultation over the Internet is effective medical services that increase the accessibility of healthcare services to remote areas. However, the quality of auscultation's sounds transmitted over the Internet is the most critical issue, especially in real-time service. Packet loss and packet delay variations are the main factors. There is little knowledge of these factors affecting auscultation's sounds transmitted over the Internet. In this work, we investigate the effects of packet loss and packet delay variations, in particular, heart and lung sounds with auscultation's sound over the Internet in real-time services. We have found that both sounds are more sensitive to packet delay variations than packet loss. Lung sounds are more sensitive than heart sounds due to their timing interpretation. Some different levels of packet loss can be tolerated, e.g., 10% for heart sounds and 2% for lung sounds. Packet delay variation boundary of 50 msec is recommended. In addition, we have developed the real-time tele-auscultation prototype that tries to minimize the packet delay variation. We have found that real-time waveform of auscultation's visualization can help physician's confident level for sound interpreting. Some techniques for quality of service improvement are suggested, e.g., noise reduction and user interface (UI).

Keywords: tele-auscultation, e-stethoscope, e-health, tele-medicine, packet loss and delay variations, heart and lung sounds

1. Introduction

Quality of healthcare services in rural areas is a critical issue. Most developing countries are actively on improving the quality of healthcare services with the short and long term policy, increasing healthcare staffs and implementing new technologies are the two wildly example policies [1–3].

Generally, people who live in rural areas receive healthcare services at primary care unit as the first choice. However, a rural healthcare unit has some limitations such as infrastructure, healthcare staff and good/advanced medical equipment. Thus, referral of patients to the secondary or tertiary care unit is used for solving these problems, which lead to cost on traveling and waste of time. The effective care at the primary care units is one of the significant keys, which can improve a quality of healthcare services in rural areas. Telemedicine is one of the main keys, and telemedicine applications can enhance the accessibility of healthcare services through the collaborations between primary care unit and cooperation unit [4–8].

Interactive consulting over the Internet is a cost-effective way between physician and specialist. The real-time applications such as Skype [9–12], Google Hangout [13, 14], FaceTime [15, 16], and WebRTC [17–19] can make good experience to participants like a face-to-face communication. However, the real-time consulting between physician and specialist requires some specific information and equipment which depend on consultation's topic such as stethoscope for listen the body sounds on auscultation process. However, when data are transmitted over the Internet, loss and delay can be occurred, especially its sensitivity in a real-time application. Packet loss [20] and packet delay variations [21] are the two main factors that reduce sound quality in real-time communication, e.g., body sounds from the stethoscope.

In our work, we investigate the effects of using e-stethoscope caused by packet loss and delay in the real-time tele-auscultation system over the Internet.

Significance: There is a little knowledge on the effects caused by packet loss and delay to the real-time tele-auscultation system over the Internet. This work deeply investigates these effects on lung and heart sounds, to see the impacts and factors that influence the quality of tele-auscultation services. We discuss what effects will happen, their causes, and results by varying a number of packet loss, delay variations, and types of lung and heart sounds. It is significantly different from human conversation sounds. We have suggested the percentage of packet loss and packet delay variations to meet some confident level of sound interpreting which can increase the success rate and effective outcomes.

The rest of chapter is organized as follows: Section 2 describes an overview of tele-auscultation including the differences between traditional auscultation and tele-auscultation, system compositions, and types of services. Section 3 presents our prototype system design and development. Section 4 shows the analysis result of the effects of packet loss and packet delay variations of heart and lung sounds over the Internet service. Finally, we conclude of our work in Section 5.

2. Overview of tele-auscultation

Tele-auscultation is a system for providing a remote auscultation to another place. The main challenge for this service is how to find the suitable mechanism to transmit the auscultation's sound over the Internet effectively with an acceptable quality of auscultation's sounds and to find other related supporting systems.

2.1. Differences between traditional auscultation and tele-auscultation

Auscultation is the medical method for sound listening inside the patient body, on detecting and identifying the abnormal sounds [22, 23]. A tele-auscultation provides the medical examination method similar to the traditional one, but the key of tele-auscultation that steps over the traditional auscultation is the mechanism for transmission the auscultation's sounds on long distance. Internet technology and electronic stethoscope are the keys for driven tele-auscultation service. Moreover, experiences on using tele-auscultation may differ from the traditional one, it is not face-to-face and may experience some delay of body sound sent from the remote site. This awareness should be raised when using this service. **Table 1** summarizes the differences between traditional stethoscope and e-stethoscope.

2.2. Compositions of tele-auscultation system

In our study, tele-auscultation can be summarized in three main compositions: stethoscope, client application, and application server. In terms of processes, they are: capturing, processing, transmission, and display. The system overview of tele-auscultation structure is shown in **Figure 1**.

In **Figure 1**, the first component is stethoscope. It is an instrument to capture the sounds in the body, and is used widely in auscultation process [24, 25]. Currently, an e-stethoscope (electronic stethoscope) is a new generation of auscultation's device. It can improve the quality of auscultation sounds [26], as summarized in **Table 1**, and it is a source for transmitting the sounds from the body to the next component. The next component, client application, is software that captures the sounds sent by e-stethoscope. There are two techniques of sound capturing: the modern one is receiving directly from e-stethoscope via the transmission module embedded in the device [27–30], and the older one is receiving from stethoscope's ear tip via audio input device such as microphone [31]. Moreover, the client application is the main processing function for the auscultation's sounds such as improving sound's quality, sounds volume control, encoding, filtering, waveform rendering, transmitting/receiving sound between cooperated components, and sound play out. The last component, application server, is a center for managing the

Properties	Electronic stethoscope	Acoustic stethoscope
Record and playback	Yes/no	No
Volume control & amplification	Yes	No
Noise reduction	Yes	No
Power supply	Batteries	No
Transmission technologies	Bluetooth, RF, USB	No
Chest piece	Single side tunable, button and screen	Single side tunable, dual side tunable (bell and diaphragm)
Tubing	Similar	
Headset		
Sound signal	Digital	Analog

Table 1. Comparison between electronic stethoscope and acoustic stethoscope.

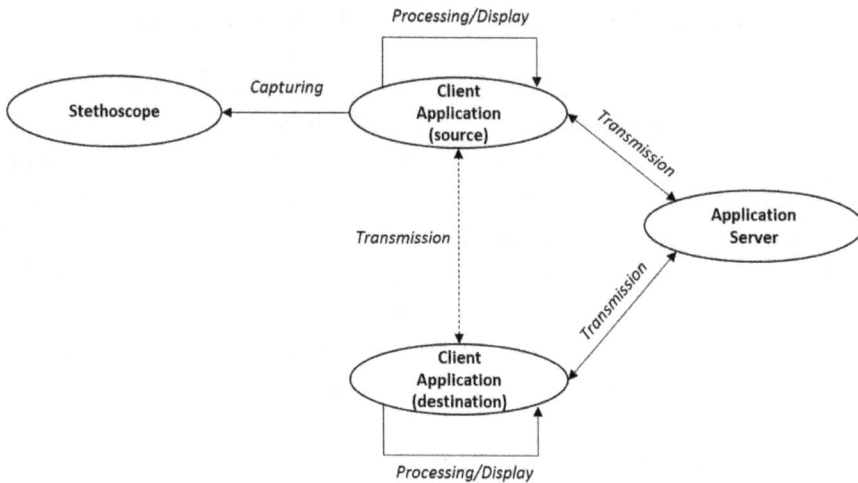

Figure 1. Overview of tele-auscultation architecture.

sessions, signaling, user accounts, forwarding the sounds (for client–server-service model). It should be noted that apart from client-server model, peer-to-peer service model may be considered. However, the server in this latter case may have less service requirements, e.g., for communication establishment, not for media streaming between client and server.

2.3. Types of tele-auscultation services

Synchronous and asynchronous (store-and-forward) are the two main communication types that describe the characteristic of each tele-auscultation service. Synchronous service is an interactive communication between participants [27–31], and auscultation' sound during the live session must be sent and played out immediately. While asynchronous service will store auscultation' sound in the middleware first, and then participants make a request and receive the data later [28, 29]. It seems that today technology with high speed Internet, asynchronous service may have small time delay while sending stored auscultation sounds to the remote site. However, since synchronous service is live session, physician can request different auscultation's sounds (from different body positions) from a patient or healthcare staff immediately to improve healthcare service level. For example, physician may ask healthcare staff to move the stethoscope up/down/left/right from the current position in place, to follow up the result from the sound interpretation, to capture a better sound quality (unclear sound). This will make the service quality of real-time tele-stethoscope much better over asynchronous one. However, the service requires some certain level of QoS, e.g., high speed link capacity. In conclusion, both services have different significant impacts to tele-auscultation services, and it depends on the purpose of usage and what practice scenarios are for of healthcare services.

2.4. Communication models

Client/server and peer-to-peer are the two widely used communication models that describe the characteristic of systems for sharing the media between source unit and destination unit.

In peer-to-peer model, it has no central server for managing the media stream. Each node directly communicates to each other. This will minimize the processing time at the central server as well as communication link time delay. Conversely, client/server model has a central server for managing almost everything, e.g., all information must be passed to the server first. However, for time-based information sharing, the client/server model will be useful. For tele-auscultation services, both models are used: client/server based model [29, 30], and peer-to-peer based model [28].

3. Design and development of a real-time tele-auscultation

We design and develop a real-time tele-auscultation application covering both communication models: peer-to-peer and client/server based models. The model consists of two main components. First component is client application that includes stethoscope controller, session controller, real-time audio waveform, and audio player. Another component is application server that comprises of account management and session management. The server is used for user authentication and session initiation between two client applications. Some more details are as follows:

3.1. Electronic stethoscope

In prototype demonstration, 3 M™ Littmann® Electronic Stethoscope Model 3200 [32] is utilized. The e-stethoscope provides a digital audio which in linear pulse-code modulation (LPCM) format, 4000 Hz of sampling rate and 16 bits per sampling.

As 4000 samples per second is not a standard voice sampling, we need to up-sample to 8000 times per second before putting in Real Time Transport Protocol (RTP) [34]. As a result, the sound quality is improved, but the bandwidth is increased to twice.

3.2. Auscultation's sound capturing

Stethoscope controller performs a connection to e-stethoscope by Bluetooth stack for capturing the auscultation's sound and handling some optional messages of e-stethoscope and other components. In our experiment, we captured the auscultation's sound every 50 msec, which created 400 bytes of audio data per packet. These audio packets will be transmitted to the destination node over the Internet for play-out at the destination.

3.3. Session and audio transmission

The handshaking mechanism is the important signal in peer-to-peer networks. Our prototype uses session initiation protocol (SIP) [33] and non-SIP (Web based signaling) for an initial protocol for real-time session establishing between participants. After completing the connection, the auscultation's sounds will be conveyed in RTP packets. There is no need for the central server participating in the media session.

4. Effects of packet loss and packet delay variations

In this section, study and analysis of auscultation's sounds quality affected by packet loss and packet delay variations in real-time communication over the Internet will be presented.

In our work, we focused and studied the characteristics of two body sounds: cardiac auscultation and lung auscultation. For the first one, cardiac auscultation, it is a method for screening heart sounds and heart murmurs [35]. In cardiac auscultation process, patient positions (left lateral recumbent, sitting and supine) and body locations (aortic area, pulmonic area, tricuspid area, and mitral area) can affect the quality of heart sounds. Particular positions and locations are important to the quality of listening to the specific heart sounds or heart murmurs [36–38]. Heart murmurs are the critical sounds related to the valvular heart disease. Intensity (grade), pitch, timing, and location have described the characteristic of each murmur [36–38]. For the second one, lung auscultation, it is a method for screening abnormal sounds over the lung's areas including front and back of the patient body [39]. Listening to the sounds of inspiration and expiration, together with comparing the intensity and pitch of each breath are the fundamental process for diagnosis the lung sounds [39, 40].

As noted above, a real-time auscultation service over the Internet should ensure a feasible and reliable. Packet loss and packet delay variations are the critical factors that significantly damage the heart and lung sound quality.

4.1. The packet loss and packet delay variation generator

We developed the software that can generate the difference level of packet loss and packet delay variation patterns, to study and analyze the effects to heart and lung sound quality. The software components are described in **Figure 2**.

- Sender: It sends auscultation's sound with a packet size of 400 bytes, 50 msec packet interval time. The following original three heart sounds [41] and five lung sounds [42] are observed, as shown in **Table 2**.

The waveforms of each sound are shown in **Figures 3** and **4**.

- Controller: It is a component for generating the patterns of packet loss and packet delay variations. The loss patterns were generated based on Gilbert-Elliot model [43–45] with 2, 5, 10, and 20% of loss values. The packet delay variation patterns were generated based on Poisson distribution [46] with 50, 60, and 70 msec time delays.

- Receiver: It is a component for converting the received packets to the play out format (LPCM, 4000 Hz, 16 bits, and 1 Mono-channel), with a controlled jitter buffer.

In this experiment, we measured the packet loss and delay variations between different network services. For example, Ethernet network was the Intranet in our experiment site which has a big bandwidth, the 3G/4G network was a service provided by local mobile operators, and ADSL in the remote area was the Internet connection provided by a local service provider. We collected test information for a week at different time. **Table 3** shows the average

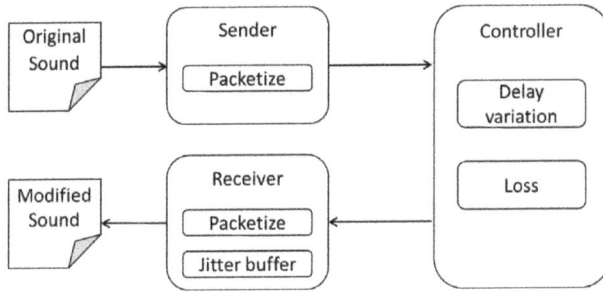

Figure 2. Software components for packet loss and packet delay variations generator.

Heart sounds	Lung sounds
1. Normal heart sound (75 bpm),	1. Coarse crackles (27 bpm),
2. Early systolic murmur (75 bpm),	2. Inspiratory stridor (23 bpm),
3. Pan-systolic murmur (75 bpm).	3. Normal vesicular (16 bpm),
	4. Pleural friction (19 bpm),
	5. Wheezing (27 bpm).

Table 2. The property of heart sounds and lung sounds.

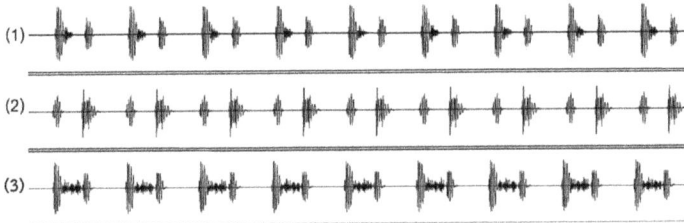

Figure 3. The original heart sounds (1) early systolic murmur, (2) heart normal, and (3) pan-systolic murmur.

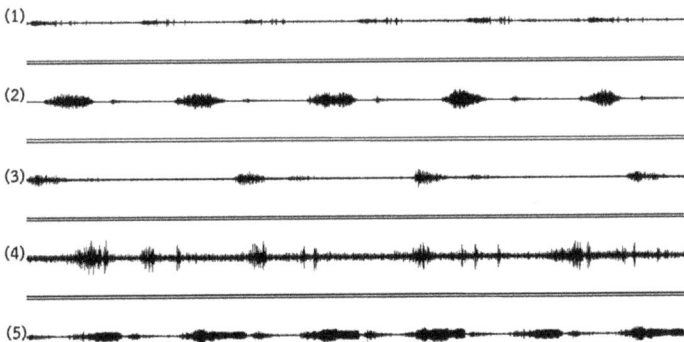

Figure 4. The original lung sounds (1) coarse crackles, (2) inspiratory stridor, (3) normal vesicular, (4) pleural friction, and (5) wheezing.

of packet loss and delays when information was sent across different network services. We noticed that the Intranet gave lowest packet loss and delays while ADSL in the remote area gave higher packet loss and larger delays.

Network types	Packet loss (%)		Packet delay variations (msec)	
	Range	Average	Range	Average
1) Sender: Ethernet network Receiver: Remote area via 3G/4G	0–3	2	10–70	55
2) Sender: Ethernet network Receiver: Ethernet network	0	0	0–5	2
3) Sender: Ethernet network Receiver: Remote area via ADSL	0–30	20	10–150	70

Table 3. Packet loss and delays between different network connection services.

4.2. Distortions of heart and lung sounds

Signal distortion is the alteration in the pulse of heart sound and the breath on lung sound. In our experiment method, we summarize the number of distortion pulses and breaths in a minute duration. Sample pulses of heart sound and breath of lung sound are shown in **Figures 5** and **6**, respectively.

4.2.1. Packet loss

In packet loss experiment, the heart and lung sound with 2, 5, 10, and 20% of packet loss are used.

Of replication five times, the signal distortions of three heart sounds and five lung sounds by comparing the pulse and breathing of each sound with its original sound. The following results are given:

Figure 7 shows the results of packet loss by varying from 2, 5, 10, and 20% for pan-systolic murmur. We can see that shape and position losses are randomly occurred from time to time where a higher value of packet loss gives more damage of shape and position. We tested all other given heart and lung sounds in **Table 2**.

Figure 8 shows sound damage positions of pan-systolic murmur randomly from five times of experiment where 20% of packet loss is applied. We can see that shape and position losses are randomly occurred from time to time. This will make the receiver node in hard condition for the result interpretation.

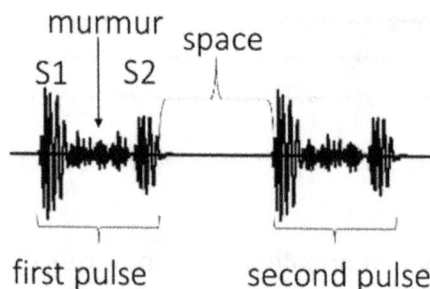

Figure 5. The pulse of hear sound.

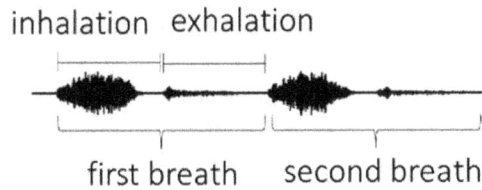

Figure 6. The breath of lung sound.

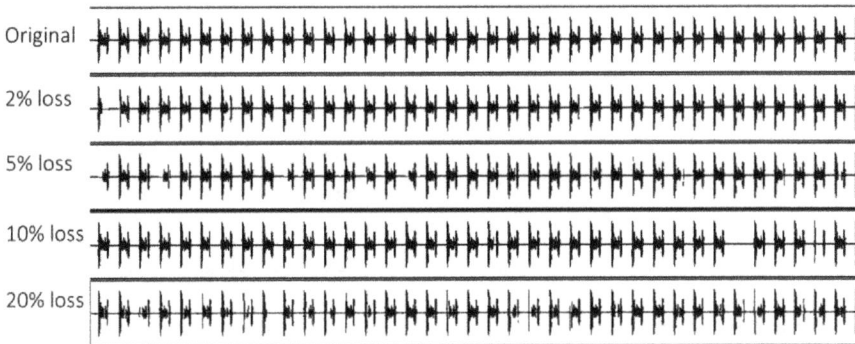

Figure 7. Packet loss varying from 2, 5, 10, 20% for pan-systolic murmur.

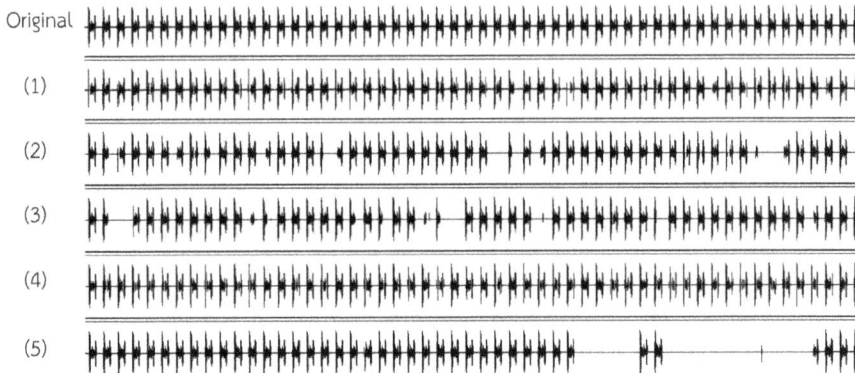

Figure 8. Randomly sound distortions and positions of pan-systolic murmur at 20% packet loss.

Of replication five times, with 2, 5, 10, and 20% of packet loss, the distortions are summarized in **Table 4**. The figures in the table are the percentage of distortions of each sound beats.

From **Table 4**, the increase of packet loss gets along with short-range distortions on heart sounds, but fluctuates and has long-range distortion of lung sounds. All of heart sounds and all of packet loss levels, the percent of distortions are less than 50%. On the other hand, for 2 and 5% of packet loss, the percent of distortions on lung sounds are less than 50%. However, when packet losses are 10 and 20%, the distortions go over 70%.

4.2.2. Packet delay variations

In packet delay variations experiment, the heart and lung sounds are investigated with three different levels of average packet delay variations; 50, 60, and 70 ms. Each delay was tested

Sounds	Packet loss			
	2%	5%	10%	20%
Heart sound				
Early systolic murmur	3	13	28	48
Heart normal	3	16	36	43
Pan-systolic murmur	6	24	27	48
Lung sound				
Coarse crackles	11	25	68	86
Inspiratory stridor	13	48	71	91
Normal vesicular	23	27	69	94
Pleural friction	25	46	68	98
Wheezing	20	37	79	85

Table 4. Percent of distortions among various heart and lung sounds on each level of packet loss.

for five times. **Figure 9** shows sample results of replication five times, the distortions of three heart sounds/five lung sounds by comparing the pulse and breathing of each sound with its original sound are shown in **Table 2**.

Of replication five times, the distortions of three heart sounds/five lung sounds by comparing the pulse and breathing of each sound with its original sound are shown in **Table 5**.

From **Table 5**, the packet delay variations at 50 msec get a short-range distortion on both heart and lung sounds and high distortion on both heart and lung sounds at 60 to 70 ms of packet delay variations. We can see that increasing a small delay variation, e.g., from 50 to 60 msec, significantly impact the sound distortion.

4.3. Evaluation of sound quality by assessor: packet loss

Ten medical professionals (they are medical doctors and nurses) who experience on auscultation operation at least 2 years participated in this evaluation. All of them are binding tests. Each person listens to three heart sounds/five lung sounds at packet loss of 2, 5, 10, and 20% without knowing which sound he or she is listening. According to the listening results, they

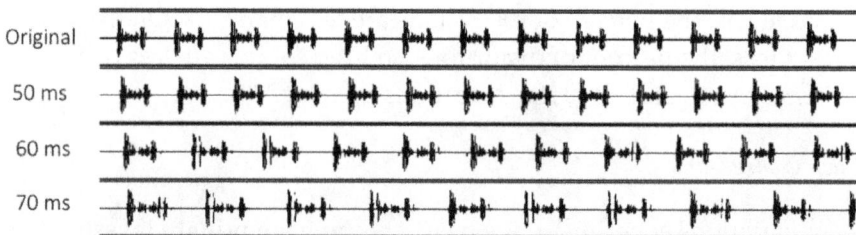

Figure 9. The result of packet delay variations for pan-systolic murmur.

Sounds	Packet delay variations (msec)		
	50	60	70
Heart sounds			
Early systolic murmur	3	83	100
Heart normal	3	72	100
Pan-systolic murmur	0	100	100
Lung sounds			
Coarse crackles	4	100	100
Inspiratory stridor	0	100	100
Normal vesicular	13	100	100
Pleural friction	5	100	100
Wheezing	15	100	100

Table 5. Percent of distortion among various heart and lung sounds on each level of packet delay variations.

indicated the type of sound with the confident level. The test result is shown in **Table 6**. It seems that most of them can detect normal heart, pan-systolic murmur, early systolic murmur, and normal vesicular sounds when a small packet loss is applied, e.g., less than 10%. More than 90% can correctly detect all heart sounds at 2–20% of packet loss. Percentage of correct detection on lung sounds depends on the type of lung sounds and level of packet loss.

4.4. Analysis of the effects of packet loss and packet delay variations

From the experiment of packet loss and packet delay variations, we analyzed the results as follows:

Sounds	Packet loss			
	2%	5%	10%	20%
Heart sounds				
Heart normal	100	100	100	90
Pan-systolic murmur	100	100	100	90
Early systolic murmur	100	90	90	90
Lung sounds				
Normal vesicular	100	100	90	60
Wheezing	100	90	80	30
Coarse crackles	70	60	40	70
Inspiratory stridor	90	80	50	70
Pleural friction	60	60	50	50

Table 6. Percent of correct detection on each sound.

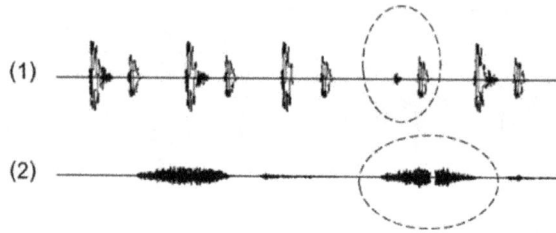

Figure 10. Sound discontinuity by packet loss, (1) early systolic murmur and (2) inspiratory stridor.

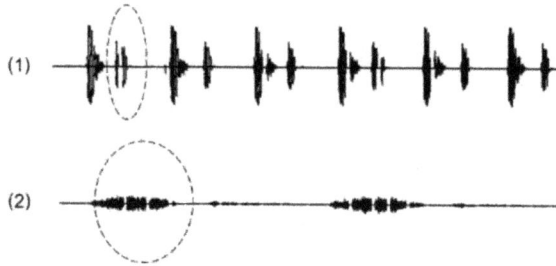

Figure 11. Sound discontinuity by packet delay variations, (1) early systolic murmur and (2) inspiratory stridor.

4.4.1. Sound missing and splitting

Auscultation method requires continued sound on each cycle to recognize the rhythm, pitch, and intensity. Packet loss and packet delay variations destroy the sounds continuity in different patterns randomly. Packet loss makes missing in some positions of sound, as shown in **Figure 10**, and packet delay variation makes split in some positions of sound, as shown in **Figure 11**.

Sound missing consists of two patterns: (1) either pulse or breath missing, and (2) some parts of pulse or breath missing, as shown in **Figure 12**. A pulse or breath missing is caused by burst loss on transmission process which is narrow range damage to heart and lung sounds. For another pattern, some parts of pulses or breaths missing, it is caused by uncertain pattern loss on transmission process. This pattern is wide range damage to heart and lung sounds. The increase of packet loss level cannot specify the pattern of sound discontinuity; it can only increase the missing sound.

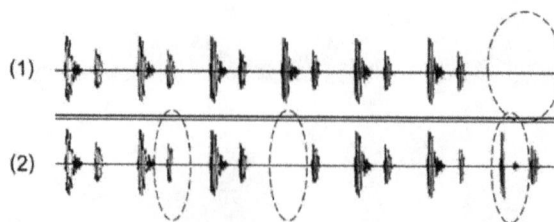

Figure 12. Behaviors of sound discontinuity on early systolic murmur after packet loss occurred, (1) a pulse and (2) some part of pulse.

4.4.2. *Pulse transformation*

Transformation is the effect caused by packet loss. When the sound missing in some positions like murmur shape, it may lead to transformation to another type, and pulse transformation

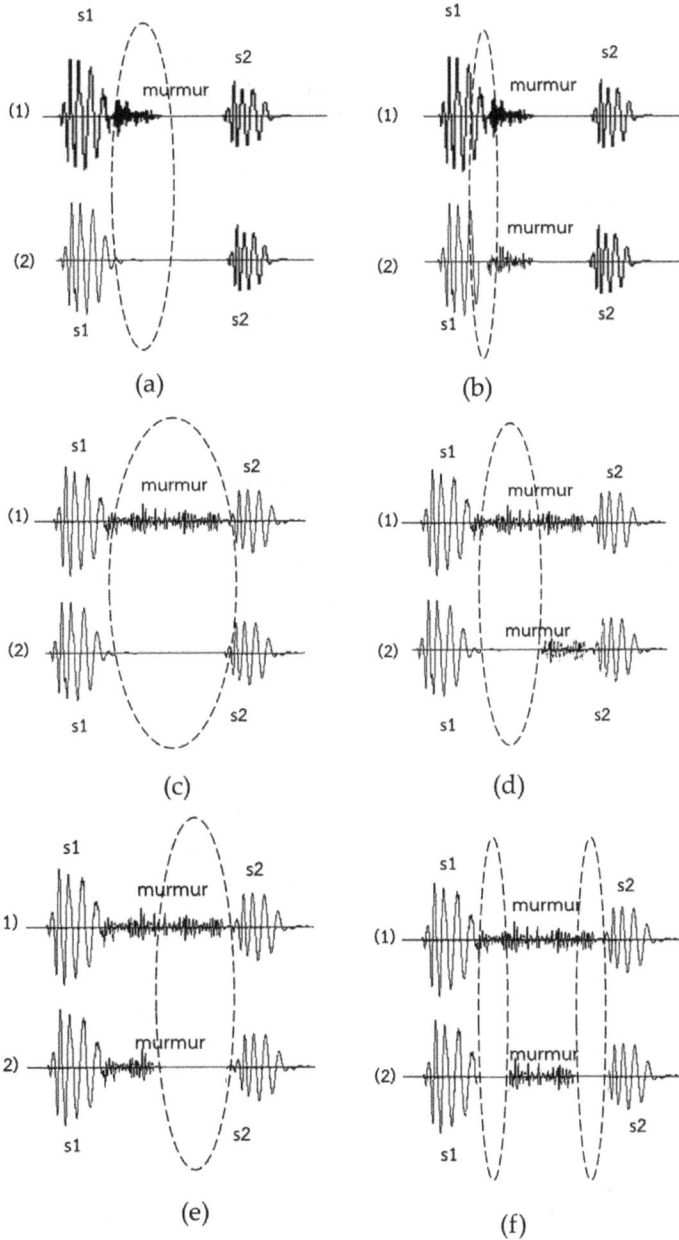

Figure 13. Samples of pulse transformations. (a) Early systolic murmur to heart normal (1) early systolic murmur (2) heart normal, (b) early systolic murmur to mid systolic murmur (1) early systolic murmur (2) mid-systolic murmur, (c) pan-systolic murmur to heart normal (1) pan-systolic murmur (2) heart normal, (d) pan-systolic murmur to late systolic murmur (1) pan-systolic murmur (2) late systolic murmur, (e) pan-systolic murmur to early systolic murmur (1) pan-systolic murmur (2) early systolic murmur, (f) pan-systolic murmur to mid systolic murmur (1) pan-systolic murmur (2) mid systolic murmur.

does not happen every pulse. The following result analysis of pulse transformation, as some examples, are as follows: Early systolic murmur sound transforms to normal heart sound, is a result of missing of the murmur shape but S1 and S2 are still remaining, as shown in **Figure 13(a)**. Transformation of early systolic murmur to mid-systolic murmur is a result of missing of the beginning part of murmur shape, as shown in **Figure 13(b)**. Transformation of pan-systolic murmur to normal heart sound is a result of missing a murmur shape, as shown in **Figure 13(c)**. Transformation of pan-systolic murmur to late systolic murmur is a result of missing of the first half of murmur shape, as shown in **Figure 13(d)**. Transformation of pan-systolic murmur to early systolic murmur is a result of missing of the second half of murmur shape, as shown in **Figure 13(e)**. Transformation of pan-systolic murmur to mid systolic murmur is a result of missing of the beginning part and tail of murmur shape, as shown in **Figure 13(f)**.

5. Design for improving the quality of service

Voice quality factors have been known for a long time, e.g., ITU guideline and standards [47], in tele-medicine applications, we do need to re-apply some techniques for this particular situation. The following design and implementation should be considered:

- ITU provides PLC (Packet loss concealment) technique for digital voice communications. However, waveform substitution (one technique in PLC) may not be appropriate. Zero insertion or silent insertion (another one in PLC) is more appropriate,

- Jitter buffer: jitter adaptation technique is deployed to reduce the effect of delay fluctuation due to the late or early arrival of voice packets (**Figure 14**). This will help the receiver-end hears sound in more comfortable level. However, due to real-time communication session condition, the buffer of delay absorption should be limited; we can have a small jitter buffer, e.g., few hundreds of milliseconds. In our experiment, 500 msec buffering (or 10 packets buffering) seems to be good enough. This will be traffic engineering choice to vary this figure.

- Noise removing: as mentioned, the device is operated remotely, and we noticed that moving of stethoscope creates a lot of noise. This creates an uncomfortable situation to the remote side. We have applied two stages noise filtering technique. The first stage looks at noise within a single voice packet (50 msec time interval), while the second stage evaluates the average noise energy for three consecutive packets. This will help a doctor in remote side working in convenience and comfortable way.

We have shown above that packet loss and delay will affect the quality of hearing, as a result, symptom determining may be hesitated. According to our prototype testing, most physicians at the remote side are happy with an e-stethoscope signal showing on the screen. This will help the interpretation confidence level after they are familiar with. We tested UI with packet loss and delay indicator, as shown in **Figure 15**, to raise awareness of a doctor during interacting operation. The levels of packet loss and delay can be easily noticed, for example, green color means there is no packet loss and delay (or very few, e.g., 1%), yellow color means there a few packet loss and delay (e.g., 5%), red color means there are high packet loss and delay

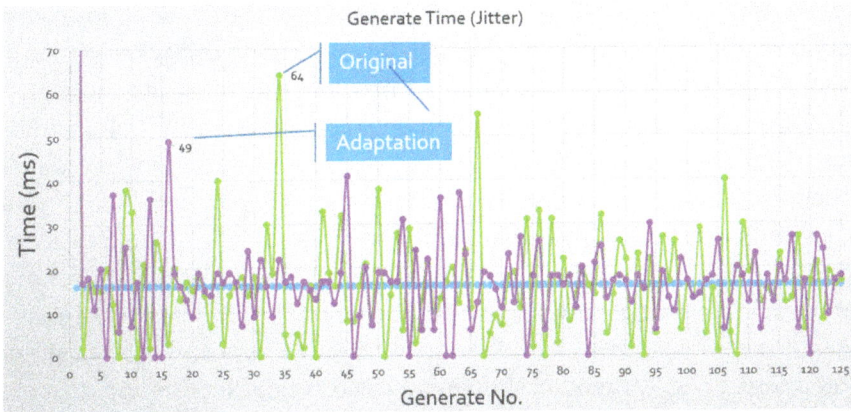

Figure 14. Jitter adaptation for time delay variation reduction.

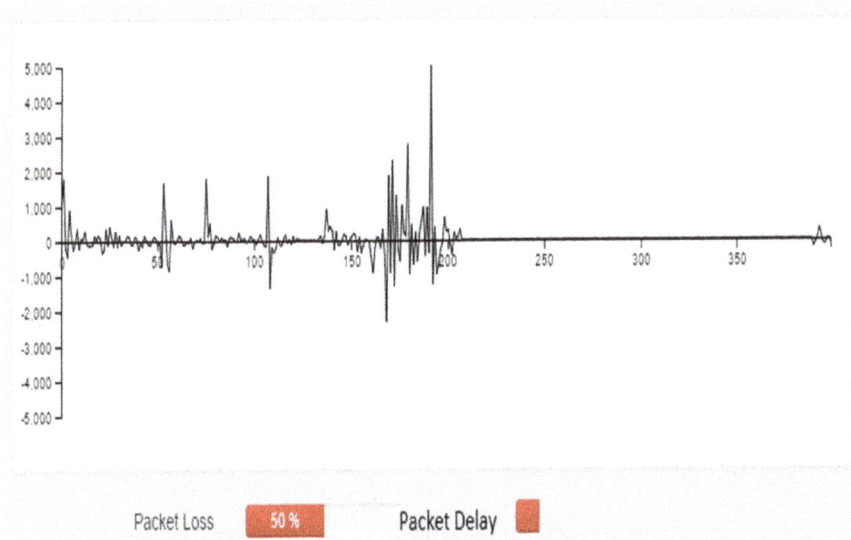

Figure 15. Real-time e-stethoscope signal with packet loss and packet delay indicators.

(e.g., more than 10%). We have concluded that with this UI designed, it helps for awareness of doctor's confidential level. Moreover, packet loss and delay pontificating levels can be adjusted according to the doctor experience.

6. Conclusion

This work studies the effects of packet loss and packet delay variations to real-time tele-auscultation services over the Internet. We categorize communications models of tele-auscultation services to asynchronous and synchronous, client/server and peer-to-peer. Some important compositions of tele-auscultation are drawn out with prototype software demonstration. We then focus and study the characteristics of two body sounds: cardiac auscultation and lung auscultation when these sounds are transmitted on the Internet in real-time applications.

From our experiment results, based on medical professional staff verification, we have found that both sounds are more sensitive to packet delay variations than packet loss. Lung sound is more sensitive than heart sound due to its timing interpretation, to recognize the rhythm, pitch, and intensity. Some different levels of packet loss can be tolerated for both sounds, e.g., 10% for heart sounds, 2% for lung sounds. However, packet delay variation boundary of 50 msec is recommended. Based on our analysis, sound missing and split, and pulse transformations are the two factors that affect the sound quality. The pulse transformation result may lead to misinterpreting of abnormal sounds. We have also found that making distinct normal sounds is more accurate than abnormal sounds. In addition to our prototype software, we have concluded that real-time waveform of auscultation's visualization can help physician confident level for sound interpreting. Moreover, showing the ratio of packet loss and delay variations in clear icon will raise awareness and increase the success rate and effective outcomes.

Acknowledgements

This work is supported by the Higher Education Research Promotion and National Research University Project of Thailand, Office of the Higher Education Commission (under the funding no. MED540548S at Prince of Songkla University).

Author details

Sinchai Kamolphiwong[1]*, Thossapon Kamolphiwong[1], Soontorn Saechow[1] and Verapol Chandeeying[2]

*Address all correspondence to: sinchai.k@psu.ac.th

1 Department of Computer Engineering, Faculty of Engineering, Prince of Songkla University, Hatyai, Songkla, Thailand

2 Faculty of Medicine, University of Phayao, Muang, Phayao, Thailand

References

[1] World Health Organization. Increasing Access to Health Workers in Remote and Rural Areas Through Improved Retention: Global policy recommendations. World Health Organization; 2010

[2] Dummer TJB, Cook IG. Exploring China's rural health crisis: Processes and policy implications. Health Policy. 2007;**83**(1):1-16

[3] Agyepong IA, Adjei S. Public social policy development and implementation: A case study of the Ghana National Health Insurance scheme. Health Policy and Planning. 2008;**23**(2):150-160

[4]   World Health Organization. Telemedicine: Opportunities and Developments in Member States: Report on the Second Global Survey on eHealth. World Health Organization; 2010

[5]   Kijsanayotin B, Kasitipradith N, Pannarunothai S. eHealth in Thailand: The current status. Studies in Health Technology and Informatics. 2010;**160**(Pt 1):376

[6]   Ekeland AG, Bowes A, Flottorp S. Effectiveness of telemedicine: A systematic review of reviews. International Journal of Medical Informatics. 2010;**79**(11):736-771

[7]   Dávalos ME, French MT, Burdick AE, Simmons SC. Economic evaluation of telemedicine: Review of the literature and research guidelines for benefit–cost analysis. Telemedicine and e-Health. 2009;**15**(10):933-948

[8]   Eron L. Telemedicine: The future of outpatient therapy?. Clinical Infectious Diseases. 2010;**51**(Supplement no 2):S224-S230

[9]   Armfield NR, Bradford M, Bradford NK. The clinical use of Skype—For which patients, with which problems and in which settings? A snapshot review of the literature. International Journal of Medical Informatics. 2015;**84**(10):737-742

[10] Nield M, Hoo GW. Real-time telehealth for COPD self-management using skype™. COPD: Journal of Chronic Obstructive Pulmonary Disease. 2012;**9**(6):611-619

[11] Reynolds HN, Rogove H, Bander J, McCambridge M, Cowboy E, Niemeier M. A working lexicon for the tele-intensive care unit: We need to define tele-intensive care unit to grow and understand it. Telemedicine and e-Health. 2011;**17**(10):773-783

[12] Brecher DB. The use of Skype in a community hospital inpatient palliative medicine consultation service. Journal of Palliative Medicine. 2013;**16**(1):110-112

[13] Engle X, Aird J, Tho L, Bintcliffe F, Monsell F, Gollogly J, Noor S. Combining continuing education with expert consultation via telemedicine in Cambodia. Tropical Doctor. 2013:0049475513515654

[14] Lee JF, Schieltz KM, Suess AN, Wacker DP, Romani PW, Lindgren SD, Kopelman TG, Dalmau YCP. Guidelines for developing telehealth services and troubleshooting problems with telehealth technology when coaching parents to conduct functional analyses and functional communication training in their homes. Behavior Analysis in Practice. 2015;**8**(2):190-200

[15] Armstrong DG, Giovinco N, Mills JL, Rogers LC. FaceTime for physicians: Using real time mobile phone–based videoconferencing to augment diagnosis and care in telemedicine. Eplasty. 2011;**11**

[16] Brandt R, Hensley D. Teledermatology: The use of ubiquitous technology to redefine traditional medical instruction, collaboration, and consultation. The Journal of Clinical and Aesthetic Dermatology. 2012;**5**(11):35

[17] Cola C, Valean H. E-health appointment solution, a web based approach. In: Proceedings of E-Health and Bioengineering Conference (EHB), IEEE; 2015. p. 1-4

[18] Vidul AP, Hari S, Pranave KP, Vysakh KJ, Archana KR. Telemedicine for emergency care management using WebRTC. In: Proceedings of Advances in Computing,

Communications and Informatics (ICACCI), International Conference on, IEEE; 2015. pp. 1741-1745

[19] Jang-Jaccard J, Nepal S, Celler B, Yan B. WebRTC-based video conferencing service for telehealth. Computing. 2016;**98**(1-2):169-193

[20] Bolot Jean-Chrysotome. End-to-end packet delay and loss behavior in the internet. In: ACM SIGCOMM Computer Communication Review. Vol. 23, No. 4. New York, NY, USA: ACM; 1993. pp. 289-298

[21] Demichelis C, Chimento P. "IP Packet Delay Variation Metric for IP Performance Metrics (IPPM); 2002

[22] Dorland's Medical Dictionary for Health Consumers. S.v. "auscultation". Available from: http://medical-dictionary.thefreedictionary.com/auscultation [Accessed: February 10, 2016]

[23] The American Heritage® Medical Dictionary. S.v. "auscultation". Available from: http://medical-dictionary.thefreedictionary.com/auscultation, [Accessed: February 10, 2016]

[24] Miller-Keane Encyclopedia and Dictionary of Medicine, Nursing, and Allied Health. 7th edition. S.v. "stethoscope". Available from: http://medical-dictionary.thefreedictionary.com/stethoscope. [Accessed: February 10, 2016]

[25] McGraw-Hill Concise Dictionary of Modern Medicine. S.v. "stethoscope". Retrieved February 10 2016 from: http://medical-dictionary.thefreedictionary.com/stethoscope

[26] Myint WW, Dillard B. An electronic stethoscope with diagnosis capability. In System Theory, 2001. In: Proceedings of the 33rd Southeastern Symposium on, IEEE; 2001. pp. 133-137

[27] Johanson M, Gustafsson M, Johansson L-A. A remote auscultation tool for advanced home health-care. Journal of Telemedicine and Telecare. 2002;**8**(2):45-46

[28] Xu, Lisheng, Ying Wang, Yue Wang, Ning Geng, Yao Jiang, Guanxiong Wang, Jiajin Liu, and Cong Feng. "The design and implementation of telemedical consulting system for auscultation." In: Proceedings of 2011 IEEE International Conference on Information and Automation, IEEE; 2011. pp. 242-247

[29] McMechan, Christian, Irina Morozov, Aaron Patten, and Poman So. "Tele-auscultation system." In: Proceedings of Broadband and Wireless Computing, Communication and Applications (BWCCA), 2011 International Conference on, IEEE; 2011. pp. 478-481

[30] Foche-Perez I, Ramirez-Payba R, Hirigoyen-Emparanza G, Balducci-Gonzalez F, Simo-Reigadas F-J, Seoane-Pascual J, Corral-Peñafiel J, Martinez-Fernandez A. An open real-time tele-stethoscopy system. BioMedical Engineering. 1186;**11**(2012):57

[31] Lu B-Y, Hsu L-Y, Wu H-D, Hsueh M-L, Sing S-S, Tang R-H, Su M-J, Wang J-C, Lai J-S. Real-time mobile-to-mobile stethoscope for distant healthcare. In: Proceedings of Advanced Communication Technology (ICACT), 2014 16th International Conference on, IEEE. 2014. pp. 151-156

[32] 3M™ Littmann® stethoscope. Electronic Stethoscope Model 3200. Internet: http://solutions.3m.com/wps/portal/3M/en_US/Littmann/stethoscope/electronic-auscultation/model-3000-series/ [Accessed: June 10, 2015]

[33] Rosenberg, Jonathan, Henning Schulzrinne, Gonzalo Camarillo, Alan Johnston, Jon Peterson, Robert Sparks, Mark Handley, and Eve Schooler. SIP: Session Initiation Protocol. Vol. 23. RFC 3261, Internet Engineering Task Force; 2002

[34] Jacobson V, Frederick R, Casner S, Schulzrinne H. RTP: A transport protocol for real-time applications. IETF RFC. 2003:3550

[35] Miller-Keane Encyclopedia and Dictionary of Medicine, Nursing, and Allied Health. 7th Edition. S.v. "cardiac auscultation". Available from http://medical-dictionary.thefreedictionary.com/Cardiac+auscultation [Accessed: June 10, 2015]

[36] Tavel ME. Cardiac auscultation a glorious past—And it does have a future! Circulation. 2006;**113**(9):1255-1259

[37] Chizner MA. Cardiac auscultation: Rediscovering the lost art. Current Problems in Cardiology. 2008;**33**(7):326-408

[38] Mangione S, Nieman LZ, Gracely E, Kaye D. The teaching and practice of cardiac auscultation during internal medicine and cardiology training: A nationwide survey. Annals of Internal Medicine. 1993;**119**(1):47-54

[39] Bohadana A, Izbicki G, Kraman SS. Fundamentals of lung auscultation. New England Journal of Medicine. 2014;**370**(8):744-751

[40] Scott PR. Lung auscultation recordings from normal sheep and from sheep with well-defined respiratory tract pathology. Small Ruminant Research. 2010;**92**(1):104-107

[41] 3M™ Littmann® stethoscope. Basic Heart Sounds Course. Available from: http://www.littmann.ca/wps/portal/3M/en_CA/3M-Littmann-CA/stethoscope/littmann-learning-institute/heart-lung-sounds/heart-sounds/. [Accessed: June 10, 2015]

[42] 3M™ Littmann® stethoscope. Listen to Lung Sounds. Available from: http://www.littmann.ca/wps/portal/3M/en_CA/3M-Littmann-CA/stethoscope/littmann-learning-institute/heart-lung-sounds/lung-sounds/. [Accessed: June 10, 06]

[43] Gilbert EN. Capacity of a burst-noise channel. Bell System Technical Journal. 1960;**39**(5):1253-1265

[44] Elliott EO. Estimates of error rates for codes on burst-noise channels. Bell System Technical Journal. 1963;**42**(5):1977-1997

[45] Haßlinger G, Hohlfeld O. The Gilbert-Elliott model for packet loss in real time services on the internet. In: Proceedings of Measuring, Modelling and Evaluation of Computer and Communication Systems (MMB), 14th GI/ITG Conference. 2008. pp. 1-15

[46] Saaty TL. Elements of Queueing Theory: With Applications. New York: McGraw-Hill; 1961

[47] ITU-T Recommendations G.114 (05/2003). Available from: https://www.itu.int/rec/T-REC-G.114/en [Accessed: June 10, 2015]

2

An mHealth Technology for Chronic Wound Management

Marcia R. Friesen, Bennet Gigliotti and
Tik Wai (Kiral) Poon

Abstract

Increasingly, mobile consumer electronic devices are able to make meaningful applications in healthcare, and this chapter discusses the development of a mHealth app called SmartWoundCare, designed to document and assess chronic wounds on smartphones and tablets. Pressure ulcers (bedsores) were selected as the application area for SmartWoundCare due to their pervasiveness in healthcare and their associated impacts on patients' quality of life and mortality, and electronic documentation is considered as an important intervention in pressure ulcer prevention and treatment. The chapter reviews the design of SmartWoundCare on Android and iOS platforms. Its benefits over paper-based charting include automatically generated wound histories in graph and text formats, alerts and notifications for user-set conditions, wound image galleries, and positioning for telehealth consultation by transmitting wound data across sites. The mobile app was implemented in a user trial in a long-term care facility in Winnipeg, Canada, and the user trial illuminated that a key benefit of SmartWoundCare was the ability to take wound photographs. This feature had benefits for patients as well as caregivers. Consequently, algorithms were developed to analyse wound images for size and colour to provide additional indicators of wound progression.

Keywords: wound care, pressure ulcers, wound management, mHealth, mobile app

1. Introduction and background

Increasingly, mobile consumer electronic devices are able to make meaningful applications in mobile health or mHealth, defined as the delivery of healthcare and healthcare support through mobile devices. For example, there are apps that allow users to track diet and fitness, health condition monitoring (e.g. diabetes [1]; arthritis [2]), and using mobile devices to replace paper records and share information between multiple healthcare providers [3].

This chapter overviews the development of a mHealth app called SmartWoundCare, designed to document and assess chronic wounds on Android and iOS smartphones and tablets. The chapter reviews the design of SmartWoundCare, the results of a user trial in a long-term care facility in Winnipeg, Canada, and the subsequent development of algorithms to provide automated analysis of wound images for wound size and colour.

The initial application area is pressure ulcers, which is also known as bedsores. However, the app is easily applicable to other wounds as well, such as venous leg ulcers, diabetic foot ulcers, and surgical wounds.

1.1. Pressure ulcers as the application area

Decubitus ulcers are more commonly referred to as pressure ulcers or bedsores. They are injuries to the skin, or skin lesions which may extend to underlying tissues. Pressure ulcers typically occur over bony areas of the body as a result of skin pressure and friction when an individual sits or lies in one position for a long time. As such, pressure ulcers often occur in the elderly population and people who may be relatively immobile due to other illness or injury. Bedsores are preventable, but easily aggravated with heat and humidity at the wound site once they are present. Bedsores are also regrettably common, with the incidence of pressure ulcers reported to be as high has 30% in non-acute care settings, with an average incidence rate of 25% over all types of healthcare facilities [4, 5].

Pressure ulcers have numerous negative impacts on patients, both in immediate comfort and well-being and in long-term quality of life. When they develop after a patient is admitted to hospital for other conditions, they can lengthen the patient's overall stay and complicate their overall healing. There are also numerous quality of life impacts reported including the psycho-emotional impacts of chronic pain and the negative impacts of social isolation when patients' movements are significantly impaired. A pressure ulcer starts as a seemingly minor skin wound and obscures its significant risk. Pressure ulcers are noted to be the second leading iatrogenic cause of death. From an institutional perspective, pressure ulcers treatment is also costly to the healthcare system [6–11].

There are many standard patient treatments used to prevent pressure ulcers in patients who are known to be at risk. These include regularly turning patients, optimizing diet and nutrition, caring for skin before pressure ulcers occur, and using pressure mattresses, pillows, and other supports to relieve pressure [12]. However, studies have also identified that due to the chronic and often long-term duration of pressure ulcers, significant information about the wound over time can become obscured when documentation is not standardized, when risk assessments are not integral to the regular wound assessment protocol, or when assessments are incomplete or lack detail. In part, standardized forms – designed to capture all possible types of pressure ulcers – often become too unwieldy for healthcare workers with heavy patient loads to use effectively [13–15].

In many other areas of healthcare delivery, electronic health (eHealth) is being examined for its promise to increase the overall efficiency of a healthcare system and to improve patient outcomes. As eHealth grows in scope and maturity, its potential includes improvements and enhancements to patient safety, health outcomes, financial efficiencies, and communication between multiple healthcare providers.

When considering the health burden of pressure ulcers, the area of electronic medical records (EMR) within eHealth is of particular interest. In the research literature, EMRs are reported to have positive impacts on the quality of care and to reduce the reliance or use of care [16].

Several studies examined the impact of EMRs relative to chronic wounds specifically. In one, an EMR system simplified wound evaluation and treatment. In this case, the impact is highly dependent on a standardized protocol for taking pictures of the wound [17]. In another study, the financial benefits of home telehealth in treating bedsores were examined. The findings indicated low-cost technologies did lead to cost savings, whereas high-cost technologies did not have that benefit. The study also determined that home telehealth could decrease the prevalence of advanced stage pressure ulcers [18]. However, not all EMR systems for wound care are effective. Other research identified that common problems with wound EMRs included redundancy or the opposite situation where the platform was not flexible or detailed enough to consider all potential types of wounds. Other issues included the lack of standard vocabulary, and custom-built EMRs which were not transferable to include or integrate with other medical records or across facilities [19].

While EMRs and other forms of electronic documentation are not a panacea, there is emerging evidence that when properly designed, they can potentially lead to better communication, better patient information and wound charting, and ultimately improved patient care and health outcomes. The work outlined in this chapter follows this anticipation that better compliance in documenting wound care, higher consistency in how a wound is documented, and the added intelligence provided by the app relative to alerts and information presentation can influence health outcomes.

2. Mobile apps for wound management

To date, many eHealth technologies have been and are being developed; however, they are not well-catalogued. Relative to wound care, MediSense, WoundRounds, and How2Trak offer web-based and/or mobile interfaces for wound management. In 2013, WoundMAP Pump, Ulcercare, and Wound Mender entered the stage of wound care apps in various stages of development [20].

2.1. SmartWoundCare system design

SmartWoundCare is similarly a mobile app for Android and iOS devices, developed in a computer engineering research lab at the University of Manitoba, Canada. SmartWoundCare was designed to replace the paper chart used in the Winnipeg Regional Health Authority

(WRHA) for pressure ulcer management. The WRHA is a publicly funded system which includes both services and facilities. It serves over 700,000 people and supports referral services to another 500,000 people outside of its boundaries in hospitals, personal care homes, as well as a home care program. Over 28,000 people are employed by the WRHA in over 200 facilities.

As its core functionality, SmartWoundCare allows nurses and other healthcare providers to replicate the information that would be entered on a paper chart. A user can create a new patient record, view an existing patient's record, enter new wounds, and assess existing wounds using the Pressure Ulcer Scale for Healing (PUSH tool) [21], Braden Scale [22], and the Bates-Jensen tool [23]. Several configurations were considered, in that one device could be associated with a given patient, and each nurse or other healthcare provider who cares for that patient would enter information on that patient's unique device. However, the model chosen was to associate the device with an individual nurse or other healthcare provider, who would use the device with all of their patients on that shift, and then transfer the device to the healthcare provider on the next shift.

As with all software, some general design objectives were established. These included keeping the user interface as simple as possible, using colours and other cues to focus the user's attention on important information, minimizing the steps needed to complete tasks, aligning the flow of information with emerging standard expectations from users ("look and feel"), and using the user's input to guide them to the applicable areas (and conversely, using the user's input to skip over areas not relevant for the particular patient or the particular wound). In light of the small screen size of a smartphone or tablet device, free-form comments in data entry are discouraged by design. Entering data from pre-set menu options is designed to reduce errors and to enable better comparisons between assessments, even when completed by different people. In a large-scale rollout within a facility or a healthcare region, attention would also need to be given to battery life of the device, protocols for infection control, and the EMR as part of the legal medical record.

Beyond the duplication of paper-based charting, SmartWoundCare was designed for several intended benefits:

1. *Data sharing between multiple healthcare providers:*the potential to seek consultation between multiple healthcare providers, including wound clinicians, physicians, allied health professionals (e.g. occupational therapy), and other specialists as needed. This potential reduces the need to transport the patient between facilities, saving the patient considerable discomfort and stress, and saving cost in the overall wound treatment. Just as significantly, the timeliness of interventions and changes in the direction of care can be improved. Information sharing (i.e. a telehealth framework) can occur within a given facility, within the same community, or between major centres and remote communities where remote communities do not have specialized health services. In Canada, with a small population living in a large geographical area, this is of particular relevance.

2. *Data organization and interpretation:*

    • Alerts: When logging into SmartWoundCare, the user will see a list of alerts, including wounds that are due for re-assessment and wounds that are deteriorating. The specific parameters for the alerts (days between assessments, criteria used to determine deterioration) can be set by the user.

- Because users have individual preferences on how they best understand data, Smart-WoundCare presents wound histories in three formats: text, graph, and photographs. Text histories allow a user to scroll through a summary of the main wound parameters from one assessment to the next. Graph histories plot an overall wound score (e.g. generated from the PUSH tool) against time. Using the smartphone or tablet devices' built-in cameras, users can also add wound photographs to the record, and scroll through the images in a chronological gallery for each individual wound.

By design, the benefit of SmartWoundCare is its potential as an EMR, either on a stand-alone basis or integrated into a wider EMR system within a facility or region. As such, privacy of data is a non-negotiable concern. In its current form, SmartWoundCare requires each user to set up a unique user ID and password to facilitate a secure login and the login is restricted to that device. When envisioning a fully networked application within a facility or wider region, SmartWoundCare access rights would be confirmed by a secure connection to a server storing all information. Connections would be via cellular or Wi-Fi, relying on all standard Internet security protocols. In that case, all login IDs and passwords would be managed centrally by a server-side application rather than a device-based login. An additional benefit of a central server, which could be facility-specific or shared between several facilities, is the potential for additional data analysis in a Big Data framework. For example, when large datasets are available centrally in standard formats, they can be examined for anomalies, trends, and correlations that ultimately feed into the body of knowledge for pressure ulcer treatment.

Selected screenshots of SmartWoundCare (iOS version) are shown in **Figures 1–5**.

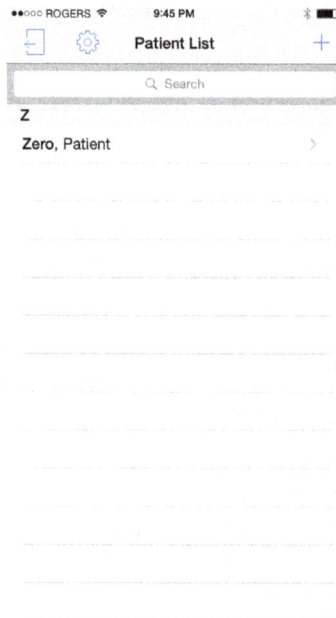

Figure 1. Patient list upon login (iOS).

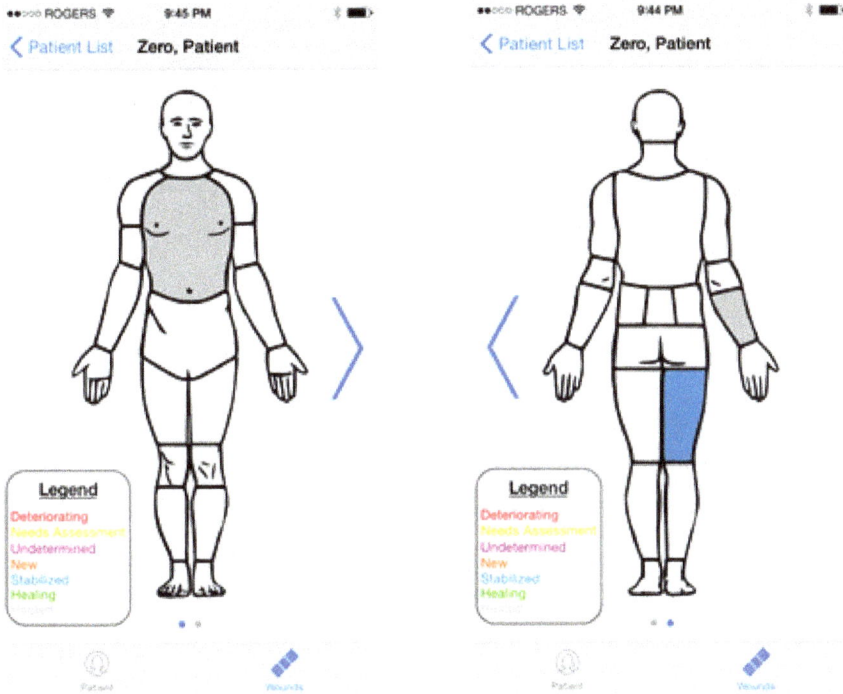

Figure 2. Wound locations and status (iOS).

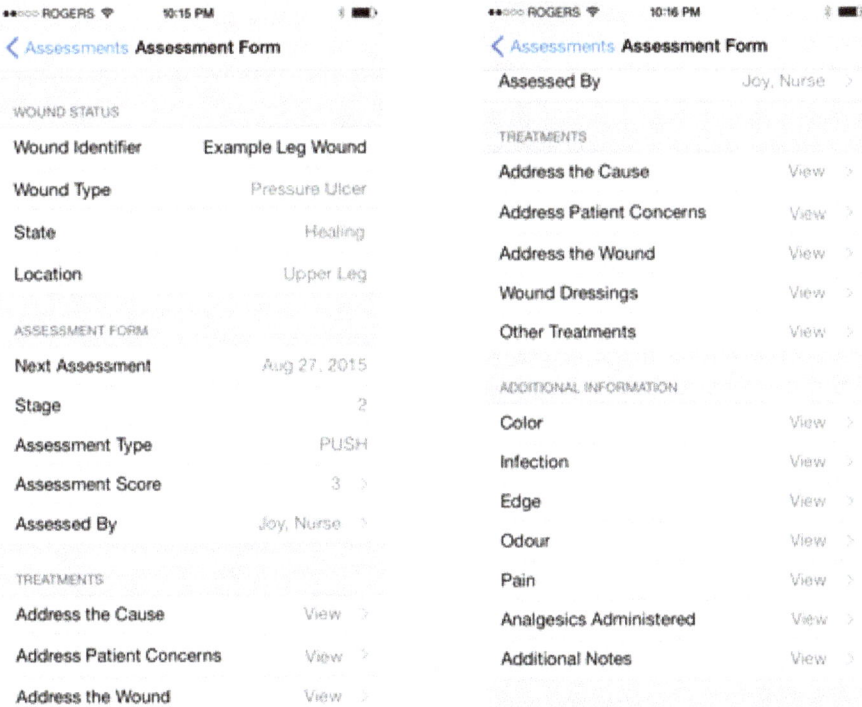

Figure 3. Assessment data entry screen (iOS).

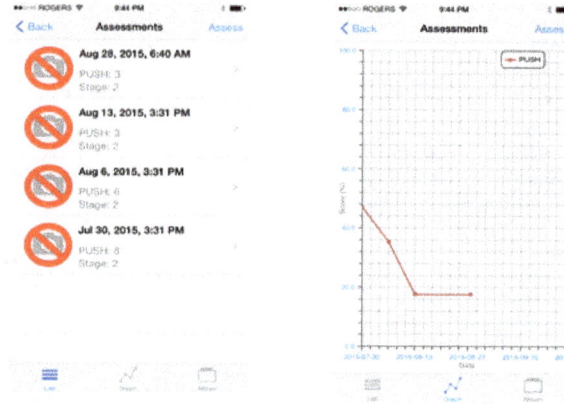

Figure 4. Single wound summary in list and graph format.

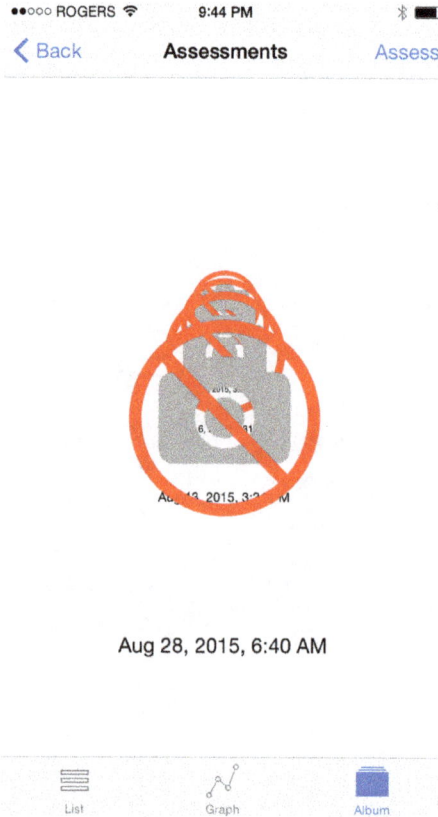

Figure 5. Chronological wound image gallery (iOS).

2.2. User trial – SmartWoundCare on Android

SmartWoundCare in a prototype Android version was subject to a small-scale user trial. Voluntary participants were nurses in a personal care home in Winnipeg, Canada, and they used the mobile app with their patients. The objective was to obtain nurses' impressions on the app's design, its functionality, and how it performed as a part of their daily clinical experiences in treating patients' wounds. Investigating patients' experiences and patients' health outcomes with the app was beyond the scope of the user trial.

The user trial took place in Riverview Health Centre (RHC) in Winnipeg, Canada. Riverview Health Centre provides rehabilitation, palliative, and long-term care. The facilities consist of hospital and personal care home units with almost 400 beds overall, as well as community programs and outpatient services. Riverview specializes in geriatric rehabilitation, brain injury, and stroke rehabilitation, palliative care, and complex long-term care.

All nurses at RHC were invited to participate in the user trial. Approximately 12 nurses expressed interest, and after timelines and the scope of the nurses' participation were established, eight nurses (three men and five women) remained willing to participate. Their participation was entirely voluntary and was not financially compensated. The nurses all had regular duties caring for patients with pressure ulcers or other wounds, and they were full-time employees of RHC. The participants had a range of experience, ranging from less than 10 years nursing experience to over 20 years in a personal care home settings specifically, and ranged from 30 to 60 years in age.

Participants were also asked to judge themselves on their comfort with technology. Four participants judged themselves to be "very tech-savvy" while the other four judged themselves to be "comfortable with common features of phones and tablets". Participants' confidence with smartphone/tablet interfaces and with touch screens was self-assessed at 4.57/5.00 (range=4.0–5.0; SD=0.53) and 4.71/5.00 (range=4.0–5.0; SD=0.49), respectively.

To preserve anonymity, the characteristics of participants were intentionally not cross-referenced with one another.

The nurses received a new Nexus 4 smartphone (four nurses) or a new Nexus 7 tablet (four nurses) with SmartWoundCare loaded and a training manual for the wound care app. They were given a 90-minute training and demonstration of the app. After this training session, the nurses took the mobile devices home and familiarized themselves with SmartWoundCare further before beginning the user trial.

The nurses used SmartWoundCare (Android version) during their nursing shifts. Smart-WoundCare was only used for patients who had pressure ulcers and who had consented to participate in the user trial. Given the patient population, patient consent was provided either directly or through a designate such as a family member. Participants used SmartWoundCare for at least seven shifts. At times, vacation schedules interrupted data collection over consecutive shifts. In most cases, participants were able to use SmartWoundCare for a longer period (more than seven shifts), enhancing the depth and scope of their feedback. All data collection was completed within two-and-a-half months of the start of the user trial.

Using SmartWoundCare in nursing practice was an additional workload over the participants' regular nursing duties, because it did not replace but rather it duplicated the paper chart that forms the patient's official medical record.

Once the nurses had been using SmartWoundCare for approximately 3 weeks, the nurses completed an anonymous on-line survey. This data collection instrument was timed to gain participants' immediate opinions and experiences of SmartWoundCare's functionality and design. The survey was administered via Surveymonkey and included open- and closed-ended questions on SmartWoundCare features, content, look and feel, usability, navigation between screens, assessment of its intended advantages over paper-based charting, as well as overall qualitative impressions of how well SmartWoundCare fits into nursing practice. An important part of the survey was for participants to assess the commensurability of the wound data entered into SmartWoundCare relative to data entered on paper-based forms (scope and format), as this forms the basis of the integrity of the app.

Six weeks later and after an initial analysis of the survey results, a focus group session was held with the participants and the researchers. The focus group was used to probe into the survey results. In that way, the findings of the user trial include both the immediate and the long-term impressions of the app's features and intended benefits, both of which are valuable to assess functionality. The research design complied with qualitative research norms, in which data and interpretations of data are validated by using triangulation and member checks.

The findings were then used to identify the key design issues for ongoing development of both the Android and a subsequent iOS version of SmartWoundCare.

2.2.1. Findings

The objectives of the survey and the focus group were to obtain feedback on the design and functionality of the app and to investigate the nurses' experiences in using the app. The main numerical findings discussed in this section are summarized in **Table 1**.

Survey parameter *All parameters are ranked on a Likert-type scale from 1.0 (low) to 5.0 (high)*	Mean score	Range	Standard deviation
How well-matched is the scope and depth of the software application to the Braden Scale tool?	4.60	4.0–5.0	0.55
How well-matched is the scope and depth of the software application to the PUSH tool?	4.57	4.0–5.0	0.53
Ease of entering a new patient record	4.57	4.0–5.0	0.53
Ease of finding my existing patient's / resident's wound record	4.71	4.0–5.0	0.49
Ease of adding a new wound to the patient's record	4.50	3.0–5.0	0.84
Ease of assessing a new wound for the first time	4.57	3.0–5.0	0.79
Ease of assessing an existing wound that had been previously assessed	4.29	2.0–5.0	1.11
Screens were presented in an expected and logical order	4.17	3.0–5.0	0.75

Survey parameter *All parameters are ranked on a Likert-type scale from 1.0 (low) to 5.0 (high)*	Mean score	Range	Standard deviation
Text history: this presentation is easy to understand	4.50	4.0–5.0	0.55
Text history: this presentation is helpful in understanding wound progression	4.50	4.0–5.0	0.55
Text history: this presentation adds to my understanding of the history of the patient's/resident's wounds and wound care, compared to not having this text-based history available	4.50	4.0–5.0	0.55
Graph history: this presentation is easy to understand	3.67	2.0–5.0	1.03
Graph history: this presentation is helpful in understanding wound progression	3.83	3.0–5.0	0.75
Graph history: this presentation adds to my understanding of the history of the patient's/resident's wounds and wound care, compared to not having this graph-based history available	3.67	2.0–5.0	1.03

Table 1. Numerical findings of a user trial on the android version of SmartWoundCare.

In general, findings over the user trial indicated that SmartWoundCare was easily learned and used in the participants' nursing duties, and that it was well-matched to the PUSH and Braden Scale tools. The benefit of the smartphone was that it was easily carried in the pocket of a uniform; however, a drawback was that the text size was difficult to read. On the other hand, tablet devices were more difficult to carry and store but had the advantage of readability.

The user trial used an Android version of the SmartWoundCare prototype, and as a custom-built software application, it did not always conform to users' expectations of the look and feel of software and how one navigates through software. Areas that caused some initial confusion included cross-navigation between different parts of the app, and confirming saves and deletions of data. Subsequent development on the Android version and later the iOS version of SmartWoundCare was a marked shift to the expected "look and feel" of mobile apps, as opposed to a custom interface.

As an important part of validating the robustness of SmartWoundCare for its intended application, nurses confirmed a strong commensurability in content and data entry between SmartWoundCare and paper versions of the PUSH and Braden Scale tools. Participants reported that the intuitive guidance accurately reflected the fields necessary for a given patient and their wound condition.

However, SmartWoundCare was developed to do more than duplicate a paper chart, and the user trial also investigated the nurses' perceptions of the added intelligence in the app. Although the user trial took place over a relatively short period of time, the nurses indicated that they appreciated and recognized the potential of the wound histories. The text histories were met with slightly better perception than the graph histories (**Table 1**), although not to an extent of statistical significance ($p = 0.05$).

A suggestion for additional features in SmartWoundCare is centred on developing a glossary of specialized terms. This was identified as a useful feature even for experienced wound care nurses.

Another feature of SmartWoundCare over and above paper charts are the alerts that display to the user upon login. These alerts received mixed reviews by the users, with the primary complaint being that the alerts needed a more prominent place within the app rather than their location within a menu with five other menu options. In the subsequent iOS version, alerts follow a more standard format for iOS mobile apps.

2.2.2. Wound images as the key benefit

The strongest finding of the user trial was the value and benefit of wound images (photographs) in SmartWoundCare. Through both the survey and the focus group, nurses identified numerous benefits for the nurse at the bedside, for the patient and their family, and for the physician and allied health professionals. Nurses appreciated the ability to photograph the wound and the associated ability to show the wounds to the patient on the device.

There are several benefits of wound images. At times, wounds are located on body parts that a patient cannot directly observe, such as buttocks, heels, or the soles of feet. The wound photo allowed them to see the wound and get a sense of its size and severity. Often, this led to a better understanding for patients and their families regarding the importance of wound hygiene and treatments.

Another reported benefit is the time saved with each wound assessment, which could add up to significant time during a shift. It can take up to 20 minutes to undress, treat, and re-dress a wound. If another healthcare provider (e.g. physician, physical therapist, wound clinician) asks to see the wound, the dressings need to be removed and the wound redressed after consultation. As a first option, the nurses could show the wound photograph to others in the healthcare team, and then a judgement was made as to whether the wound needed to be undressed or whether the photograph met the needed information within the healthcare team. A further advantage is when the healthcare team is consulting on a wound, the additional information that the wound photograph provided in comparison to solely having a verbal or written description of the wound.

Overall, the ability to add a wound history from photographs to the patient record was recognized for its potential to reduce the number of dressing changes and thus promote healing. The finding also supported SmartWoundCare's potential impact in telehealth.

The findings of the user trial also corresponded to other research findings related to the value of wound photograph, which is contingent on the quality of camera equipment, photomicrography (the art of photographing small objects in large scale), the orientation of the camera lens relative to the wound, flash settings relative to consistent lighting, and duplicate photographs [17]. Two separate studies examined measurements of wounds taken in traditional ways compared to measurements taken from photographs. In those studies, the wounds were venous leg ulcers and diabetic foot ulcers, respectively [24, 25]. The conventional technique to measure wounds is to lay a transparent film over the wound, to trace the wound margin on the film, and then to lay the film over graph paper and count the number of squares. When comparing this technique to measurements derived from digital images, the latter method resulted in improved accuracy, lower inter-observer variations, and improved ease of use. Because the film physically touches the patient's wound and can cause irritation, the digital photograph also had the advantage of being a non-contact method. Another study explored the potential of telehealth, specifically videoconferencing, compared to in-person assessment for pressure ulcer assessment. Both procedures led to very similar assessment of the stage of the wound. However, the telehealth approach led to an overestimate of wound size and volume when compared to in-person assessment [26].

3. Algorithms for wound image analysis: wound size and colour

Given the key finding of the user trial of the significant value of wound photographs, further work focussed on developing algorithms that would add intelligence to SmartWoundCare relative to image analysis.

The objective of the image analysis work was to develop algorithms to determine the size of the wound in both relative and absolute terms, and to analyse the colour breakdown of a wound, all from an image of the wound taken by a smartphone or tablet camera. Further, this objective was to be carried out without any peripheral or ancillary devices. Such devices, as seen in related literature, might include templates or positioning boxes by which the user would help the patient to position themselves and the wound, or it may include ultrasonic transducers and additional lenses for the mobile device. Carrying out the image analysis independent of any ancillary devices contrasts work by other researchers which, for example, control the lighting and wound position with an image capture box when performing image analysis of diabetic foot ulcers [27].

The application represented a general objective applicable to other fields, in that the work was intended to produce non-contact measurements of irregularly-shaped images taken with a smartphone or tablet camera, where the target range for error is <10% for images taken from distances of up to 30 cm. Relying only on the internal smartphone sensors to generate high-accuracy measurements brings novelty to the work and specifically to the field of wound management.

Each new smartphone and tablet that comes to market generally has a higher-resolution camera than the previous version of the device, and these progressions are often evident in short to medium timeframes of 6–18 months. Nonetheless, consumers are still hesitant to rely on on-board cameras for any application that requires high precision and accuracy. In prior work, the state of image analysis from photographs was reviewed [28]. At first instance, several mobile apps were identified which claim to measure objects and distances in the 0.5–20 m range [29, 30], as well as ultrasonic-transducer that ranges for measurements in the 1–6 cm range [31], and infrared distance measurements in the 4–30 cm range [32]. Depth-of-field cameras were also considered [33–35]. That early research also explored one method for determining distance from the camera to the wound and two algorithms to determine the size of the wound. Although both methods are promising, the specifications for error were not met [28].

It is foreseeable that smartphones with dual-lens camera will enter the market within a timeframe of 6–24 months [36]. This development would create new and significant potential for high-resolution images and subsequent analysis for accurate and precise characterization. The analysis techniques would build on the existing work in other fields, such as stereoscopic cameras in manufacturing. Google's Project ARA, a collaborative effort to develop modular smartphone hardware may also provide a future framework by which to include dual-lens cameras in mobile devices.

3.1. Overview

Three components of the image analysis work are outlined in the following sections. In the first component referred to as Mask Image, the objective is to obtain the relative dimensions of an object in the image (in this case, a wound), in which the size determination is relative to the previous image of the same object. The second component, referred to as Camera Calibration, reconstructs an image taken on an angle and references it back to a two-dimensional (2D) plane, in this way facilitating a measurement of the absolute or actual size of the object in the image. The third algorithm determines the range of colours present in an image. The algorithm separates the image into three component colours by extracting components from the red-green-blue (RGB) format of the image, and by doing so, makes possible an inference of the wound stage.

The software framework (**Figure 6**) in a high level abstraction consists of modules including acquisition of the wound image, pre-processing of the wound image, segmentation of the wound image, recognition of the wound type, and classification of the wound. In reference to the three major components of the analysis indicated previously, the Mask Image component lies within the image acquisition module. Grabcut (a segmentation method [37]) and the

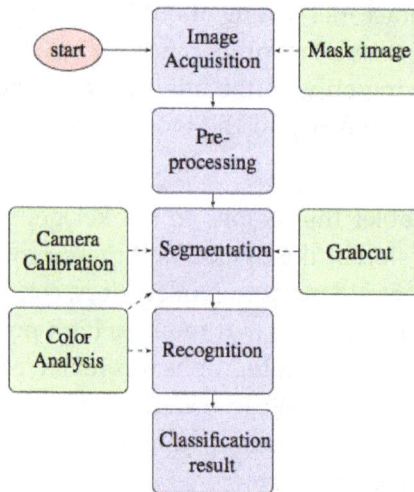

Figure 6. Basic application model.

Camera Calibration component both lie within the segmentation module, and the colour analysis component lies within both the segmentation and the wound recognition modules.

Although the wound photographs are taken with the cameras built into a mobile device (smartphone or tablet as per **Table 2**) or a webcam, all of the processing takes place on a computer. Computation times are generally in the order of seconds. Further work to have the processing take place on the mobile device itself is ongoing, and comes with the usual challenges of carrying out computation- and memory-intensive processes on mobile devices.

Processing the photograph on a computer allows for both static and dynamic environments. In this case, a static environment denotes an environment where both the camera setup relative to the wound position is fixed (e.g. known, constant distance and angle, often with the use of staging devices) and the light source is stable. A dynamic environment refers to a mobile camera (i.e. smartphone or tablet) and/or the wound in a natural position at varying distances and angles to the camera and in varying lighting conditions.

With a series of photographs taken in a static environment, the Camera Calibration component, which corrects for angle by reconstructing an image in three-dimensional (3D) space back to a 2D plane, only needs to be done once and the correction can be applied to the entire series of photographs. In a dynamic environment where distance and angle between the wound and the camera vary with each photograph, the Camera Calibration component needs to be done for each image.

Table 2 summarizes the hardware and software specification applied in this work.

Nexus 4 (LG-E960)	MacBook Pro
Krait Quad-core 1.5 GHz	Processor 2.6 GHz Intel Core i7
Display resolution 1280 × 768	Memory 8 GB 1600 MHz DDR3
Camera resolution 8MP (3264 × 2448)	Graphics Intel Iris Pro 1024 MB
High Performance Adreno 320 GPU	Software OS X 10.9.5 (13F34)
Bluetooth 3.0 BLE	
Wi-Fi 802.11 a/b/g/n	**Software**
	Android 4.2 (Jelly Bean)
Samsung Galaxy S4	Android NDK r9d
ARM Cortex-A15 Quad-core 1.9 GHz processor	OpenCV 2.4.9 Android SDK
Display resolution 1080 × 1920	Python 2.7.10
13+ megapixel camera	Numpy
Bluetooth 4.0	Matplotlib
802.11 a/b/g/n	OpenCV 3.0.0
	Matlab

Table 2. Hardware and software specifications.

3.2. Mask image for relative size

The first two components of the image analysis work, Mask Image and Camera Calibration, are used to determine the relative size and the absolute size of a wound, respectively, from the wound photograph. **Figure 7** expands the first two modules of basic software framework in **Figure 6**, specifically the image acquisition module and the image pre-processing module. The Mask Image component is situated within these modules.

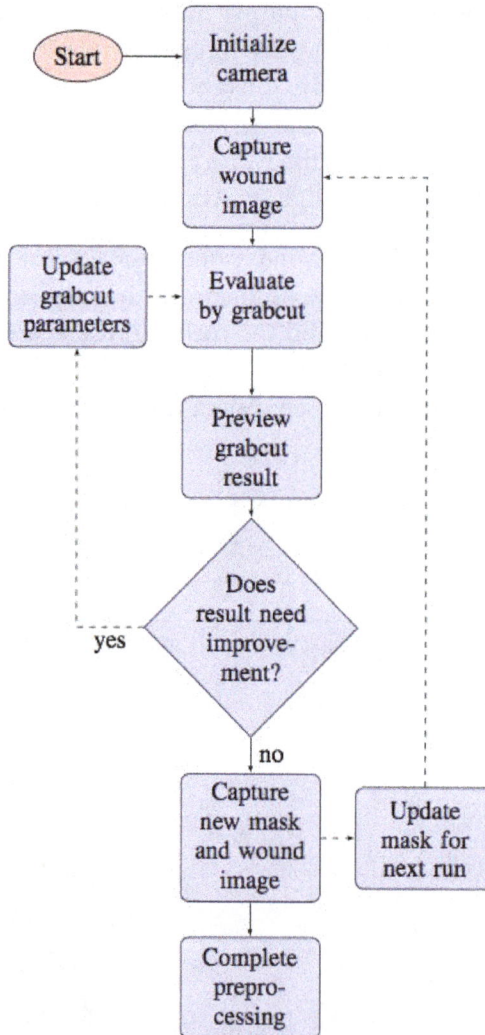

Figure 7. Image acquisition and pre-processing flowchart.

Wounds are generally three-dimensional, with volume below the skin surface. Wounds can also exhibit undermining, which refers to a wound that is larger at its base (below the skin) than the opening at the surface of the skin suggests, creating a cavity below the surface of the skin. Tunnelling refers to wounds, similar to undermining, which have channels (rather than cavities) below the skin surface.

As noted earlier, conventional methods to measure wound dimensions and/or area often use contact methods, in which adhesive strips or transparent films are laid around or on the wound, respectively, and wound edges are noted on the strips or films. The strips or films are then read directly for size or overlaid on to graph paper or rulers for measurement. The depth is generally measured with a cotton-tipped applicator to the deepest part of the wound.

Two approaches in the literature to automatically determine the size of a wound include grid capture and scanner capture. Grid capture is a hybrid of conventional contact methods and digital image analysis. In this case, a transparent film with a marked grid is placed on the wound and the wound perimeter is traced on to the film. The film with the tracing on a known grid is then the basis from which the dimensions and area of the wound can be calculated with a software application [38]. This approach has the advantage of basing the calculation on a real tracing of the wound perimeter and a known grid, thus capturing the near-real orientation of the wound. However, the disadvantage remains the potential for discomfort to the patient when the film rests on the wound.

In another approach denoted as scanner capture, a box with two internal mirrors is constructed as a template. The box has openings for a mobile device and an LED light source. In the scanner capture approach developed by others, a box with two mirrors inside is placed at 45 degrees relative to the horizontal, with openings for a smartphone and an LED light source [27]. The patient rests their foot in the box, and in this way, the setup maintains a constant distance between camera and wound and constant lighting conditions. While the computation remains intensive, the advantage of this method is that these two conditions serve to simplify the image processing requirements. The disadvantage of this method is the reliance on ancillary staging devices, and the setup will be impractical for certain areas of the body.

In this work, the objective of the Mask Image component is to obtain the comparative dimensions of an object in the image relative to a previous image of the same wound. An initial photograph is taken, from which a transparent digital 'mask' of the wound is created. The user then overlays or aligns this digital mask to the wound for the subsequent assessment and photograph (**Figures 8** and **9**). While most of the perimeter is expected to align between the mask image and the wound in its current state, one can reasonably anticipate that if the wound is either healing or deteriorating, portions of the perimeter between the digital mask and the wound in its current state will differ. The algorithm compares the digital mask to the current wound image, recognizing and aligning wound perimeter, and estimating the relative size difference. From this size difference, either healing, deterioration, or no change is inferred. The result is given as a percentage change in the area of the most current image relative to the previous digital mask image.

The mask image or mask overlay essentially serves to provide a point of reference when aligning the wound for the current assessment with its previous condition. As such, the point of reference does not necessarily need to be the transparent mask overlay. A medical tattoo could also act as a point of reference. In this case, it would be either a temporary or permanent skin marker or pattern (e.g. three dots) close to the wound. This marker or pattern would be used each to create a digital overlay which would provide the point of reference when aligning the camera for all subsequent photographs.

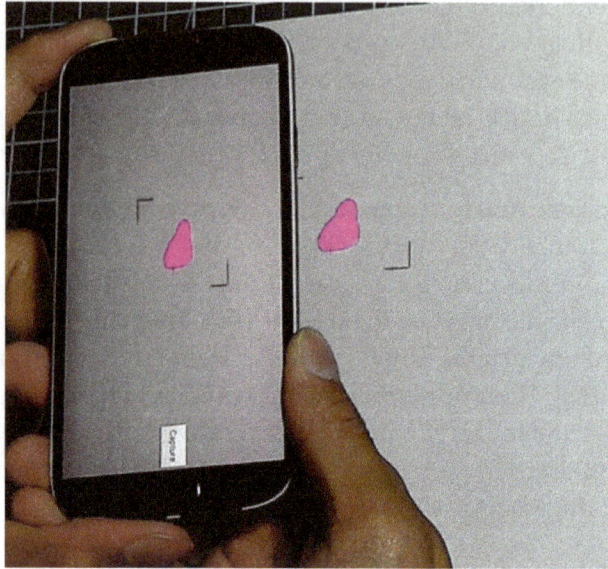

Figure 8. Creating a mask image from the wound.

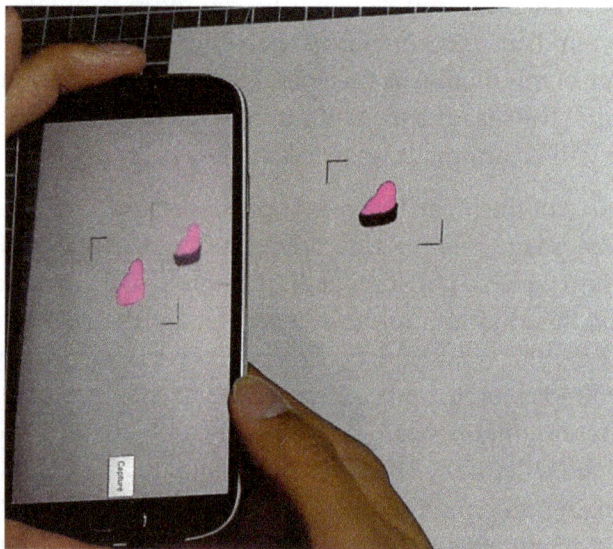

Figure 9. Overlay of mask image to new wound.

The Mask Image component of the work provides the relative size of the wound from one assessment to the next. Users can choose to create one digital mask and compare all subsequent photographs to the initial digital mask; alternately, users can create a new digital mask at each wound assessment so that wound size comparison is always to the most recent assessment. A combination of the two methods is also possible. The advantage of the method is the absence of direct contact with the wound, thus preventing patient discomfort. Another advantage is that no additional devices to the camera or to the patient (e.g. props) are required. The error inherent in the approach is largely determined by the user's dexterity in aligning the digital mask over the current wound. A limitation of the method is that wound depth is not considered in the calculation. A further limitation of the method is that the outcome is a relative size of the wound rather than an absolute size. When an absolute size of the wound is desired, the Camera Calibration component is implemented.

3.3. Camera calibration for absolute size

Figure 10 shows the Camera Calibration component within the basic software framework outlined in **Figure 6**.

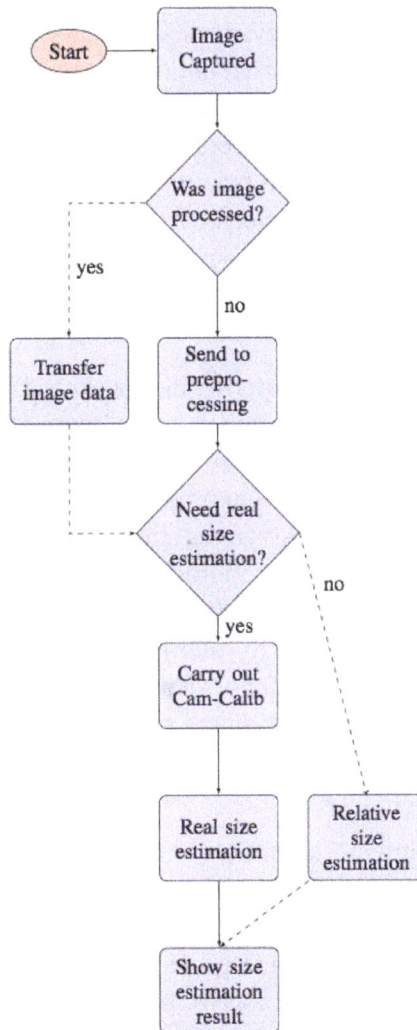

Figure 10. Size estimation with segmentation flowchart.

Grabcut, a segmentation method used to differentiate an object (in this case, a wound) in the foreground from its background (in this case, the surrounding skin or body part), is applied in this module. Grabcut accomplishes this by using colour information to compare side by side pixels and also by using edge or contrast information to identify an object in an image. Further, Grabcut uses progressive iteration and runs the process multiple times to optimize the results. The result is a segmented image (the foreground object, in this case, a wound). This segmented image is then used in the Camera Calibration component as well as the third component of colour analysis. While other segmentation algorithms are available, Grabcut is considered an efficient algorithm and has the benefit of minimal user interaction [37], which was a requirement in this work. An example of Grabcut applied to wound photographs is found at https://youtu.be/Iyvochswrws.

The purpose of the Camera Calibration component is to take an image photographed on an angle and reconstruct or reference it back to a two-dimensional plane. Essentially, the Camera Calibration module computationally achieves one of the objectives of the scanner capture box [27] in terms of aligning the wound to known and fixed positions relative to the camera. The Camera Calibration component uses a known pattern with 13 or more fixed reference points, and applies the Tsai2D algorithm [39, 40] to obtain a reconstructed image of the wound. Since the distance between the points are known from the calibration model, the view angle can be calculated and the image can be reconstructed on a 2D plane. From here, the size of the wound can be calculated. Like the Mask Image component, the Camera Calibration component also does not identify depth or volume of wounds. This is a known limitation, given that surface size and area alone are an incomplete descriptor of wounds.

A chessboard pattern was chosen as the pattern. This was found to be effective for photographs taken in static and dynamic conditions. Similar to the conventional approach of placing an adhesive ruler near the wound to measure size, the chessboard pattern is placed close to the wound and then photographed. The inherent assumption is that the wound and the pattern are in the same two-dimensional plane. Given that the chessboard pattern is known and fixed, the planar orientation of the pattern in the photograph can be calculated and then the image corrected accordingly. This approach has been shown to be effective in calculating the dimensions of a soccer field, in which a top (plan) view of the field was reconstructed from images taken on an angle, using Camera Calibration [41]. In this work, the chessboard pattern is used for calibration to obtain the extrinsic matrix of the wound. The extrinsic matrix provides information on the camera location and the view direction, allowing for translation and rotation to the two-dimensional plane.

Figure 11 demonstrates the Camera Calibration sequence at a high level. The red lines denote the objects which were detected, i.e. the dark squares. The algorithm finds the centre of each square and applies the Tsai 2D algorithm to process the coordinates. The blue lines show the scanning sequence. The green lines are the re-projected lines from the model points to the real world coordinates, as an indication of the success of the Camera Calibration algorithm. If the green lines were curved or otherwise irregular, this would indicate that the projection back to a two-dimensional plane was not successful.

Figure 12 shows the Camera Calibration component applied to a wound. The wound was photographed at an angle and then re-projected on a two-dimensional plane at 90 degrees to the viewer.

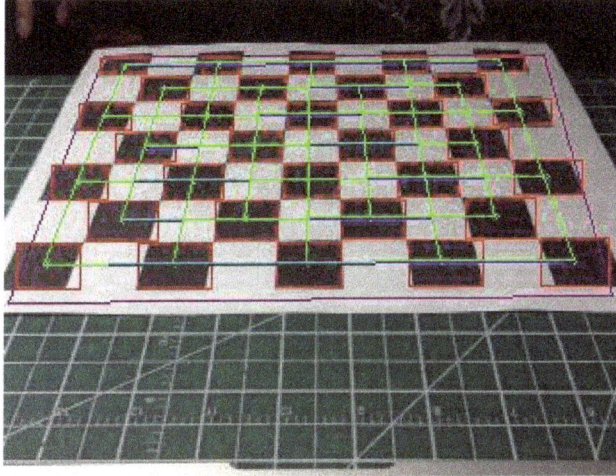

Figure 11. Original and re-projected planes.

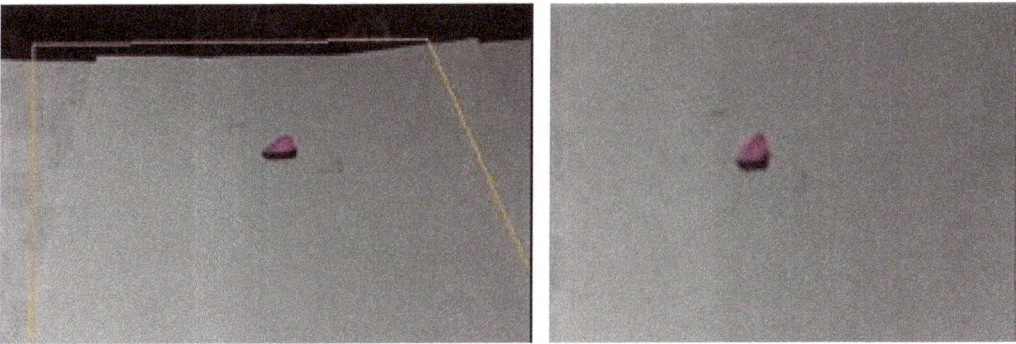

Figure 12. Wound image before (left) and after (right) reconstruction.

While the Mask Image component results in a relative size of the wound and the Camera Calibration component results in a corrected orientation and an absolute size of the wound, taken together, they allow for more accurate calculations. When applied to a Canadian dollar coin (26.5 mm diameter with eleven edges), the actual size was determined with an error of <1%.

A demonstration of the Camera Calibration module is available at https://youtu.be/ OiJk3nMymSE.

3.4. Colour analysis

The third algorithm focuses on colour analysis of the wound. It determines the range of colours present in an image, separating the image into three component colours by extracting components from the red-green-blue (RGB) format of the image and presenting them in a histogram. These data can then be fed into an expert system to infer the stage of the wound. **Figure 13** shows the Colour Analysis component within the software framework outlined in **Figure 6**.

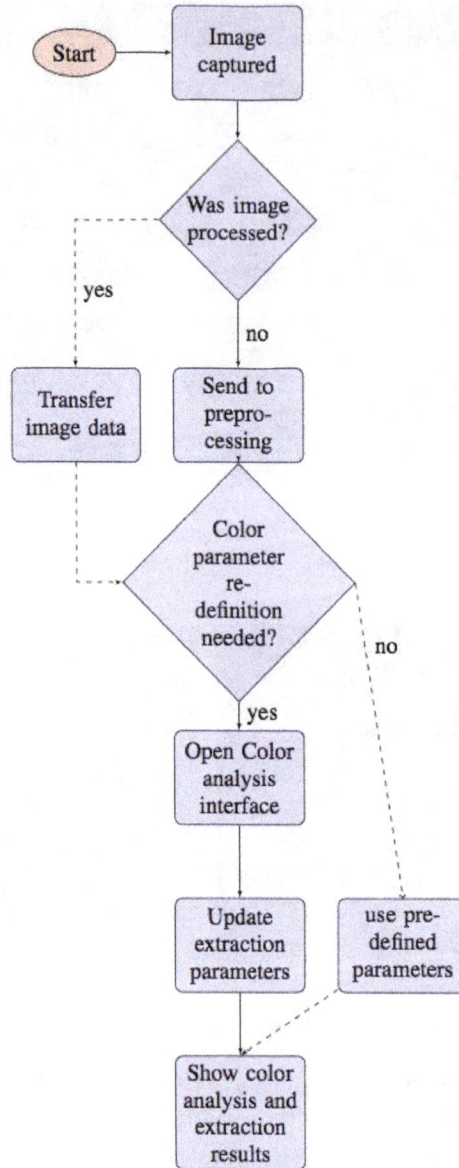

Figure 13. Colour analysis flowchart.

Pressure ulcers will be assessed as one of six stages (stage I through IV, Suspected Deep Tissue Injury, and Unstageable) [42]. Because the current work is unable to calculate the depth of the wound, the last two categories (both of which are wounds with some depth below the skin surface) have been combined as Unstageable. In addition to wound depth, other factors that determine the stage of a wound include skin condition (intact or broken), tissue loss, the colour of the skin, tissue, and wound bed, and the presence and nature of discharge.

To analyse the colour of a wound, the algorithm uses an RGB format of the image and determines the presence of the three component colours. Each component colour has a defined range, although the user can adjust that range or calibrate the range for variable lighting conditions.

While segmentation is not mandatory, the results of the colour analysis component are much more accurate if done on a segmented image, as this allows the algorithm to disregard the background (**Figure 14** images taken from http://reference.medscape.com/features/slideshow/ pressure-ulcers).

Users can also consider hue, saturation, value (HSV) and red-yellow-black (RYB) formats for colour analysis. Hue, saturation, value (HSV) format responds to lighting, and as such, it may be a good option when one wants to tune the colour more specifically. RYB (red-yellow-black) has a fitting relationship to wound stages, and RGB results can be converted to RYB. The approximate ratios of red, yellow, and black correlated to wound stages are shown in **Figure 15**. Wound stages I and II rely only on red, but are differentiated on the intensity of the red in the image. The subsequent wound stages are differentiated on the proportions of each of the three colours in the image. The error inherent in this method depends to some extent on the definitions of colours set by the user. A recommendation is to associate this component with a machine learning component, once a large enough data set is collected. In this way, colour parameters can be more precisely defined.

Finally, expert systems can be developed to determine wound stages from the RGB and/or RYB data. This again relies on collecting a sufficiently large data set. Alternatively, support vector machine (VSM) or another machine learning algorithm can be applied to determine the

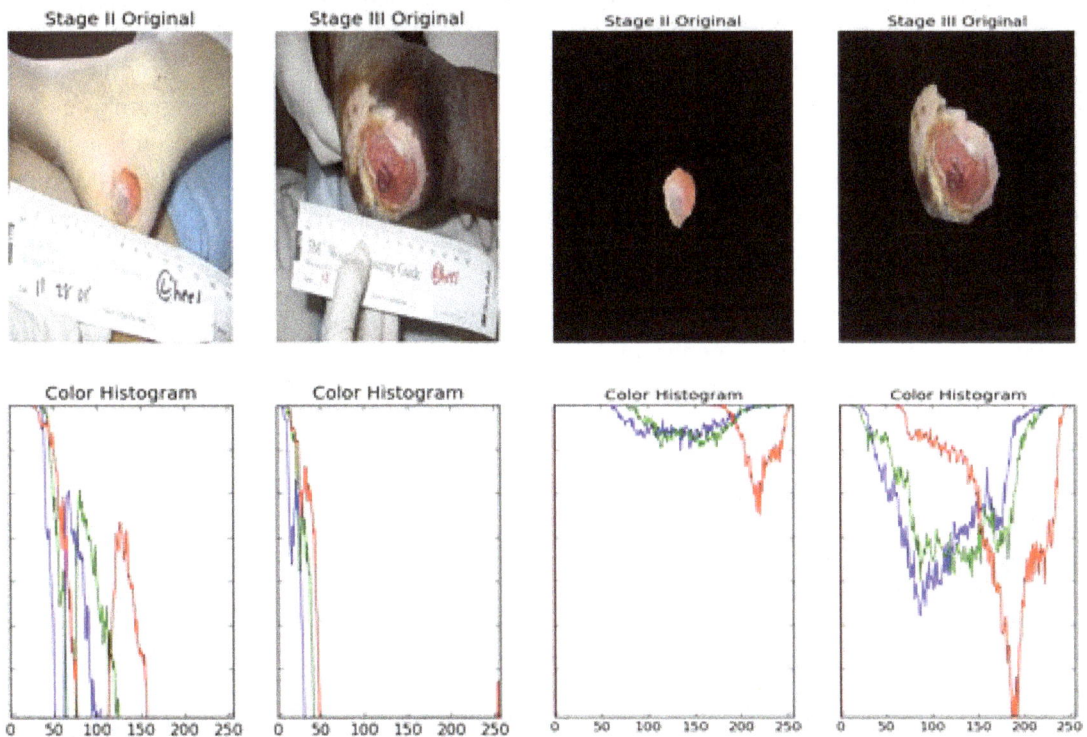

Figure 14. Histogram results before and after segmentation.

stages of a wound. In the current work, the framework for an expert system is in place. The next step is to collect and populate the expert system with training data.

An example of the colour analysis on wound photographs can be viewed at https://youtu.be/Iyvochswrws.

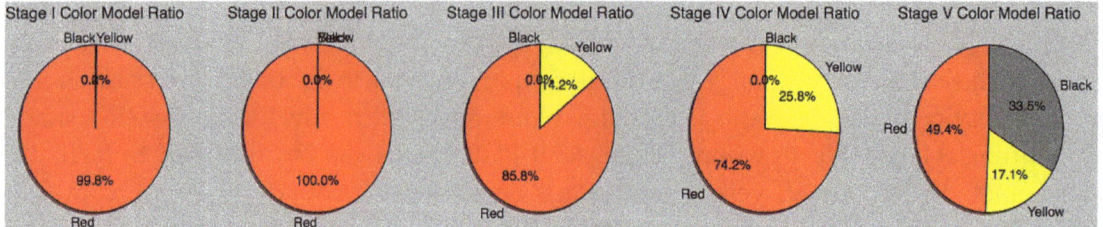

Figure 15. RYB output correlated to wound stage.

4. Conclusion

SmartWoundCare as a mobile wound management prototype demonstrates the wide relevance of mHealth for applications within healthcare facilities and their integration with larger EMR and eHealth systems, as well as the application of telehealth to connect underserved communities. Community health and home-based care is an equally important and in some way a more urgent implementation. For example, nurses of the Winnipeg Regional Health Authority alone carry out 450,000 wound visits per year in its Home Care program in clients' homes. Particularly in home-based care, the integration of SmartWoundCare with a suite of mHealth tools is a natural extension. A logical partner app for SmartWoundCare is diabetes monitoring, as well as novel pre-emptive applications such as an early warning system for injury or damage to diabetic feet due to neuropathy [43].

SmartWoundCare and other mHealth applications also illuminate opportunities in Big Data, in which a community of users generate data – in this case, a wound database – from which relevant trends in wound diagnosis and healing can be extracted and form part of the body of knowledge in wound care.

Author details

Marcia R. Friesen*, Bennet Gigliotti and Tik Wai (Kiral) Poon

*Address all correspondence to: marcia.friesen@umanitoba.ca

Electrical & Computer Engineering, University of Manitoba, Winnipeg, Manitoba, Canada

References

[1] Cafazzo JA, Casselman M, Hamming N, Katzman DK, Palmert MR. Design of an mHealth app for the self-management of adolescent type 1 diabetes: A pilot study. Journal of Medical Internet Research. 2012;14(3): e70. DOI: 10.2196/jmir.2058

[2] RheumMate [Internet]. Available: http://gvu.gatech.edu/research/projects/rheummate [Accessed 2015-06-15].

[3] Health Outcomes Worldwide [Internet]. Available: http://healthoutcomesww.com [Accessed 2015-06-15].

[4] Canadian Association of Wound Care [Internet]. Available: www.cawc.net [Accessed 2015-07-15].

[5] Woodbury MG, Houghton PE. Prevalence of pressure ulcers in Canadian healthcare settings. Ostomy Wound Management. 2004;50: 22–38.

[6] Gorecki C, Brown J, Nelson A, Briggs M, Schoonhoven L, Dealey C, Defloor T, Nixon, J. Impact of pressure ulcers on quality of life in older patients: A systematic review. Journal of the American Geriatrics Society. 2009;57: 1175–1183.

[7] Groeneveld A. The prevalence of pressure ulcers in a tertiary care pediatric and adult hospital. Journal of Wound, Ostomy Continence Nursing. 2004;31: 108–120.

[8] Reddy M, Gill SS, Rochon PA. Preventing pressure ulcers: A systematic review. JAMA. 2006;296: 974–984.

[9] Landi F, Onder G, Russo A, Bernabei R. Pressure ulcer and mortality in frail elderly people living in community. Archives of Gerontology and Geriatrics. 2007;44: 217–223.

[10] Allman RM, Goode PS, Burst NBS, Bartolucci AA, Thomas DR. Pressure ulcers, hospital complications, and disease severity: Impact on hospital costs and length of stay. Advances in Wound Care. 1999;12: 22–30.

[11] Allman RM. Pressure ulcer prevalence, incidence, risk factors, and impact. Clinics in Geriatric Medicine. 1997;13: 421–436.

[12] Keast DH, Parslow N, Houghton PE, Norton L, Fraser C. Best practice recommendations for the prevention and treatment of pressure ulcers: update 2006. Wound Care Canada. 2006;4: 31–43.

[13] Van Gilder C. Results of nine international pressure ulcer prevalence surveys: 1989–2005. Ostomy and Wound Management. 2008;54: 40–54.

[14] Gallagher P. Prevalence of pressure ulcers in three university teaching hospitals in Ireland. Journal of Tissue Viability. 2008;17: 103–109.

[15] Gunningberg L, Stotts N. Tracking quality over time. What does pressure ulcer data show? International Journal for Quality in Health Care. 2008;20: 246–253.

[16] Chaundry B, Wang J, Wu S, Maglione M, Mojica W, Roth E, Morton SC, Shekelle PG. Systematic review: Impact of health information technology on quality, efficiency, and costs of medical care. Annals of Internal Medicine. 2006;144: 742–752.

[17] Rennert AB, Golinko M, Kaplan D, Flattau A, Brem H. Standardization of wound photography using the wound electronic medical record. Advances in Skin and Wound Care. 2009;22: 32–38.

[18] Smith MW, Hill ML, Hopking KL, Kiratli, BJ, Cronkite RC. A modeled analysis of telehealth methods for treating pressure ulcers after spinal cord injury. International Journal of Telemedicine and Applications. 2012. Volume 2012, January 2012, Article ID 729492, 10 pages. DOI : 10.1155/2012/729492. Epub 2012 Aug 28.

[19] Harrison J, Harrison DG. It is possible to standardize wound ostomy continence documentation with a mobile app. Journal of Wound, Ostomy, and Continence Nursing. 2013;40: 537.

[20] mHealthNews [Internet]. Available: http://www.mhealthnews.com/news/onc-names-winners-pressure-ulcer-app-challenge [Accessed 2015-10-25].

[21] PUSH Tool [Internet]. Available: http://www.npuap.org/resources/educational-and-clinical-resources/push-tool [Accessed 2015-12-24].

[22] Prevention Plus: Home of the Braden Scale [Internet]. Available: http://www.braden-scale.com/index.htm [Accessed 2015-11-04].

[23] Harris C, Bates-Jensen B, Parslow N, Raizman R, Singh M. The Bates-Jensen Wound Assessment Tool (BWAT): Development of a pictorial guide for training nurses. Wound Care Canada. 2009;7: 33–38.

[24] Samad A, Hayes S, French L. Digital imaging versus conventional contact tracing for the objective measurement of venous leg ulcers. Journal of Wound Care. 2002;11(4): 137–140.

[25] Rajbhandari SM, Harris ND, Sutton M. Digital imaging: An accurate and easy method of measuring foot ulcers. Diabetic Medicine. 1999;16(4): 339–342.

[26] Hill ML, Cronkite RC, Ota DT, Yao EC, Kiratli BJ. Validation of home telehealth for pressure ulcer assessment: A study in patients with spinal cord injury. Journal of Telemedicine and Telecare. 2009;15(4): 196–202.

[27] Wang L, Pedersen PC, Strong DM, Tulu B, Agu E, Ignotz R. Smartphone-based wound assessment system for patients with diabetes. IEEE Transactions on Biomedical Engineering. 2015;62(2): 477–488. DOI: 10.1109/TBME.2014.2358632

[28] White PJF, Podaima BW, Friesen MR. Algorithms for smartphone and tablet image analysis for healthcare applications. IEEE Access. 2014;2(1): 1–10. DOI: 10.1109/ACCESS.2014.2348943

[29] Multi Measures; TapeMeasure! [Internet]. Available: https://play.google.com [Accessed 2014-12-20].

[30] SmartMeasure; Ruler. [Internet]. Available: https://itunes.apple.com [Accessed 2014-12-18].

[31] Robot Electronics – Ultrasound Rangers [Internet]. Available: http://www.robot-electronics.co.uk/products/sensors/ultrasonics.html [Accessed 2015-10-07].

[32] Active Robots – IR Distance Measuring [Internet]. Available: http://www.robot-electronics.co.uk/products/sensors/infrared-range.html [Accessed 2015-10-07].

[33] Lytro – "You'll never think about pictures the same way" [Internet]. Available: https://www.lytro.com/camera [Accessed 2015-10-24].

[34] Toshiba putting focus on taking misfocusing out of photos [Internet]. 2012. Available: http://ajw.asahi.com/article/economy/business/AJ201212270054. [Accessed 2015-11-25].

[35] Dent S. Nokia's Refocus Lens camera app promises infinite depth of field control [Internet]. 2013. Available: http://www.engadget.com/2013/10/22/nokias-refocus-lens-camera-app/. [Accessed 2015-11-24].

[36] Pinto S. Dual-Lens smartphone camera: Killer feature or just a gimmick? [Internet]. 2014. Available: http://www.techtree.com/content/news/5615/dual-lens-Smartphone-camera-killer-feature-gimick.html. [Accessed 2015-11-24].

[37] Rother C, Kolmogorov R, Blake A. GrabCut interactive foreground extraction using iterated graph cuts. Microsoft Research, Cambridge, UK [Internet]. Available: http://cvg.ethz.ch/teaching/cvl/2012/grabcut-siggraph04.pdf [Accessed 2015-11-24].

[38] Foltynski P, Ladyzynski P, Wojcicki JM. A new smartphone-based method for wound area measurement. Artificial Organs. 2014;38(4): 346–352.

[39] Zhang Z. A flexible new technique for camera calibration. IEEE Transactions on Pattern Analysis and Machine Intelligence. 2000;22(11): 1330–1334. Available: http://research.microsoft.com/en-us/um/people/zhang/Papers/TR98-71.pdf [Accessed 2015-04-20].

[40] Tsai RY. A versatile camera calibration technique for high-accuracy 3D machine vision metrology using off-the-shelf TV cameras and lenses. IEEE Journal of Robotics and Automation. 1987;3(4): 323–344. DOI: 10.1109/JRA.1987.1087109

[41] Anderson J, Baltes J. A pragmatic global vision system for educational robotics. In: AAAI Spring Symposium: Semantic Scientific Knowledge Integration; 2007. Available: www.aaai.org/Papers/Symposia/Spring/2007/SS-07-09/SS07-09-001.pdf [Accessed 2015-07-18].

[42] NPUAP Pressure Ulcer Stages/Categories [Internet]. Available: http://www.npuap.org/resources/educational-and-clinical-resources/npuap-pressure-ulcer-stagescategories/ [Accessed 2015-08-08].

[43] Jegede OD, Ferens K, Griffith B, Podaima BW. A smart shoe to prevent and manage diabetic foot diseases. In: Proceedings of the 2015 International Conference on Health Informatics and Medical Systems; 26–30 July 2015; Las Vegas, NV, USA. p. 47–54.

3

Exploring the Interrelationship of Risk Factors for Supporting eHealth Knowledge-Based System

Geletaw Sahle Tegenaw

Abstract

In developing countries like Africa, the physician-to-population ratio is below the World Health Organization (WHO) minimum recommendation. Because of the limited resource setting, the healthcare services did not get the equity of access to the use of health services, the sustainable health financing, and the quality of healthcare service provision. Efficient and effective teaching, alerting, and recommendation system are required to support the activities of the healthcare service. To alleviate those issues, creating a competitive eHealth knowledge-based system (KBS) will bring unlimited benefit. In this study, Apriori techniques are applied to malaria dataset to explore the degree of the association of risk factors. And then, integrate the output of data mining (i.e., the interrelationship of risk factors) with knowledge-based reasoning. Nearest neighbor retrieval algorithms (for retrieval) and voting method (to reuse tasks) are used to design and deliver personalized knowledge-based system.

Keywords: knowledge-based system, eHealth, pattern discovery, data mining, association rule

1. Introduction

In Africa, on average there are nine hospital beds per 10,000 people in comparison to the world average of 27. In sub-Saharan Africa, the physician-to-population ratio is the lowest in the world [1, 2]. Countries like Ethiopia set a strategic plan to improve access and equity to preventive, essential health interventions at the village and household levels to ensure healthcare coverage in rural areas [3, 4].

On the one hand, because of the limited resource setting, the healthcare services have not got the equity of access to the use of health services, the sustainable health financing, and the quality of healthcare service provision. The physician-to-population ratio is below the World Health Organization (WHO) minimum recommendations [1, 2]. Still, pneumonia, diarrhea, acute upper respiratory tract infection, acute febrile illness, and malaria account for 64% under five morbidity [5].

> About 68% of the country's total population living in areas at risk of malaria, 75% of the country is vulnerable to malaria (defined as areas <2000 m, those areas are fertile and suitable for agriculture and accounts for up to 17% of outpatient consultations, 15% of admissions and 29% of inpatient deaths. [6, 7]

On the other hand, it has been more than four decades the computer program reasons (e.g., MYCIN was developed in the early 1970s) and uses knowledge to assist the domain experts and minimize routine activities. To prevent and control the crisis of malaria, different scholars and responsible bodies have made remarkable efforts by conducting researches, implementing strategies, and policies [6, 7]. A predictive data mining model has been constructed using Ethiopian WHO malaria database, metrological database, and national mapping database [8]. The model is accurate to determine the occurrence of death, and it is good enough to identify the cases.

However, the system is looking a mechanism to assist routine healthcare activities, administrative and medical cost, demographic challenges, and equitable health distribution. For instance, the health extension workers (HEWs) assist peripheral health services by bridging the gap between the communities and health facilities [3, 4]. Each kebele has two HEWs responsible for providing outreach services. A kebele is the smallest governmental administrative unit and on average has a population of 5000 people. The HEWs teach the community house to house for each and every person in the kebele in order to create and promote healthy lifestyles. In all, the healthcare system is searching a mechanism for teaching, alerting, and recommendation system to support the daily routine activities.

To alleviate those issues, creating a competitive eHealth knowledge-based system (KBS) is the main goal of this work which will bring unlimited benefit in low resource setting. As a case study, we choose malaria (malaria dataset) because malaria prevention and control at the community level face numerous challenges because of the climate condition (temperature, rainfall), epidemiological, and genetic, poverty, malaria outbreak, over prescription for positive result and so on. Knowing the pattern and interrelationship of risk factors is important for supporting knowledge-based system as well as prediction of malaria death occurrences/cases. An attempt is made for exploring the degree of association between malaria risk factors (related to the malaria death occurrence and case identification). Investigating the degree of interrelationship among risk factors will have a great contribution toward eradicating the outbreak of malaria. The outcome of the study helps to mitigate the severity through investigating the association of risk factors and building of a competitive knowledge-based system.

2. Literature review

Knowledge-based systems is aimed to understand or bring human-level intelligence through simulating or acting one or more of intelligent behaviors (such as thinking, problem-solving, learning, understanding, emotions, consciousness, intuition and creativity, language capacity, etc.). On the one hand, KBS is advantageous when there is shortage of expert, decision-making for problem-solving needs an intelligent assistant, expertise is needed to be stored for future use, and so on. On the other hand, KBS faces a lot of challenges due to the abstract nature of knowledge, limitation of cognitive science, and other scientific methods [9, 10].

Knowledge representation and inference engine are the two building blocks of KBS. The knowledge acquired from experts, documents, books, and other resources has been organized using knowledge representation. The inference engine gets the knowledge and instructs how to use the knowledge to solve problems using rule- or case-based reasoning. Rule-based reasoning is a technique that reasons out about a problem based on the knowledge that is represented in the form of rules [11]. Case-based system represents situations or domain knowledge in the form of cases, and it uses case-based reasoning technique to solve new problems or to handle new situations [12].

Knowledge-based system (in health and medical domain) has made a remarkable effect through providing a reliable diagnostic and cost-effective service. Several systems have been implemented in different medical areas like cancer therapy, infections, blood diseases, general internal medicine, glaucoma, and pulmonary function tests [13, 14]. Such systems can be designed to exhaustively consider all possible diseases in a domain, which could outperform human experts to achieve a rapid and accurate diagnosis. Integrating and updating domain knowledge with knowledge discovery are relevant to increase the interestingness and user belief (such as matching discovered pattern with existing knowledge) [15]. Integrated eHealth knowledge-based system based on acquiring health knowledge will support users in exchange of knowledge and accessibility for the users through data collection, care documentation, and knowledge extraction [16].

Following and implementing a hybrid (integrated) intelligent system for medical data classification is good to produce effective knowledge-based system [17]. A promising result is scored through integration to improve the quality of knowledge-based system [17, 18]. For instance, integrating the result (rule) of the PART classification algorithm with the knowledge-based system has delivered a favorable result for the diagnosis and treatment of visceral leishmaniasis [19]. The paper by Seera and Lim has experimented and used fuzzy min-max neural networks to learn incrementally from sample data, classification, and regression tree for prediction and random forest model to achieve high classification performance [17]. Kerdprasop and Kerdprasop also tried to automate data mining model by focusing on post data mining process to step of automatic knowledge deployment using induced knowledge and formalization classification rules [20].

However, the need to work more in providing explanatory rules and handling missing data in real-world application is expected. A mechanism for handling irrelevant rule (result) is required in case of inductive experiment system and so on. To alleviate those issues, in our case study, we tried to explore the pattern and the interrelationship of risk factors for supporting the knowledge-based system as well as prediction of malaria death occurrences/cases. The result will increase the interestingness and belief of eHealth knowledge-based system which will bring unlimited benefit in low resource setting.

2.1. Research aim and objectives

Investigating the potential applicability of exploring the interrelationship of risk factors using data mining to create a competitive eHealth knowledge-based system is the main goal of this work.

2.2. Methodology

Cross industry standard process for data mining (CRISP-DM) methodology is adopted to investigate the interrelationship of malaria risk factors. Then, to design eHealth knowledge-based system, nearest neighbor retrieval algorithms (for retrieval) and voting method (to reuse tasks) are used. The technique is easy in exploring relevant cases and provides an opportunity to retrieve partially matching cases [21–24].

The malaria data is collected from a zonal health facility in each of the 86 zones of Ethiopia. To understand the problem domain, we used observation, interviewing with experts and data managers and reviewing documents, reports, and literatures. This helps us to select and integrate decisive attributes from different sources. The data selected from the WHO (World Health Organization) database is integrated with the decisive attributes (like temperature, rainfall, and altitude) extracted from the Ethiopian National Meteorological Agency and Mapping Agency in order to find the association of risk factors.

Exploratory data analysis is performed to get familiar with the data and prepared for investigating the degree of interrelationship. The data mining task is finding the internal association between data elements that will determine the occurrence of death/case. To maintain the quality of the data, preprocessing tasks such as data cleaning (handling missing values, noisy, and outer values), data integration tasks, and data transformation tasks are performed.

The collected Ethiopian WHO malaria database contains five basic attributes (more than 37,000 records) that provide information about the geographic location and period of coverage. These attributes include country name, region (administrative regions from which malaria information is collected), zone and health facility name, year, and month. The detailed information of the attributes is categorized based on the WHO standards and explicitly represents the detailed information about malaria in each zone of the region across Ethiopia. These categories contain age (less than, equal, or greater than 5 year), malaria type (*P. vivax* and *P. falciparum*), cases (inpatient and outpatient), inpatient cases (cases and deaths), severe anemia (inpatient malaria cases less than 5 years and greater than 5 years), and uncomplicated lab-confirmed malaria less than 5 years and greater than 5 years (*P. vivax* outpatient cases and *P. falciparum* outpatient cases). Each attribute is preprocessed and statistically summarized into address, patient profile, weather, and altitude. For example, **Table 1** presented the statistical summary of uncomplicated malaria less than 5 years of lab-confirmed *Plasmodium falciparum*.

In order to extract hidden patterns and relationships within the data, from the initial dataset, a number of attributes are constructed. As shown in **Table 2**, from malaria with severe anemia, attributes such as age, malaria type, cases, and malaria visits, as well as the number of cases and deaths, are constructed.

Summary of the datasets compiled for association rule discovery with their possible nominal values and description is depicted in **Figure 1**. The malaria dataset used for this study consists

Uncomplicated Malaria <5 years P.FALCIPARUM Lab Confirmed				
Cases	Yes	No	Missing Value	Noisy Value
Frequency	105	4555	43	1
Percent	2.232%	96.832%	0.914%	0.021%

Table 1. Summary of uncomplicated malaria less than 5 years.

Initial Dataset Attribute	Target Dataset (Attribute Constructed)
Inpatient malaria with severe anemia < 5 years cases	- Age
Inpatient malaria with severe anemia < 5 years deaths	- Type of cases - Type of malaria
Inpatient malaria with severe anemia > 5 years cases	- Type of malaria visits - Number of cases
Inpatient malaria with severe anemia >5 years deaths	- Number of deaths

Table 2. Malaria with severe anemia and list of attributes constructed.

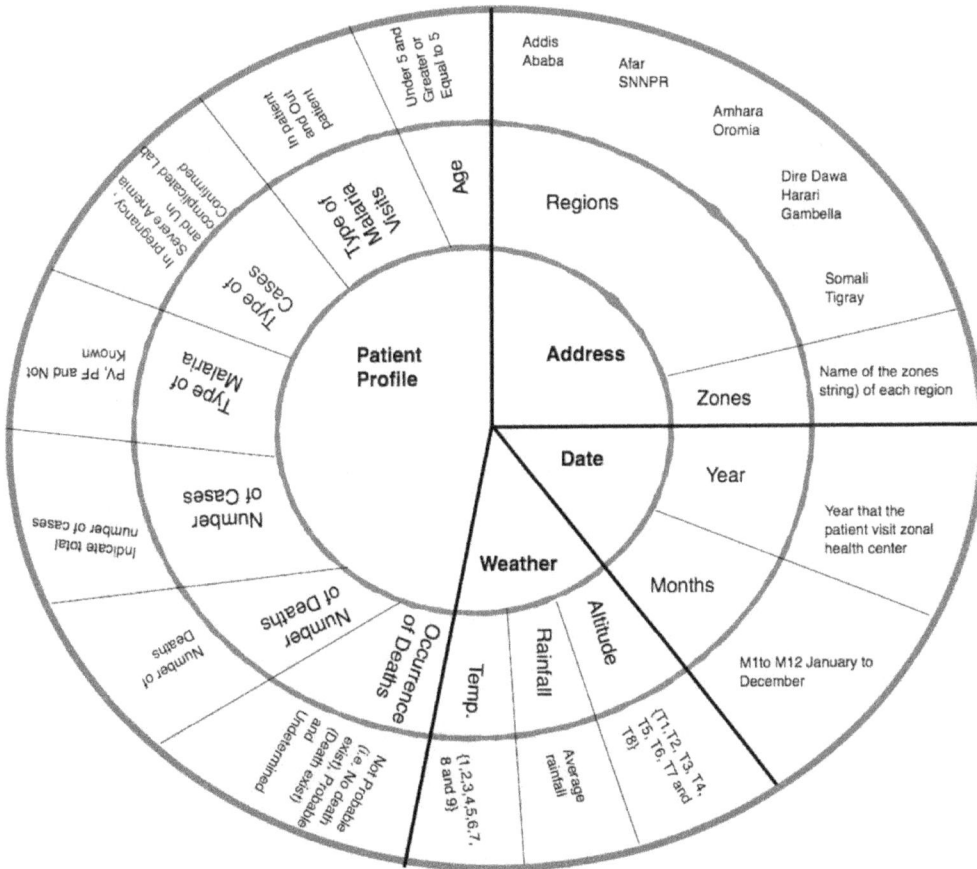

Figure 1. Summary of attributes and their transformed values.

of 14 attributes. The first inner part mainly presents the category of the attributes (i.e., profile, weather, address, and date), the second inner part presents the list of attributes constructed from category, and the last inner part indicates the value of each attribute. The region and zones contain all administrative regions in Ethiopia and the locations where the patients live. The date (year and month) indicates the year and the months that the patients visit the zonal health center. The age indicates the category of patients usually classified under 5 and greater or equal to 5. The type of malaria visits is classified into inpatient and outpatient malaria visits. The attribute type of case indicates the category of cases called in pregnancy, severe anemia, and uncomplicated lab-confirmed malaria. The type of malaria attributes contains PV, PF, and not-known values. In case of severe anemia and in pregnancy, the type of malaria is not known or determined in the dataset. A number of cases and deaths indicate the total number of cases and deaths, respectively. The attribute occurrence of deaths contains not probable (i.e., no deaths exist), probable (deaths exist), and undetermined values. The rainfall attribute contains a numeric value to represent average rainfall. In the case of outpatient visit, in pregnancy and uncomplicated lab-confirmed malaria, death is not known or listed in the dataset. The transformed temperature values 1, 2, 3, 4, 5, 6, 7, 8, and 9 represents $0–5^{0c}$, $5–10^{0c}$, $10–15^{0c}$, $16–20^{0c}$, $21–25^{0c}$, $25–30^{0c}$, $31–35^{0c}$, $35–40^{0c}$, and $>40^{0c}$, respectively. The transformed altitude values T1, T2, T3, T4, T5, T6, T7, and T8 represent >3500 m, 2500–3500 m, 2000–2500 m, 1500–2000 m, 1000–1500 m, 500–1000 m, 0–500 m, and <zero values, respectively.

3. Apriori method

The Apriori algorithm (a well-known association rule discovery method) takes a dataset with a list of items that can be easily transformed into a transaction form by creating an item for each attribute value pair that exists in the dataset [25–27]. Minimum support and minimum confidence thresholds are also defined to enable Apriori algorithms identify frequent items that are strongly associated. **Table 3** presented the step-by-step procedure to mine and extract frequent items using Apriori methods.

Given a support threshold (S), sets of X items that appear in greater than or equal to S baskets are called frequent item sets. Find all rules on item sets of the form X→Y with minimum support and confidence. For example, if-then rules about the content of the baskets {i1, i2,...,ik} → j means "if a basket contains all of i1,...,ik then it is likely to contain j." A typical question of Apriori is to "find all association rules with support ≥ S and confidence ≥ C." In

> - *Initially, scan database once to get frequent 1-itemset*
> - *Generate candidate k+1 itemsets from frequent k itemset. For each k, we construct two sets of k –tuples:*
>   - *C_k = the set of candidate k – tuples*
>   - *L_k = the set of truly frequent k –tuples.*
> - *Test the candidates against DB*
> - *Terminate when no frequent or candidate set can be generated*

Table 3. Apriori methods.

general, support of an association rule is the frequency of occurrence of the set of items it mentions, and confidence of this association rule is the probability of j given i1,...,ik. It is the number of transactions with i1,...,ik containing item j. This will measure the strength of associations between i1, i2,...,ik, and j.

The key concepts are frequent item sets (the set of items which have minimum support, denoted by Li for ith-item set), a priori property (any subset of frequent item set must be frequent), and join operation (to find Lk, a set of candidate k-item sets are generated by joining Lk-1 with itself). Once frequent item sets are obtained, it is straightforward to generate association rules with confidence larger than or equal to a user-specified minimum support and minimum confidence. The next top quality of the Apriori algorithm is to implement its achievement of good performance by reducing the size of candidate sets that are considered and selected for frequent k-item set [28].

A class implementing an Apriori-type algorithm iteratively reduces the minimum support until it finds the required number of rules with the given minimum confidence [29].

For mining Weka (Waikato Environment for Knowledge Analysis), knowledge discovery tool using Java is used. In Weka 3.7.3, if class association rule (car) property is enabled, the class association is mined instead of (general) association rules. Class classification generates rules that are frequently happening to the probable occurrence of malaria cases. In many studies, associative classification has been found to be more accurate than some traditional classification methods, such as C4.5 [25]. Associative classification can search strong associations between frequent patterns (conjunctions of attribute-value pairs) and class labels. Because association rules explore highly confident associations among multiple attributes, this approach may overcome some constraints introduced by decision tree induction, which considers only one attribute at a time. In all, in association of rule mining, finding all the rules that satisfy both a minimum support and a minimum confidence threshold is important so as to generate strong and interesting rules from the frequent patterns.

4. eHealth knowledge-based system

Knowledge-based systems are computer programs that try to solve problems in a human expert-like fashion by using knowledge about the application domain (knowledge base) and problem-solving techniques (inference method). The rule-based reasoning technique can be used with other reasoning techniques in order to make a knowledge-based system more efficient. For example, case-based and rule-based reasoning can be used together. Rule-based system is an example of knowledge-based system that uses rules for knowledge representation and rule-based reasoning for reasoning techniques. The development of knowledge-based systems in medical areas has made it possible to provide reliable and thorough diagnostic services with a minimum cost. Such systems can be designed to exhaustively consider all possible diseases in a domain, which could outperform human experts to achieve a rapid and accurate diagnosis. Several systems have been implemented in different medical areas like cancer therapy, infections, blood diseases, general internal medicine, glaucoma, and pulmonary function tests [13, 14].

Figure 2 presented the detail architecture of the proposed system. In this research we tried to integrate the output of data mining (i.e., the interrelationship of risk factors) with a knowledge-based system. Apriori algorithm using CRISP-DM methodology is adopted to create the interrelationship of risk factors and used for knowledge acquisition to develop a knowledge-based system. Nearest neighbor retrieval algorithms (for retrieval) and voting method (to reuse tasks) are used to design the eHealth knowledge-based system. The knowledge is represented using "IF a certain situation holds, THEN take a particular action," and the knowledge acquired (interrelationship of risk factors) from Apriori algorithm are rules. An

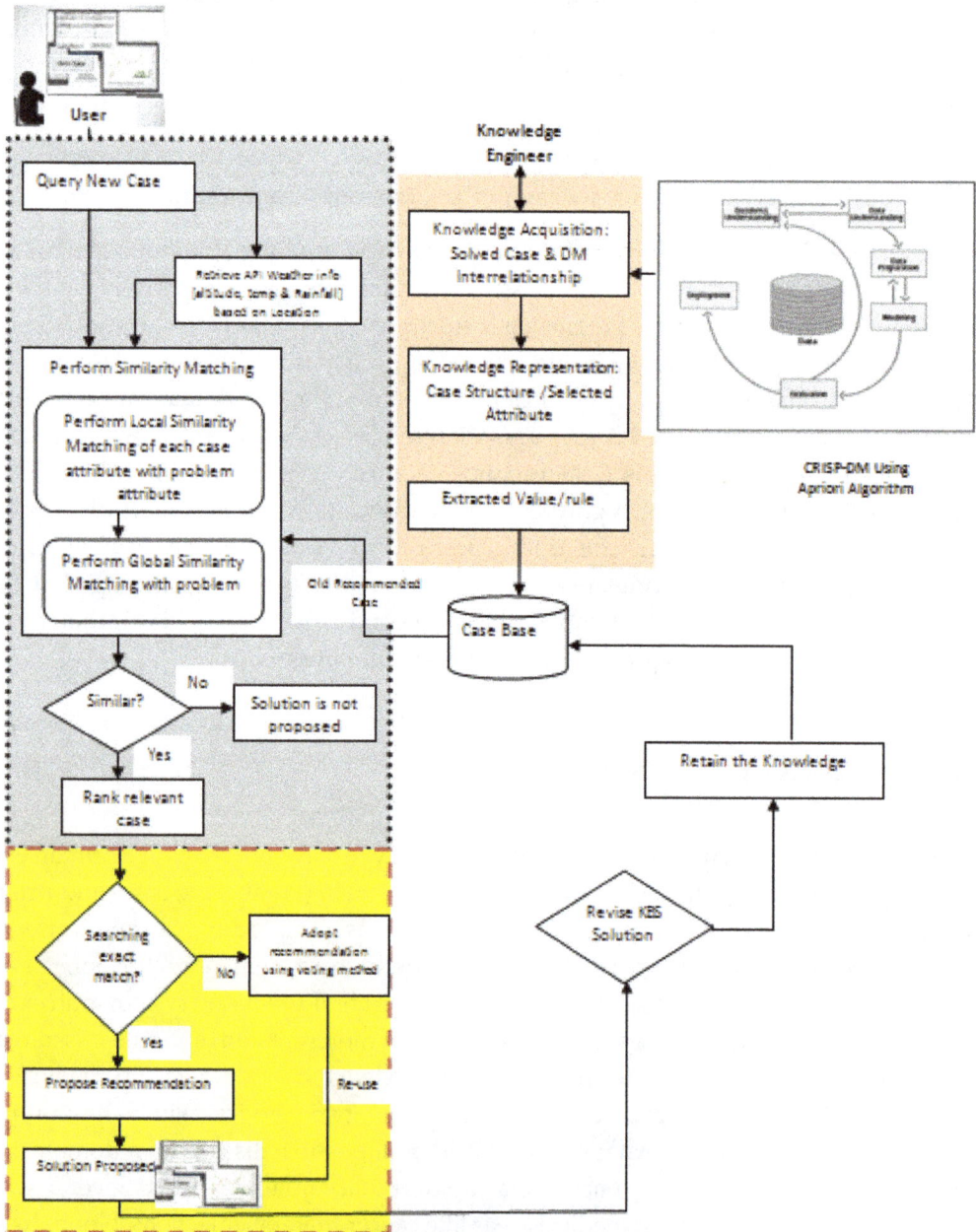

Figure 2. Adopted and proposed architecture for supporting eHealth KBS [19, 23, 24].

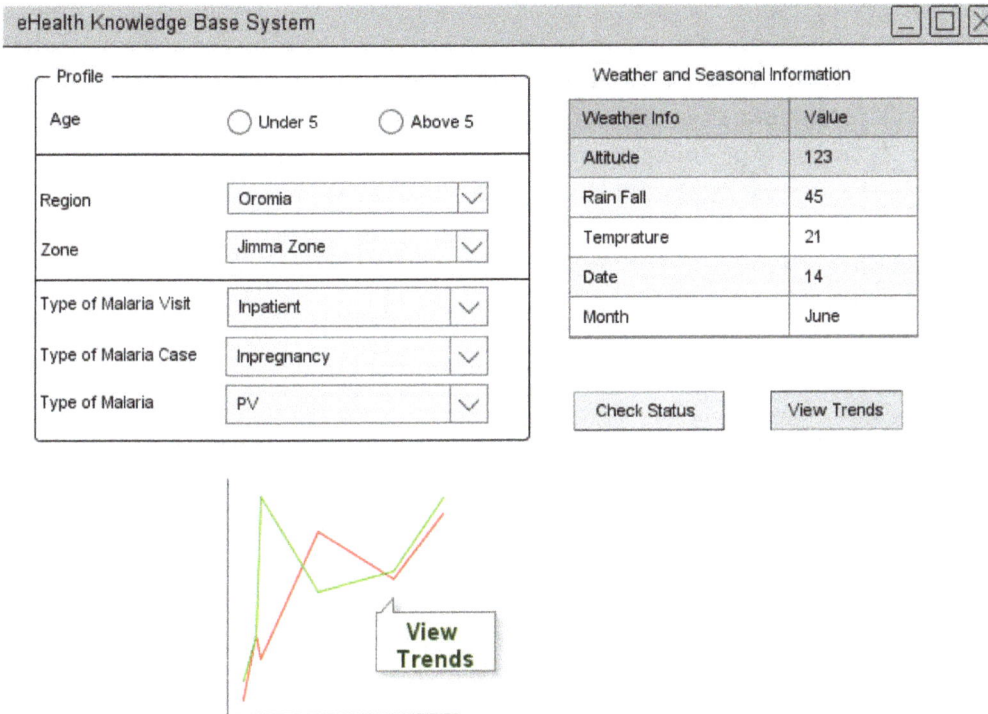

Figure 3. Graphical user interface.

inference engine of the knowledge-based system can derive the conclusion by looking the possible scenario and recommendations. The goal of the case study is to provide a personalized knowledge-based system solution using the support of interrelationship of risk factors. The user interfaces provide a communication between the user and the system.

Figure 3 presents the graphical user interface. The user tries to use the system or initiate queries by selecting profile and address information. Based on the desired location (using region and zone), weather information such as altitude, rainfall, and temperature are filled automatically from external weather API. Then, similarity matching is performed using the new queries to retrieve and recommend the proposed solution. However, if similarity matching is unsuccessful, voting technique is applied to select the relevant cases. Finally, to select or recommend the solution, the domain expert will evaluate and validate the new case. The knowledge-based system will use the validated case for future purpose.

5. Experimental results and discussions

The study tried to explore the interrelationship of risk factors for supporting eHealth knowledge-based system. We have used malaria dataset as a case study to discover the association among the various malaria risk factors using associative rule discovery data mining, and we integrate it with the eHealth knowledge-based system.

5.1. Experimental setup

A general and a class association rules are used to discover interesting association patterns. A total of 120 experiments executed using Apriori algorithm (60 experiments using general association rule and 60 experiments for class association rule mining) as depicted in **Table 4**. The confidence level is the most important parameter to attain the required objective. By considering this, the experiment is done at different confidence levels of 100, 90, 80, 70, 60, and 50%. Each confidence level is also experimented with a lower bound support of 10–100%. In both scenarios the min support of the upper bound is 100%.

Confidence level	No. of experiments	Min support lower bound	Experiment result		
			No. of association/ interrelationship rules generated	No. of cycles performed	Min support used to generate the rules
100%	5	60–100%	None		
	1	50%	7	10	50%
	1	40%	7	12	40%
	3	10–30%	10	11	35%
90%	4	70–100%	None		
	1	60%	2	8	60%
	1	50%	7	10	50%
	1	40%	7	12	40%
	3	10–30%	10	13	35%
80%	4	70–100%	None		
	1	60%	2	8	60%
	5	10–50%	10	10	50%
70%	4	70–100%	None		
	1	60%	2	8	60%
	5	10–50%	10	10	50%
60%	4	70–100%	None		
	1	60%	2	8	60%
	5	10–50%	10	10	50%
50%	4	70–100%	No rule generated		
	1	60%	2	8	60%
	5	10–50%	10	10	50%
Total exp.	60				

Table 4. Scenario and result of general association rule experiment.

5.2. Generated association rules

From the experiment, we observed that the class association mining supports the rules generated in general association mining. It also discovers interesting interrelationship (with 100% confidence level) related with the type of visit, age, altitude, temperature, and malaria type. With 100% confidence level and 60% support, outpatient cases are more closely related to the undetermined occurrence of death specifically when the age group of malaria patient is greater than 5. On the one hand, the result noted that occurrence of death is mostly related to outpatient case instead of the inpatient one. This shows that health workers offer great attention and intensive care for inpatient visits. On the other hand, most of outpatient visits are uncomplicated lab-confirmed malaria. However, the occurrence of death is undetermined and probable when the type of malaria visit is outpatient and the age of the patients is greater than 5. This may be because of lack of qualified health workers and the patients are not properly prescribed as confirmed by Ndiaye et al. [30] in Senegal that the lay health workers made negative diagnostic test.

6. Discussions

Table 5 illustrates the summary of experimental results. It is difficult to determine the occurrence of death for outpatient cases, and the experimental result revealed that the occurrence of death is related with the increment of malaria case. Roca-Feltrer et al. [31] noted that the increment of malaria cases is related with the transmission intensity, seasonality, and age that lead to a probability of occurrence of deaths. For instance, the experimental result in west Gojjam (specifically in November) supports the probability of occurrence of deaths related with the increment of malaria cases.

Knowing the seasonality of malaria helps to provide proper intervention to eradicate occurrence of death and cases [31]. Roca-Feltrer et al. [32] relate the transmission intensity, seasonality, and the age pattern of malaria and confirm that younger age groups are with increasing transmission intensity. Our experimental result also confirmed that occurrence of death is undetermined if the altitude is 1500–2000 m and when the age of the person is greater than 5 with a confidence level of 62 and 60%, respectively. This happens because of high transmission intensity. With 100% confidence level, if the type of malaria visit is outpatient and age is below 5, it is difficult to predict occurrence of deaths. Interestingly, occurrence of malaria death is related with severe anemia rather than pregnancy. As discussed by Knoblauch et al.

- If temperature is between 15 and 200°C, the type of malaria visits is outpatient, and the type of cases is uncomplicated lab-confirmed malaria, then the occurrence of death is undetermined.
- If the type of malaria is PV, then occurrence of death is undetermined, and if the type of malaria is PF, then occurrence of death is undetermined.
- If age is under 5 years and the type of malaria visits is outpatient, then occurrence of death is undetermined.

Table 5. Summarized experimental rules.

58

[33], anemia is prevalent in the 6- to 59-month-old children, and the association of anemia with a child age, underlying with iron requirements, is related to growth rate, and hence iron demand declines with age. Further, the algorithm associated (with 100% confidence level) with the type of malaria is unknown for inpatient malaria visits.

However, some unexpected or interesting interrelationship is prevailed such as with 100% confident level, and it is difficult to determine the occurrence of death for both PV and PF malaria types. This needs further investigation to verify whether it is unrelated or expected.

In all, the study presents the association of malaria risk factors using climate, elevation, location, type of malaria, type of malaria visits, number of cases, and death attributes. Both general and class association minings are done using Apriori techniques for discovering the association or patterns between the occurrence of deaths with the type of cases and malaria visits. And then, integrate the output of data mining (i.e., the interrelationship of risk factors) with knowledge-based reasoning. Nearest neighbor retrieval algorithms (for retrieval) and voting method (to reuse tasks) are used to design and deliver personalized knowledge-based system.

6.1. Evaluations

The evaluation of the result is executed by combining both an expert and testing tool approaches. An overall measure of pattern values, combining novelty, usefulness, and simplicity, to achieve a predefined goal is evaluated to measure the interestingness of the interrelationship. We have used different multitudes of measurement in the evaluation such as accuracy, support level, confidence, confidence level, and complexity with a 10fold cross validation. We adopted the four measures such as sensitivity, specificity, prediction accuracy, and precision to evaluate the correctness of interrelationship and validate the system through performance testing. Tenfold cross validation is used in the experiment to predict the error rate [34, 35]. The basic measure is accuracy, which computes the percentage of correctly classified instances in the test set. The accuracy of a test compares how close a new test value is to a value predicted by if-then rules [36].

The interrelationship of risk factors (association rules) was evaluated in terms of the number of rules and meaning of patterns generated at different minimum support and confidence thresholds for measuring interestingness of the rules. Association (interrelationship) was analyzed in terms of different criteria. The criteria include the number of rules generated at different minimum support and confidence thresholds. The minimum support and confidence thresholds varied from 0.1 to 1 and 0.5 to 1, respectively. As depicted in **Table 4**, at 90% confidence level with min support of 60 and 20%, the techniques generate 2 and 10 rules, respectively. Furthermore, we investigate the following indicators of the quality of the rule ranking induced by the interestingness measures of the mining algorithm in the average rank of the first rule that covers a test instance and the average rank of the first rule that covers and correctly predicts a test instance.

The performance of eHealth knowledge-based system prototype is evaluated using test case. Thus, the effectiveness of the retrieval process of eHealth knowledge-based system reasoning is measured by using recall and precision. Precision and recall are useful measures of retrieval performance [34]. Recall is the percentage of relevant cases for the query (new case) that are retrieved, whereas precision is the percentage of retrieved cases that are relevant to the query [34, 36, 37]. Accuracy is used to measure the performance of the reuse process [34, 36].

The case similarity testing shows that when the query is made up of attribute values that have the same value with the case from the case base, the result of the global similarity becomes 1.0. But when there is a difference in the attribute values of the query and the case in the case base, the global similarity value decreases. Therefore, adding cases in the case base improves the performance of knowledge-based reasoning system in solving problems (new cases).

The nearest neighbor algorithm, which is used to develop the retrieval process of the proto-type, uses distance to compute the similarity between the query and cases by representing the cases in N dimension vector. However, the recommendation doesn't have clear boundaries as it has subjectivity and depends on the experience of the domain experts as tested and adopted in [19, 23, 24]. In addition, the importance value that is assigned to the attributes of the case structure is done manually with the help of the domain experts, as there is no research that is conducted for the importance value of the attributes in malaria case management. This could affect the result of the retrieval and the reuse performance of the prototype. However, it needs user acceptance testing (using measuring usability with the system usability scale) in real-world scenarios to measure whether the potential users would like to use the proposed system frequently or not. So that, eHealth knowledge-based system for retrieving relevant cases and proposing solution will attain promising user acceptance, accuracy, and domain expert evaluation.

7. Conclusion and future work

The experimental result presents the association of risk factors (with relation to the malaria occurrence of death and type of case identification in Ethiopia) using climate, elevation, location, type of malaria, type of malaria visits, number of cases, and death attributes. Both general and class association minings are done using Apriori techniques for discovering the association or patterns of risk factors. The results noted the existence of strong association between occurrence of deaths, type of malaria visits, age, and type of cases. More interestingly, it discovers occurrence of malaria deaths, which are mostly related with severe anemia cases rather than pregnancy. It is also important to precede usability and user acceptance testing of eHealth knowledge-based system in real time and perform testing to compare and contrast with domain experts. So, health institutions have to give great attention to provide the necessary diagnosis and treatment for anemia, especially in regions that are more vulnerable for malaria. It also provides a significant contribution to design an optimal strategy in support of malaria prevention and control program within the country.

Acknowledgements

First and foremost I would like to thank God and the Holy Mother. Then, I would like to express special thanks for Worku Birhane who provided me proofreading and valuable comments.

Author details

Geletaw Sahle Tegenaw

Address all correspondence to: gelapril1985@gmail.com

Faculty of Computing, Jimma Institute of Technology, Jimma University (JU), Ethiopia

References

[1]   ESTA, OSHD. Health in Africa Over the Next 50 years. 2013. www.afdb.org

[2]   AfricaNext Investment Research. The future of African broadband: Economics, business models and the rise of 3G. 2010;(5)

[3]   Federal Ministry of Health. Health Extension Program in Ethiopia. Addis Ababa, Ethiopia: Health Extension and Education Center; 2007

[4]   Family Health Department. National Strategy for Child Survival in Ethiopia. Addis Ababa, Ethiopia: Federal Ministry of Health; 2005

[5]   http://www.moh.gov.et/factsheets {Accessed: August 2017]

[6]   Federal Democratic Republic of Ethiopia Ministry of Health. Ethiopia National Malaria Indicator Survey 2007 Technical Summary; 2008

[7]   Ministry of Health. Malaria Prevention Control Program. 2014. http://www.moh.gov.et/malaria [Accessed: June 2014]

[8]   Sahle G, Meshesha M. Uncovering knowledge that supports malaria prevention and control intervention program in Ethiopia. Electronic Journal of Health Informatics. 2014;8(1):e7. www.eJHI.net

[9]   Sajja PS, Akerkar R. Knowledge-based systems for development. Advanced Knowledge Based System: Model, Application & Research. 2010;1:1-11

[10] Tan C. A prototype of knowledge-based system for fault diagnosis in automatic wire bonding machine. Turkish Journal of Engineering and Environmental Sciences. 2008;32:235-244

[11] Hayes-Roth F. Rule-based systems. Communications of ACM. September 1985;28(9):921-932. DOI: 10.1145/4284.4286

[12] Engelmore RS, Feigenbaum E. Knowledge-Based Systems in Japan. Japanese Technology Evaluation Center. Maryland: Loyola College; 1993. http://www.wtec.org/loyola/kb/toc.htm

[13] Abdelhamied K, Hafez S, Abdalla W, Hiekal H, Adel A. A rule-based expert system for rapid problem solving in crowded outpatient clinics in Egypt. IEEE. 1988;3:1419-1420

[14] Pandey J, Bajpai D. Developmental design of a rule based expert system for diagnosis. In: Proceedings of the First Regional Conference, IEEE Engineering in Medicine and Biology Society and 14th Conference of the Biomedical Engineering Society of India. New Delhi: An International Meet; 1995. pp. 1/41-1/42. DOI: 10.1109/RCEMBS.1995.508680

[15] Pohle C. Integrating and updating domain knowledge with knowledge discovery. In: 6th International Conference for Business Informatics 2003 (WI-2003); Dresden, Germany; September 15-17; 2003

[16] Nasiri S, Fathi M. Toward an integrated e-health based on acquired healthcare knowledge. In: 2014 Middle East Conference on Biomedical Engineering (MECBME); 2014

[17] Seera M, Lim CP. A hybrid intelligent system for medical data classification. Expert Systems with Applications. 2014;**41**:2239-2249

[18] Sedighian Z, Javanmard M. The effect of data mining on expert systems used for improving efficiency of correct speech E-learning systems. Advances in Natural and Applied Sciences. 2014;**8**(10):102-106

[19] Mulugeta T, Beshah T. Integrating Data Mining Results with the Knowledge Based System for Diagnosis and Treatment of Visceral Leishmaniasis. 2015. Available at www.ijarcsse.com

[20] Kerdprasop K, Kerdprasop N. Bridging data mining model to the automated knowledge base of biomedical informatics. International Journal of Bio-Science and Bio-Technology. 2012;**4**(1):13

[21] Martin B. Instance-based learning: Nearest neighbour with generalisation [MSc thesis]. University of Waikato; 1995. Available at: http://www.cs.waikato.ac.nz/pubs/wp/1995/uow-cs-wp-1995-18.pdf [Accessed: March 27, 2011]

[22] Mishra D, Sahu B. Feature selection for cancer classification: A signal-to-noise ratio approach. International Journal of Scientific & Engineering Research. Hamilton, New Zealand: University of Waikato. 2011;**2**(4):1-7

[23] Salem AM. Case-based reasoning technology for medical diagnosis. World Academy of Science, Engineering and Technology. 2007;**31**:9-13

[24] Bekele H. A case based reasoning knowledge based system for hypertension management [MSc thesis]. Ethiopia: Addis Ababa University; 2011

[25] Han J, Micheline K. Data Mining: Concepts and Techniques. Waltham, USA: Morgan Kufman Publishers is an imprint of Elsevier; 2006

[26] Larose DT. Discovering Knowledge in Data: An Introduction to Data Mining. New Jersey, Canada: John Wiley & Sons; 2005

[27] Witten IH, Frank E. Data Mining: Practical Machine Learning Tools and Techniques. Morgan Kaufmann Series in Data Management Systems. 2nd ed. Physical Description xxxi. San Francisco: Morgan Kaufman Publishers; 2005. 525 p. ill. https://trove.nla.gov.au/version/46617902

[28] Wu X, Kumar V, Ross Quinlan J, et al. Knowledge and Information Systems. Springer-Verlag. 2008;**14**:1. https://doi.org/10.1007/s10115-007-0114-2. Print ISSN: 0219-1377. Online ISSN: 0219-3116

[29] The University of Waikato, WEKA Manual (Waikato Environment for Knowledge Analysis) for Version 3-7-4, This manual is licensed under the GNU General Public License version 2. Available at http://www.gnu.org/copyleft/gpl.html

[30] Ndiaye Y, Ndiaye JLA, Cisse B, Blanas D, Bassene J, Manga IA, Ndiath M, Faye SL, Bocoum M, Ndiaye M, Thior PM, Sene D, Milligan P, Gaye O, Schellenberg D. Community case management in malaria: Review and perspectives after four years of operational experience in Saraya district, south-East Senegal. Malaria Journal. 2013;**12**:240

[31] Roca-Feltrer A, Armstrong Schellenberg J, Smith L, Carneiro I. A simple method for defining malaria seasonality. Malaria Journal. 2009;**8**:276

[32] Roca-Feltrer A, Carneiro I, Smith L, Schellenberg JRMA, Greenwood B, Schellenberg D. The age patterns of severe malaria syndromes in sub-Saharan Africa across a range of transmission intensities and seasonality settings. Malaria Journal. 2010;**9**:282

[33] Knoblauch AM, Winkler MS, Archer C, Divall MJ, Owuor M, Yapo RM, Yao PA, Utzinger J. The epidemiology of malaria and anaemia in the Bonikro mining area, central Côte d'Ivoire. Malaria Journal. 2014;**13**:194

[34] McSherry D. Precision and recall in interactive case-based reasoning. In case-based reasoning research and development (ICCBR). Lecture Notes in Artificial Intelligence. 2001;**2080**:392-406

[35] Kohavi R. A study of cross validation and bootstrap for accuracy estimation and model selection. In: The International Joint Conference on Artificial Intelligence; 1995

[36] Junker M, Hoch R, Dengel A. On the evaluation of document analysis components by recall, precision, and accuracy. In: Proceedings of the Fifth International Conference on Document Analysis and Recognition; 1999. pp. 713-716

[37] Losee RM. When information retrieval measures agree about the relative quality of document rankings. Journal of the American Society for Information Science. 2000;**51**: 834-840

4

The Emerging Wearable Solutions in mHealth

Fang Zhao, Meng Li and Joe Z. Tsien

Abstract

The marriage of wearable sensors and smartphones have fashioned a foundation for mobile health technologies that enable healthcare to be unimpeded by geographical boundaries. Sweeping efforts are under way to develop a wide variety of smartphone-linked wearable biometric sensors and systems. This chapter reviews recent progress in the field of wearable technologies with a focus on key solutions for fall detection and prevention, Parkinson's disease assessment and cardiac disease, blood pressure and blood glucose management. In particular, the smartphone-based systems, without any external wearables, are summarized and discussed.

Keywords: wearable inertial sensors, accelerometer, gyroscope, ECG patch, classification algorithm, smartphone, fall detection and prevention, Parkinson's disease, cardiac rhythm, blood glucose, blood pressure

1. Introduction

Nowadays, dramatic advances in microelectromechanical systems (MEMS) technology have paved the way for wearable sensors to make inroads into mHealth, providing the potential for medical care and research to take place outside the standard doctor's office or hospital. A wide variety of wearable biometric sensors, such as bracelets, watches, skin patches, headbands, earphones, and clothing [1, 2], have been designed and developed. Regardless of the various forms and functions of these sensors, their unifying design focus is to allow for unobtrusive, passive, and continuous monitoring. Beyond sensing capability, another key characteristic is their ability to seamlessly connect with a mobile device to transfer all biometric data into a software application (APP) that can be shared with healthcare providers, researchers or family members. Inertial sensors, the most ubiquitous wearables, combined with dedicated algorithms are able to "count" steps (i.e., pedometers), gauge physical activity levels, indirectly estimate energy expenditure [3], and implement activity recognition [4]. Today, the Holter monitor, the most commonly used ambulatory electrocardiography device for assessing cardiac abnormalities, is one of the technologies that may soon become obsolete, since prolonged continuous rhythm monitoring is available by wearing an electrocardiogram (ECG) patch on the chest [5]. Other notable examples of sensor technologies under development which allow for a more personalized understanding of our health include cuffless blood pressure monitoring and noninvasive blood glucose tracking. Through progressively miniaturized, smartphones are equipped with comparatively advanced sensing capabilities (i.e., accelerometer, gyroscope, magnetometer, camera, and many more) and powerful computing capabilities, making it the ideal platform for remote health monitoring without the extra expense of purchasing and inconvenience of using dedicated wearables. As a result, smartphone-based solutions have emerged most recently for fall detection and prevention [6], activity recognition [7], Parkinson's disease (PD) assessment [8], and cardiac rhythm measurement in mHealth.

This chapter provides a review of recent progress in the field of wearable systems and solutions that have already entered into or have the potential to apply in mHealth. Aging of the population is a global issue, and it presents tremendous challenges to society and healthcare systems all over the world. The most common healthcare issues of the aging population include the following: (i) falls that are considered as one of the major hazards for the elderly, especially for those living alone [9]; (ii) neurological disorders that are categorized as major chronic diseases inducing motor impairments, with PD as one of the most frequently occurring conditions [10]; and (iii) cardiac disease, hypertension and diabetes are the most common chronic diseases affecting the elderly [11]. Therefore, a critical analysis of the state-of-the-art wearable solutions for these age-related care issues and chronic diseases are presented.

The remainder of this chapter can be separated into five sections. The wearable solutions for motion monitoring are discussed in Section 2. Firstly, the basic architecture of the wearable motion monitoring systems is described, followed by a summary of the state-of-the-art smartphone-based fall detection and prevention systems, with a focus on the sensor used, extracted features, the classification algorithm, and the outcomes in each system. The wearable solutions for PD are then discussed. A selection of external wearable solutions and smartphone-based systems that used pattern recognition algorithms to classify motor signs of functional activities impairment in PD are presented and compared. Section 3 illustrates the wearable solutions for cardiac activity monitoring. Several commercially available portable devices are presented. Section 4 describes the approaches for cuffless blood pressure monitoring and noninvasive blood glucose monitoring. Unfortunately, these approaches are not satisfactory to date. Finally, conclusion offered in Section 5 points out important observations and areas that need further research.

2. Wearable solutions for motion monitoring

Mirroring the increasingly widespread adoption of wearable inertial sensors in personalized healthcare is an equally remarkable development in algorithms to classify human activity [7].

As a result, inertial sensor technologies can go well beyond step counts to a wealth of person-alized activity information to help guide health and wellness. Earlier work by Bouten *et al.* [12] established a significant relationship (r=0.89) between accelerometer output and energy expenditure due to physical activity, impelling wearable sensor to become capable of estimat-ing energy expenditure in diabetes or obesity management. Subsequent work by Najafi *et al.* [13] founded a significant correlation between postural transition (PT) and falling risk using a gyroscope, which led to a variety of other works to exemplify the prominence of wearable inertial sensors in fall detection and prevention in elderly care. The activity recognition by wearable inertial sensors has also been used in the assessment and rehabilitation of many neurological diseases [14], such as Parkinson's disease (PD), stroke, cerebral palsy (CP), multiple sclerosis (MS), and Huntington's disease (HD), which can induce motor impairment. Transformations are under way in movement monitoring to provide care in the daily lives of those afflicted with these diseases as a result of all these breakthroughs.

2.1. Architecture

The basic architecture of motion monitoring systems for mHealth consists of three common phases namely, sensing, processing and communication (**Figure 1**). Feature extraction and motion classification algorithm used in the processing phase may differ greatly from system to system.

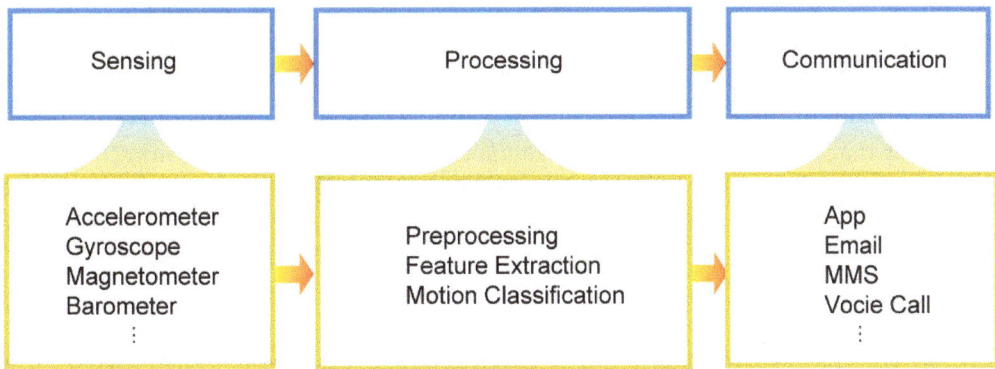

Figure 1. Basic architecture of activity tracking systems for mHealth.

2.1.1. Sensing

Multimodal MEMS sensors can be utilized to identify physical activities, including acceler-ometer, gyroscope, magnetometer, barometer, etc. The terms accelerometer, gyroscope, and magnetometer will refer to triaxial accelerometers, triaxial gyroscopes and triaxial magneto-meters, respectively, unless otherwise stated. Each type of sensor is sensitive to a kinematic quantity: accelerometer for sensing acceleration along three orthogonal directions; gyroscope for detecting angular momentum; magnetometer for gauging changes in orientation by measuring the strength of the local magnetic field along three orthogonal axes; and barometer for determining rapid changes in altitude (e.g., walking up/down stairs) by measuring absolute atmospheric pressure to infer altitude above sea level. Their combination can even estimate three-dimensional (3D) orientation and displacement.

2.1.2. Processing

The processing phase encompasses preprocessing, feature extraction and physical motion classification steps. Preprocessing needs to be first applied to the raw data collected from MEMS sensors to improve the signal-to-noise ratio. The signals are often smoothed by median filters of a short sliding window to remove spurious noise [15]. Accelerometer data are often high-pass filtered to separate acceleration caused by gravity from acceleration due to body movement [16].

After preprocessing of MEMS data, features are generally extracted from sequential epochs of time using window techniques. The most commonly used approach is the sliding window often with 50% overlap between consecutive windows [17], which is the most suitable for real-time or online applications. Statistical measures of the time domain and frequency domain features are widely used to reduce the MEMS data of each window epoch to a finite number of derived parameters from which a physical movement can be inferred.

Prior to classification, feature selection techniques [18] may be applied to find the optimal feature subset, which can best distinguish between movements, from all of the features generated. Feature selection is of particular importance as inappropriate or redundant features may deteriorate the overall classification performance. The selected features from the MEMS sensor data are exploited by the classification algorithms in the development of a model that can identify specific physical movements. Classification methods used in activity recognition include (but are not limited to) hidden Markov models (HMM), K nearest neighbors (KNN), support vector machines (SVM), discrete wavelet transform (DWT), decision tree classifiers (DTC), random forests (RFs), linear discriminant analysis (LDA) or feed-forward neural network (Bpxnc).

2.1.3. Communication

After processing, the classified motion data can then be sent to medical staff (e.g., a caregiver or a physician) for remote monitoring or back to the user or patient for self-monitoring. Once an abnormal movement (i.e., fall event) is detected, the wearable mHealth systems sent out a signal to seek help from the monitoring center or a caregiver via smartphones.

2.2. Fall detection and prevention

Falls are one of the major causes of injuries and hospital admissions of elderly people. Those who suffer from neurological diseases (e.g., stroke, PD) also give rise to increased fall risks. Falls can potentially cause severe physical injuries, such as bleeding, fracture and central nervous system (CNS) damage, and long lie times (remaining involuntarily on the ground for a prolonged period) after the fall can lead to disability, paralysis, even death. Therefore, the first line of defence against fall hazards is to prevent them and the second line of defence is to provide emergency treatment in time.

2.2.1. Smartphone-based systems

Initially, dedicated wearable kinematic sensors have been developed with the ability to assist in identifying falls [19, 20] and estimating the likelihood of future falls by monitoring activity levels or analyzing the individual's gait [21, 22]. However, their widespread adoption has been limited by the cost associated with purchasing the device and the low utilization coefficient by the user (who may often forget or refuse to wear the specially designed wearables). There has been a shift toward smartphones in recent years, as the smartphone with multimodal built-in MEMS sensors, coupled with its ubiquitous nature and increased computational power, make it the ideal platform for fall monitoring in mHealth. The first smartphone-based fall detection app iFall [23] utilized an integrated accelerometer to recognize the difference in position before and after the fall. Later in 2010, the PreFallD [24] was developed considering both the wearer's acceleration and orientation during the fall event. **Table 1** summarizes and compares the features of the existing smartphone-based fall detection and prevention systems or applications. The literatures that presented very preliminary investigations and did not declare the performance of their proposed solutions are not included here.

Arti cle	Appli cation	Sensors (Placement)	Algorithm	Performance	Notification (Information)
[23]	Detection	Accelerometer (Any)	Threshold	Demonstrated fall can be detected by smartphone.	SMS (time, GPS coordinates), audible notification.
[24]	Detection	Accelerometer & gyroscope & magnetometer (chest, waist, thigh)	Threshold	2.67% (Average *FN*), 8.7% (Average *FP*)	Audio alarm, voice call.
[25]	Detection	Accelerometer (trouser pocket)	DWT	85% (*RC*), 95% (*PR*)	SMS (GPS coordinates), email (Google map), twitter.
[30]	Detection	Accelerometer (chest, waist, thigh)	Threshold	97% (*PR*), 2.67% (average *FN*), 8.7% (Average *FP*)	Audio alarm, voice call
[26]	Detection	Accelerometer (Waist)	C4.5 DT, NB, SVM	98.85% (*AC* for DT); 86.47% (*AC* for SVM); 87.78% (*AC* for NB)	SMS
[97]	Detection	Accelerometer (waist)	Threshold	Detected 54 out of 67 simulated falls.	Email, SMS.
[31]	Detection	Accelerometer (waist)	Threshold	0.81 (*SP*), 0.77(*SE*)	SMS (time, location)

Arti cle	Appli cation	Sensors (Placement)	Algorithm	Performance	Notification (Information)
[39]	Detection	Accelerometer & gyroscope (hand, shirt, or trouser pocket)	Threshold, One-class SVM	75% (AC for hand); 77.9412% (AC for shirt pocket); 84.2857% (AC for trouser pocket)	Undisclosed
[98]	Detection	Accelerometer (waist)	Threshold	Capability of differentiate between running and falling	SMS (time, GPS coordinates)
[44]	Detection	Accelerometer (waist)	Threshold, ANN	100% success rate for a total of 500 epochs.	Message (GPS coordinates)
[6]	Detection, prevention	Accelerometer & gyroscope (waist)	Threshold	The uFall and uTUG can ran on a smartphone to realize long-term and real-time monitoring.	Audio alarm, email, SMS.
[99]	Detection	Accelerometer (shirt, or trouser pocket)	Threshold	97% (average SE), 100% (average SP)	Undisclosed
[32]	Detection	Accelerometer (Shirt pocket)	threshold	92.75% (SE), 86.75% (SP)	Text message
[40]	Detection	Accelerometer (trouser pocket)	SVM	95.7% (PR), 90% (average RC)	vibration, audio alarm, SMS (time, location)
[27]	Detection	Accelerometer & gyroscope (hand, pocket, waist)	Semisupervised learning	85.3% (SE), 90.5% (SP)	Undisclosed
[33]	Detection	Accelerometer (chest, waist, thigh)	Threshold	72.22% (SE), 73.78 (SP)	SMS
[34]	Detection	Accelerometer & gyroscope (hand, pocket)	Threshold	80% (SE), 96.25% (SP), 85% (AC)	Undisclosed
[41]	Detection	Accelerometer & Wi-Fi module (waist)	DT, SVM, NB, RSSI	100% & 75.8% (PR & RC for DT); 99.81% & 75.43% (PR & RC for SVM); 98.67% & 73.20%	SMS (name, time, location)

Arti cle	Appli cation	Sensors (Placement)	Algorithm	Performance	Notification (Information)
				(*PR* & *RC* for NB).	
[28]	Detection	Accelerometer & gyroscope & magnetometer (chest)	Fisher's discriminant ration and *J*3 criterion, hierarchical classifiers	97.63% (*AC*) for fall; 95.03% (*AC*) for total	MMS (time, GPS coordinate, map)
[35]	Detection	Accelerometer (waist)	Threshold	83.33% (*SE*), 100% (*SP*)	SMS, voice call, twitter, email, Facebook
[100]	Detection	Accelerometer (waist)	Threshold	Detected 47 out of 50 samples.	SMS (time, GPS data)
[29]	Prevention	Accelerometer & gyroscope (trouser pocket)	C4.5 DT, Hjorth mobility and complexity	99.8% (*AC*)	Message, vibration
[42]	Detection	Accelerometer (trouser pocket)	OneR, ReliefF, SCMA, K*, C4.5, NB	90% success ratio, 83.8% & 82.0% (*PR* & *RC* for NB); 83.8% & 82.0% (*PR* & *RC* for J48 DT); 88.9% & 88.6% (*PR* & *RC* for K*).	SMS (GPS coordinate)
[36]	Detection	Accelerometer (waist)	Threshold	90% (*SP*), 100% (*SE*), 94% (*AC*)	SMS
[37]	Detection	Accelerometer & encompass (pocket)	Cascaded classification	92% (*SE*), 99.75% (*SP*)	Message (GPS coordinate)
[38]	Detection	Accelerometer (side, or back pocket, arm, neck)	Threshold & orientation	95% (*PR*), 90 (*AC*), 100% (*RC*)	Undisclosed
[43]	Detection	Accelerometer (Pocket)	PNN[1], PSVM[2]	PNN: 0.9861 (mean AUC); PSVM: 0.9914 (mean AUC)	Undisclosed

[1]PNN-Personalized Nearest;
[2]PSVM-Personalized SVM.

Table 1. Smartphone-based fall detection and prevention systems.

The most common sensor used in fall detection and prevention was the accelerometer, followed by the gyroscope (**Table 1**). In most of the studies, threshold-based algorithm was adopted for fall detection due to its low complexity. The most commonly used feature for threshold-based algorithm is the magnitude vector of acceleration signal:

$$| A_T |= \sqrt{| A_x |^2 + | A_y |^2 + | A_z |^2} \tag{1}$$

where A_x, A_y, and A_z represent accelerometer signals of the x-, y-, and z-axis, respectively. The threshold value could be predefined (fixed) or adaptive (changed with user-provided physiological data, such as height, weight).

The surge in computing power has fashioned a foundation for complex machine-learning classification algorithms for fall detection and prevention to be implemented in smartphones. The classification algorithms used in the processing phase vary considerably across systems. Yavuz *et al.* [25] utilized DWT and achieved a better true-positive (TP) performance while decreasing the false positives (FP) when compared to threshold-based algorithm. Zhao *et al.* [26] implemented three machine-learning algorithms—namely C4.5 DTC, NB, and SVM and compared their performances based on recognition accuracy. Fahmi *et al.* [27] designed a semisupervised algorithm to detect a genuine fall event with smartphone. He and Li [28] employed a combined algorithm of Fisher's discriminant ratio (FDR) criterion and J3 criterion for feature selection and hierarchical classifiers to recognize 15 activities including fall events. Majumder *et al.* [29] applied Hjorth mobility and complexity to identify high-risk gait patterns, hence developed a fall prevention system called iPrevention.

Once a fall event is detected, the systems send out notifications including audible alarms, vibrations, automatic voice calls, short message service (SMS), multimedia messaging service (MMS), E-mails, Twitter messaging, etc., (**Table 1**). Notification messages may contain information regarding time and location (GPS coordinates or Google Map).

2.2.2. Performance evaluations

There is no uniform standard for outcome evaluations of fall detection or prevention systems now. The outcomes are often represented by four possible situations [24, 30]: *TP*, a fall occurred and was correctly detected; *FP*, the system declared a fall that did not occur; true negative (TN), a fall-like event was not misclassified as a fall event; false negative (FN), a fall occurred, but the system missed it. The reliability of systems is usually evaluated based on the following parameters: sensitivity *(SE)* = *TP/(TP+FN)*, which is the ratio of fallers correctly classified as fall event [27, 31–34]; specificity *(SP)* = *TN/(TP+FN)*, which is the ratio of fall-like events correctly classified as nonfallers [35–38]; accuracy = *(TP+TN)/(TP+FP+FN+TN)*, which is the ratio of true results in the whole data set [26, 28, 29, 39]. Some works measured the performance in a different way; they utilized *precision* = (∩)/and recall—namely, the number of correct results divided by the total outputs—as the performance indexes [40–42]. Some other works evaluated the proposed system by measuring the area under the receiver operating characteristic curve (AUC), where the curve represented *SE* versus *FN* [43].

2.2.3. Limitations and challenges

Despite the expanding body of evidence to support the use of smartphones for fall detection and prevention, it is important to recognize the limitations in this area of science. The prominent weakness is problems induced by the limited battery life of the smartphone. The rate at which the smartphone's battery is consumed is dependent on both internal and external factors. Internal factors are built-in sensor dependent, including the sampling rate and resolution mode. High-resolution mode can dramatically increase the rate of power consumption. External factors are related to the number of sensors used, data recording time, and complexity of the algorithms. Mellone *et al.* [6] showed that a battery could power a smartphone (Samsung Galaxy S II) for 30 h with only one sensor used and 16 h with three sensors activated. Majumder *et al.* [29] reported that a fully charged battery can only power an iPhone for 3 h at the most, when running a machine learning algorithm. Energy efficiency will continue to be an important criterion when choosing the algorithm, unless advancements in battery technology could lead to higher density energy storage.

Model	Sensors	Dynamic ranges	Resolution
Samsung S4	Accelerometer	±2 g	±0.001 ms^{-2}
	Gyroscope	$\pm500°$/s	$\pm0.057°$/s
	Magnetometer	±1200 μT	±0.15 μT (x/y axis) ±0.25 μT (z axis)
	Barometer	300–1100 hPa	±1 hPa
Samsung S3	Accelerometer	±2 g	±0.01 ms^{-2}
	Gyroscope	$\pm500°$/s	$\pm0.015°$/s
	Magnetometer	±1200 μT	±0.30 μT
	Barometer	260–1260 hPa	±0.24 hPa
Galaxy Nexus	Accelerometer	±2 g	±0.61 m·s^{-2}
	Gyroscope	$\pm2000°$/s	$\pm0.06°$/s
	Magnetometer	±800 μT	±0.15 μT (*x/y* axis) ±0.30 μT (z axis)
	Barometer	300–1100 hPa	±1 hPa
HTC One	Accelerometer	±4 g	±0.039 m·s^{-2}
	Gyroscope	$\pm2000°$/s	$\pm0.06°$/s
	Magnetometer	±4900 μT	±0.15 μT
LG Nexus 4	Accelerometer	±4 g	±0.001 m·s^{-2}
	Gyroscope	$\pm500°$/s	$\pm0.015°$/s
	Magnetometer	±4912 μT	±0.15 μT
	Barometer	0–1100 hPa	±1 hPa
iPhone 5/5s	Accelerometer	±8 g	±0.002 m·s^{-2}
	Gyroscope	$\pm2000°$/s	$\pm0.06°$/s
	Magnetometer	±1200 μT	±0.30 μT
iPhone 6/6plus	Accelerometer	±8 g	±0.002 m·s^{-2}
	Gyroscope	$\pm2000°$/s	$\pm0.06°$/s
	Magnetometer	±4900 μT	±0.15 μT
	Barometer	300–1100 hPa	±0.16 hPa

Table 2. Specifications of the built-in sensors in some currently available smartphones.

The resolution and dynamic range of the built-in inertial sensors vary considerably across smartphones (**Table 2**). Acceptable dynamic ranges for accelerometers from ±4 g to ± 16 g (g = 9.81 ms^{-2}) have been reported for fall detection applications [35, 44], which is beyond the typical dynamic ranges of most currently available smartphone accelerometers (± 2 g). The newest high-end commercially available smartphones (i.e., iPhone 6/6plus) have accelerometers with higher dynamic ranges (± 8 g), making these devices more suitable for detecting falls.

In addition, a major limitation of using smartphones to detect fall is that it requires the smartphone to be consistently located and/or oriented in the same position. It may be difficult to do so due to the multifunctional nature of smartphones. Habib *et al.* [45] showed that individuals may not place their smartphone on their body whilst at home so, that being said, it may limit the ability of the smartphone to detect fall in the home. At present, smartphone placement and usability issues should be handled carefully.

2.3. Functional activities assessment for Parkinson' s disease

For a population that is shifting toward an older age range, PD is categorized in the most common chronic neurological disorders. PD is characterized as an age-related neurodegenerative disorder due to the loss of dopamine-producing brain neurons, an important neurotransmitter involved in the regulation of movement. Progressive tremor, bradykinesia, hypokinesia, rigidity, and impaired postural control are common and disabling features of most patients with PD. The motor disorder analysis is generally performed in a clinical setting to provide subjective assessments. However, the motor fluctuation measurements in the clinical setting might not precisely reveal the real functional disability experienced by patients in natural environment. With the existing and on-going advance developments in MEMS technologies, continuous, unsupervised, objective and reliable monitoring of mobility and functional activities in natural environments is now possible, allowing for long-term, home-based intensive care and improvement of the individual healthcare and well being.

2.3.1. Wearable inertial sensor-based methods

A growing body of literature studied the use of wearable inertial sensors to detect and quantify tremor, bradykinesia and levodopa-induced dyskinesia (LID) in PD populations. Most studies were focused on finding the features derived from sensor signals that are effective for detecting differences between people with PD and healthy controls [46–49]. Results from these studies presented a range of outcomes which included the root mean square (RMS) of accelerations, the deviation of acceleration, step or stride variability, gait regularity or symmetry, FFT features, entropy and many more. Only a few works established and validated motion analysis methods or systems that used pattern recognition algorithms to classify motor signs of functional activities impairment in PD. **Table 3** provides a detailed comparison of these different methodological approaches. Leave-one-subject-out method and cross-validation method were used for validating the approaches.

Arti cle	Sensors (Placement)	Algorithm	Features	Performance	Validity
57	Accelerometer & gyroscopes (shanks, trunk)	Logistic regression model with Mamdani fuzzy rule-based classifier	Duration of transition, amplitude, range, minimum value, maximum value, relative time.	Differentiate between sit-to-stand and stand-to-sit transitions with 83.8% *SE*.	Cross-validation
52	Accelerometer (limbs, trunk, belt)	KNN, Parzen, Parzen density, binary decision tree, Bpxnc, SVM.	RMS, range.	Detect the severity of bradykinesia with an *AC* range of 70–86% depending on the algorithm.	Cross validation
55	Accelerometer & gyroscopes (wrist, thigh, foot, sternum)	DT	IAA[1] and change in thing inclination per second (thigh); differentiate an upright position from a horizontal one (trunk, thigh); AAM[2] (wrist); peak detection (foot).	98.9% (overall *AC*); Detect significant changes in rest and kinetic tremor with an *AC* range from 78.8–94.1% depending on the activity performed.	Leave-one-subject-out method
53	Accelerometer & gyroscopes (shoes)	Boosting with decision stump, LDA and SVM with linear and RBF kernel.	Step duration, entropy, variance, energy ratio, 0.5–3 Hz energy band.	Classify patients with PD and healthy controls using LDA with 88% *SE* and 86% *SP*; Distinguish mild from severe gait impairments with 100% *SE* and *SP*.	Leave-one-subject-out method
54	Accelerometer & gyroscopes (shoes)	LDA, AdaBoost, SVM with linear and RBF kernel.	Single steps, complete gait sequence, FFT of gait sequences.	Distinguish patients with PD from controls with an overall *AC* of 81%; Differentiate between Hoehn and Yahr III patients to controls with 91% *AC*.	Cross validation
51	Accelerometer	Supervised machine-learning models	FFT features: P_{total} between 0.5–8 Hz, $P_{locomotion}$	94.94% (*AC*), 94% (*SP*)	Undisclosed

Arti cle	Sensors (Placement)	Algorithm	Features	Performance	Validity
			on 0.5–3 Hz, P_{freeze} on 3–8 Hz, freeze index.		
56	Four accelerometers (extremity) and one accelerometers & gyroscopes (waist)	HMM (for tremor)	Time, frequency and spatial features.	87% (AC), 0.008 (MBE)	Leave-one-subject-out method
		DT (for LID)	Mean value, standard deviation, entropy, energy in specific frequency subbands, entropy.	85.4% (AC), 0.31 (MBE)	
		SVM (for Bradykinesia)	Approximate entropy, sample entropy, RMS, cross correlation, range.	74.5% (AC), 0.25 (MBE)	
		RF (for FOG)	Entropy	79% (AC), 0.79 (MBE)	

[1]IAA-Integrals of the absolute value of the accelerometer output;
[2]AAM-active arm movement.

Table 3. Wearable inertial sensor-based methods for Parkinson's disease.

These methods were founded on various machine-learning classifiers. Salarian *et al.* [50] applied a fuzzy classifier combined with a logistic regression model to categorize sit-to-stand (STS) transitions. Three inertial sensors were used to detect the kinematic features of the trunk movements during the transitions. Compared to video recordings reference system, it demonstrated the ability to differentiate sit-to-stand from stand-to-sit with a sensitivity of 83.3% in PD and 94.4% in controls. Another study by Mazilu *et al.* [51] presented the GaitAssist system to detect FoG with two ankle-mounted IMUs, streaming data via Bluetooth to an Android phone. Supervised machine-learning models, trained offline using several FFT features, were utilized with an overall FoG hit rate of 94.94% and a specificity of 94%.

Some studies, on the other hand, evaluated various classifiers to identify ambulatory activities. Cancela *et al.* [52] implemented six activity recognition algorithms, —namely KNN, Parzen, Parzen density, DTC, Bpxnc, and SVM, to detect the severity of bradykinesia and found out that the SVM revealed the best classification results with 86% sensitivity by using two features (RMS and range). Barth *et al.* [53] employed three classifiers, including boosting with decision stump, LDA and SVM, to measure gait patterns in PD to distinguish mild and severe gait impairment. The system was able to classify PDs and controls with 88% sensitivity and 86% specificity using the LDA classifier based on three activities—namely 10 m walking, heel-toe tapping, and foot circling. It reached a 100% sensitivity and specificity to distinguish mild from severe using optimal features—namely step duration, entropy, variance, energy ratio, and a

0.5–3 Hz energy band. Klucken *et al.* [54] used 694 features and three pattern recognition algorithms (LDA, AdaBoost, and SVM) to categorize patients in different stages. The developed eGaIT system, which consists of accelerometers and gyroscopes attached to shoes, was able to successfully distinguish patients from controls with an overall classification rate of 81%. The classification accuracy increased to 91% for more severe motor impairment or H&Y III patients.

Besides evaluating classifier, other works provided a complete motor assessment by analyzing the severity of several PD motor symptoms. Zwartjes *et al.* [55] used DTC to analyze motor activity and the severity of tremor, bradykinesia, and hypokinesia in patients with PD at three different levels of deep brain stimulation (DBS) treatment. An overall accuracy of 99.3% was achieved. Tzallas *et al.* [56] developed a system called PERFORM, using four accelerometers at each extremity and one accelerometer/gyroscope on the waist, to evaluate and quantify various symptom severity. The severity and type of tremor were classified by HMM classifier based on several time and frequency domain characteristics with 87% accuracy and 0.008 mean absolute error (*MBE*). The C4.5 DCT algorithm was used for LID detection and severity classification with an accuracy of 85.4% and a *MBE* of 0.31. A SVM classifier with optimum features (including approximate entropy, across correlation value, and range value) achieved 74.5% accuracy and 0.25 *MBE* for bradykinesia assessment. The detection of FoG was realized by an RFs classifier using the boot strap technique with 79% accuracy and 0.79 *MBE*. The PERFORM system also included a local base unit and a centralized hospital unit, allowing for the continuous remote monitoring and management of patients with PD.

2.3.2. Smartphone-based solutions

Given that smartphones are ubiquitous and have advanced built-in inertial sensors, research has recently sought to develop smartphone-based systems for PD assessments, which can keep the patient "connected" to his physician on a daily basis. The important features of existing smartphone-based solutions are summarized and compared in **Table 4**.

Arti cle	Sensors (Placement)	Features	Algorithm	Performance	Validity
57	Accelerometer (undisclosed)	Mean, SD[1], 25th percentile, 75th percentile, IQR[2], median, mode, range, skewness, kurtosis, mean squared energy, entropy, cross correlation, mutual information, cross entropy, DFA[3], instantaneous changes in energy, auto-regression coefficient, zero-crossing rate, dominant frequency component, radial distance, polar angle, azimuth angle.	RFs	Discriminate patients with PD from controls with an average *SE* of 98.5% and average *SP* of 97.5%.	Cross validation

Arti cle	Sensors (Placement)	Features	Algorithm	Performance	Validity
8	Accelerometer & gyroscope & touch screen & microphone	Average frequencies, RMS angular velocity, speed of movement, amplitude of dominant rhythm, CV[4], PSD, RMS values.	SVM, RFs	94.5% (*AC*), > 0.85 (AUC)	Cross validation
58	Accelerometer (hips)	Freeze index, energy, cadence variation, the ratio of the derivative of the energy.	fuzzy Logic algorithm	89% (*SE*), 97% (*SP*)	Undisclosed
60	Accelerometer & gyroscope (hand)	Magnitude of acceleration and rotational velocity, SD of acceleration, mean magnitude of rotation rate.	BagDT	82% (*AC* in patients), 90% (*AC* in controls)	Cross validation
59	Accelerometer & gyroscope (ankle, trouser pocket, waist, chest pocket)	Mean, variance, SD, entropy, energy, Fi, power, RMS, interquantile range, kurtosis, frequency domain features.	AdaBoost. M1,	86% & 84% & 81% (*SE* at the waist, in the trouser pocket and at the ankle, respectively).	Cross validation
61	Accelerometer (hand or ankle)	Hand tremor: power between 4–6 Hz, fraction of power, power ration in 3.5–15 Hz to 0.15–3.5 Hz, total power from 0–20 Hz, peak power, average acceleration.Gait: average gait cycle, average stride length, average walking speed, average acceleration, the number of steps and the speed of turning 360°.	SVM	77% & 82% (*SE* & *AC* for hand resting tremor detection), 89% & 81% (*SE* & *AC* for gait difficulty detection).	Cross-validation

[1]SD-Standard Deviation;
[2]IQR-Inter-quartile range;
[3]DFA-Extent of randomness;
[4]CV-Coefficient of variation.

Table 4. Smartphone-based solutions for Parkinson's disease.

These smartphone-based solutions use the signal from the integrated accelerometers or gyroscopes in consumer-grade smartphones and in conjunction with machine learning algorithms to quantify key movement severity symptoms (i.e., bradykinesia, FoG, hand tremor) and discriminate patients with PD from controls. Arora *et al.* [57] using an RFs classifier with a range of different time and frequency features of the acceleration time series, achieved 98.5% average sensitivity and 97.5% average specificity in differentiating patients with PD from controls. Another study by Printy *et al.* [8] developed an iPhone application using embedded hardware of a smartphone, including gyroscope, accelerometer, capacitive touch screen, microphone, and the front-facing camera, and a SVM algorithm to discriminate between more severe and less severe bradykinesia with an accuracy of 94.5%. The accurate classification of bradykinesia severity was not achieved in this work.

Some studies, on the other hand, aimed to detect FoG, a common motor impairment to suffer an inability to walk in PD patients. Pepa *et al.* [58] presented a smartphone-integrated accelerometer-based system to detect the FoG. They developed a linguistic fuzzy modelling (LFM) with Mamdani rule structure by fusing the information of freeze index, energy sum, cadency variation, and energy derivative ratio with a sensitivity of 89% and a specificity of 97%. In the smartphone-based system for FoG detection proposed by Kim *et al.* [59], data are derived from both embedded accelerometer and gyroscope. An AdaBoost.M1 classifier using several time and frequency domain features showed the best sensitivity of 86% at the waist, 84% and 81% in the trouser pocket and at the ankle, respectively.

Two other studies used the smartphone to measure the hand tremor symptom. Kostikis *et al.* [60] utilized a Breiman's RFs to classify upper limb tremor and achieved 82% accuracy in patients with PD and 90% accuracy in controls, with 0.9435 AUC. The feature metrics were derived from the acceleration vector and rotational velocity vector when patients performed two MDS-UPDRS postures—namely "Extended" and "Rest". Pan *et al.* [61] designed a prototype mobile cloud-based mHealth app on the Android platform called "PD Dr" to measure the severity of both hand resting tremor and gait difficulty, using the built-in accelerometer. The SVM classifier was used with a sensitivity of 77% and a specificity of 82% for hand resting tremor detection, and 89% sensitivity and 81% specificity in gait difficulty detection. Lasso regression approach was built to estimate the symptom severity. There was a strong correlation with PD disease stage (r=0.81), hand resting tremor severity(r=0.74), and gait difficulty severity (r=0.79).

2.3.3. Limitations and challenges

Given the relatively small number of classifier-based studies in this area and the wide variety of research questions addressed, ranging from activity classification to different symptom severity level assessment, it is currently difficult to address which classifier is ideal in PD populations for mHealth. Meanwhile, the accuracy levels of the classifiers were generalized on small sample sizes ranging from 5 to 27 subjects [50–53, 55–61]. Only one out of these studies enlisted a relatively larger sample of 92 patients with PD and 81 controls [54]. It is therefore important to evaluate the performance of classifiers according to larger, homogeneous population sets. Moreover, It is difficult to evaluate how effective or well performing of a classifier, because its performance also depends on the selected features and the properties of wearable sensors (i.e., resolution, noise level). Therefore, the effectiveness of wearable inertial-based methods in mHealth regimens still has to be further examined.

Using a smartphone for PD management seems promising in mHealth, yet there are the same issues as those in smartphone-based fall detection systems. The performance and usability of smartphone-based solutions remain limited by the relatively lower quality of embedded sensors, and the limited battery life of smartphones, as well as the need to wear the smartphone in a fixed position.

Only very few studies provided a complete overall assessment of PD [55, 56]. Most of the existing solutions with external wearables sensors or the smartphones built-in sensors have limited focus on a particular motor symptom, and lack the important characteristic for PD-monitoring services, such as long-term recording, qualitative and quantitative assessments. Therefore, more effort should be put into providing a complete tool that comprises the most common PD motor disabilities, such as tremor, bradykinesia, LID, and FoG.

3. Wearable solutions for cardiac monitoring

Heart disease, a worldwide chronic condition, is the leading cause of death in many countries. There are various parameters that capture the characteristics of cardiac activity. Among them, resting HR is one of the simplest, yet most informative, cardiovascular parameters. Heart rate variability (HRV) has been identified as a prognostic marker for cardiac abnormalities. Although the "gold standard" for assessing cardiac abnormalities remains a 12-lead Holter, a large number of innovative and versatile wearable devices, including chest strips, wrist-worn devices, earphones, and smart clothing, have emerged as alternatives, which can provide the opportunity for prolonged, continuous cardiac rhythm tracking in real-world environments. Today, several portable devices are commercially available for determining cardiac status via a single-lead ECG, either by wearing a patch for continuous rhythm tracking [5] or using a smartphone for rhythm capture whenever needed. If multiple leads are needed to increase the accuracy of arrhythmia diagnosis, there are smart shirts that allow for 3- to 12-lead ECG monitoring [2].

3.2.1. ECG patch monitor

An ECG patch monitor (EPM) attached to the skin on the chest via an adhesive carrier generally consists of electrodes, a signal-processing subsystem, and a wireless data transmission subsystem. The two most representative examples of single-lead EPM are the Zio Patch recorder [62] and NUVANT PiiX event recorder [63].

The Zio Patch can be categorized as a single-lead Holter with a memory of up to 14 days of stored rhythms. The Zio Patch has a frequency response of 0.15–34 Hz, an input impedance greater than 3 MΩ, a differential range of ± 1.65 mV, and a resolution of 10 bits. There is a button on the patch allowing the patient to mark a symptomatic episode. Once the recording period is complete, the patient mails the patch back to iRhythm Clinical Centers (iCC), where the recorded ECG data will be processed and analyzed by the Zio ECG Utilization Service (ZEUS) system with the capability of detecting up to 10 categories of rhythms. Rosenberg *et al.* [64] compared the Zio Patch with a 24-h Holter monitor in 74 consecutive patients. The mean wear time was 10.8 ± 2.8 days. Compared with the first 24 h of monitoring, there was an excellent agreement between the Zio Patch and Holter in identifying atrial fibrillation (AF) events. In another study, Turakhia *et al.* [65] evaluated the performance of the Zio Patch in 26,751 consecutive patients. The Zio Patch was well tolerated, with a mean monitoring period of 7.6 ± 3.6 days, and the median analyzable time was achieved 99% of the total wear time. The overall diagnostic yield of the Zio Patch was 62.2% for any arrhythmia and 9.7% for any symptomatic arrhythmia.

The NUVANT system consists of a 15-cm adhesive patch named the PiiX, a wireless data transmitter called zLink® and a patient trigger magnet [66]. The PiiX sensor samples the ECG signal at 200 Hz with a resolution of 10 bits. The PiiX patch that is integrated with multiple sensors cannot only continuously monitor many physiological parameters, including HR, HRV, RR, fluid status, body position, activity, and body temperature, but also automatically identify nonlethal cardiac arrhythmias [67], including bradycardia ≤40 bpm, pause ≥3 seconds, atrial fibrillation, ventricular tachycardia or ventricular fibrillation, tachycardia HR >130 bpm, a-Fib/a-Flutter (all rates), heart block, and fall-associated arrhythmia. When an arrhythmia is detected, the PiiX sends the data to zLink via Bluetooth. The zLink then transmits the data to the monitoring center or a caregiver using cellular communication. The clinical experience of the NUVANT/PiiX is currently lacking. One study with regard to patient compliance of the NUVANT system has shown no reduction in the on-patient longevity or performance of the device [66].

The ECG patch capable of recording up to three lead signals is on its way for the public's use [69]. A three-lead PEM, developed by IMEC and the Holst Center [70], integrates an ultra-low power ECG chip and a Bluetooth Low Energy (BLE) ratio, allowed to run continuously for 1 month on a 200 mAh Li-Po battery. The IMEC patch can monitor not only three channels ECG, but also the contact impedance, providing real-time information on the sensor contact quality that is important for aiding in filtering motion artifacts. The recording data are processed and analyzed locally on ECG SoC to reduce motion artifacts using adaptive filtering or principal component analysis and compute beat-to-beat HR based on discrete or continuous wavelet transforms.

PEM is considered to be a promising technology for its unobtrusive, wireless, and long-term recording capabilities. Further studies are necessary to examine the sensitivity and specificity of the recordings and long-term impact of the use of EPM in AF.

3.2.2. Smartphone-based monitor

Recently, a flood of smartphone-based monitors has been designed for heart rhythm monitoring, which falls into two broad categories, namely smartphone-only and smartphone with external sensors.

The most representative in the smartphone-only category is the camera-based apps, which measure the cardiovascular blood volume pulse (BVP) generated by repeated, rhythmic heart contractions (that can be registered by photoplethysmogram (PPG)) using the embedded camera in the smartphone. Researchers have shown that pulse rhythm and phase information regarding the BVP waveform can be deduced from the brightness change in the red (R), green (G), or blue (B) channels [68]. Several approaches to deal with the motion artifacts in the camera signals have been proposed to improve the measurement accuracy. The MIT laboratory used the blind source separation (BSS) to separate RGB color channels into independent components, which demonstrated its ability to extract the HR with digital, off-the-shelf webcams in normal ambient lighting in the presence of a limited range of motion artifacts [71, 72] Fang *et al.* [73] uncovered the underlying PPG signal from a single-channel recording using the dynamic embedding technique followed by ICA. This method relies only on the inherent temporal dynamic of the single-channel signal, making it suitable for all kinds of cameras. Thus, the built-in camera in smartphones could easily double as a heart rate monitor. Camera-based apps were subsequently brought into being based on these methods. Azumio's Instant Heart Rate app [74] is one of the most popular health apps on the market, which uses the smartphone's built-in camera and flash to compute HR and update the number through placing the tip of one's finger on the camera for about 10 sec. Many apps with advanced algorithms have also been launched for noncontact measurement of heart and respiration rate, such as a Vital Signs Camera app developed by Philips Innovation [75], extracting HR from the changes in color of the face and RR from the motion of the chest.

On the other hand, some external sensors, wired or wirelessly connecting with a smartphone, are used for sensing cardiac signals. These sensors transmit raw data to the smartphone for processing and analyzing based on computational algorithms embedded on smartphones. One example of these significant achievements is the most recent FDA approved AliveCor Heart Monitor platform [76], which supports both iPhone and Android platforms. It has been designed as a smartphone case with finger electrodes that snaps onto the back of a smartphone to measure the single-channel ECG and wirelessly communicate with the app on the phone. With secure storage in the cloud, the data can be retrieved confidentially by users themselves or their physician anytime, anywhere.

Documented clinical outcomes in the scientific literature with smartphone-based monitors is lacking at present. More work still needs to be done to examine the accuracy and sensitivity of the smartphone-based monitors.

4. Wearable solutions for other physiological parameters

There are no satisfactory wearable solutions that can provide continuous, stable, and reliable measurements for blood pressure and blood glucose at this stage [77]. Standard technology to monitor blood pressure requires an inflatable cuff to be pressurized, which may not suitable for continuous monitoring. Several approaches have been proposed for cuffless blood pressure measurement, such as arterial tonometry [78], measuring blood pressure over the radial artery by placing a pressure transducer on the wrist to capture the radial pulse waveform, or indirectly estimating blood pressure from pulse wave transit time (PTT) [79–81]. However, their consistency and reliability are still under investigation compared to the conventional method.

Currently, glucose-level measurements usually require a blood sample via the finger-pricking method. The so-called "minimally-invasive" approaches, using a disposable biosensor needle inserted under the skin on the abdomen to derive the glucose level in interstitial fluid, have been developed for continuous blood glucose monitoring. The invasiveness currently required is a high barrier to realize a practical wearable device. Many efforts targeted the field of noninvasive glucose-monitoring (NGM) techniques have been reported. Many NGM approaches—namely reverse iontophoresis [82], impedance spectroscopy [83], electromagnetic sensing [84, 85], optical methods [86–90], and photoacoustic spectroscopy [91]—have been proposed. However, key challenges to apply these technologies to wearable blood glucose monitoring are the inherent lack of specificity behind these technologies, interference from other tissue components, and poor signal to noise ratio. Other studies have aimed to develop a glucose sensor on a contact lens to monitor the glucose level in tear fluid [92–96]. Google Inc. and the University of Washington have announced a prototype of "smart" contact lenses embedded with a fully integrated sensor with signal processing circuits and a wireless coil [96]. A drawback of this technique is the glucose concentration in tears is on the sub-mm level that is almost 10 times lower than the glucose concentration in blood. A microfabricated amperometric glucose sensor, prepared by immobilizing glucose oxidase (GOx) in a titania sol-gel layer [95], can enhance sensitivity at the same level as a glucose sensor can do directly in blood.

5. Summary

The wearable technologies highlighted in this chapter can improve the accessibility and convenience of healthcare by bringing clinic and hospital quality monitoring to the point of need. The greatest potential of the continuous and ubiquitous monitoring with wearables might be in enhancing our understanding of the evolving process of poorly defined chronic conditions and allowing for more personalized or precise treatment. However, the performance and usability of current technologies and systems according to larger, homogeneous population sets are currently lacking. The high-quality clinical evidence for the use of wearable systems in mHealth to improve chronic disease management and inpatient care is very limited. Future research should be aimed at high-quality clinical evidence related to the usability, accuracy, and robustness of wearable technologies. In addition, there are still many technical issues and limitations yet to be resolved to realize high robustness and reliability in long-term recordings. These include the lack of a full range of appropriate sensors, susceptibility to motion artifacts, battery life, lack of interoperability, security and privacy issues in data communication, the low reliability and poor specificity of cuffless blood pressure and noninvasive blood glucose-monitoring methods. Despite all the potential hurdles, we envision that there will be further evolvement and improvement in this field in the upcoming years.

Author details

Fang Zhao[1*], Meng Li[1] and Joe Z. Tsien[1,2]

*Address all correspondence to: fzhao@augusta.edu

1 Brain and Behavior Discovery Institute and Department of Neurology, Medical College of Georgia, Augusta University, Augusta, Georgia, USA

2 Banna Biomedical Research Institute, Xi-Shuang-Ban-Na Prefecture, Yunnan Province, China

References

[1] Di Rienzo M., Rizzo F., Parati G., Brambilla G., Ferratini M., Castiglioni P. MagIC system: a new textile-based wearable device for biological signal monitoring applicability in daily life and clinical setting. In: Conference Proceedings IEEE Engineering in Medicine and Biology Society; 2005; Shanghai, China. IEEE; 2005. p. 7167–7169. DOI: 10.1109/IEMBS.2005.1616161.

[2] Lee Y.D., Chung W.Y. Wireless sensor network based wearable smart shirt for ubiquitous health and activity monitoring. Sensor Actuat. B-Chem. 2009;140(2):390–395. DOI: 10.1016/j.snb.2009.04.040.

[3] Jakicic J.M., Winters C., Lagally K., Ho J., Robertson R.J., Wing, R.R. The accuracy of the TriTrac-R3D accelerometer to estimate energy expenditure. Med. Sci. Sports Exerc. 1999;31(5):747–754. DOI: 00005768-199905000-00020.

[4] del Rosario M.B., Redmond S.J., Lovell N.H. Tracking the evolution of smartphone sensing for monitoring human movement. Sensors. 2015;15:18901–18933. DOI: 10.3390/s150818901.

[5] Lobodzinski S.S. ECG patch monitors for assessment of cardiac rhythm abnormalities. Prog. Cardiovasc. Dis. 2013;56(2):224–229. DOI: 10.1016/j.pcad.2013.08.006.

[6] Mellone S., Tacconi C., Schwickert L., Klenk J., Becker C., Chiari L. Smartphone-based solutions for fall detection and prevention: the FARSEEING approach. Z. Gerontol. Geriatr. 2012;45(8):722–727. DOI: 10.1007/s00391-012-0404-5.

[7] Attal F., Mohammed S., Dedabrishvili M., Chamroukhi F., Oukhellou L., Amirat Y. Physical human activity recognition using wearable sensors. Sensors. 2015;15(12): 31314–31338. DOI: 10.3390/s151229858.

[8] Printy B.P., Renken L.M., Herrmann J.P., Lee I., Johnson B., Knight E., et al. Smartphone application for classification of motor impairment severity in Parkinson's disease. In: 36th Annual International Conference Proceedings of the IEEE Engineering in Medi-

cine and Biology Society (EMBC); 26–30 Aug. 2014; Chicago, IL, USA. IEEE; 2014. p. 2686–2689. DOI: 10.1109/EMBC.2014.6944176.

[9] Elliott S., Painter J., Hudson, S. Living alone and fall risk factors in community-dwelling middle age and older adults. J. Community Health. 2009;34:301–310. DOI: 10.1007/s10900-009-9125-x.

[10] Hobert M.A., Maetzler W., Aminian K., Chiari L. Technical and clinical view on ambulatory assessment in Parkinson's disease. Acta Neurol. Scand. 2014;130(3):139–147. DOI: 10.1111/ane.12248.

[11] Topol E.J. Transforming medicine via digital innovation. Sci. Transl. Med. 2010;2(16): 16cm4. DOI: 10.1126/scitranslmed.3000484.

[12] Bouten C.V., Koekkoek K.T., Verduin M., Kodde R., Janssen J.D. A triaxial accelerometer and portable data processing unit for the assessment of daily physical activity. IEEE Trans. Biomed. Eng. 1997;44(3):136–147. DOI: 10.1109/10.554760.

[13] Najafi B., Aminian K., Loew F., Blanc Y., Robert P.A. Measurement of stand-sit and sit-stand transitions using a miniature gyroscope and its application in fall risk evaluation in the elderly. IEEE Trans. Biomed. Eng. 2002;49(8):843–851. DOI: 10.1109/TBME. 2002.800763.

[14] Steins D., Dawes H., Esser P., Collett J. Wearable accelerometry-based technology capable of assessing functional activities in neurological populations in community settings: a systematic review. J. Neuroeng. Rehabil. 2014;11:36. DOI: 10.1186/1743-0003-11-36.

[15] Karantonis D.M., Narayanan M.R., Mathie M., Lovell N.H., Celler B.G. Implementation of a real-time human movement classifier using a triaxial accelerometer for ambulatory monitoring. IEEE Trans. Inf. Technol. Biomed. 2006;10(1):156–167. DOI: 10.1109/TITB. 2005.856864.

[16] Mathie M.J., Coster A.C., Lovell N.H., Celler B.G., Lord S.R., Tiedemann A. A pilot study of long-term monitoring of human movements in the home using accelerometry. J. Telemed. Telecare. 2004;10(3):144–151. DOI: 10.1258/135763304323070788.

[17] Bao L., Intille S. Activity recognition from user-annotated acceleration data. In: Pervasive Computing. 2004;3001:1–17.

[18] Huan L., Lei, Y. Toward integrating feature selection algorithms for classification and clustering. IEEE Trans. Knowl. Data Eng. 2005;17:491–502. DOI: 10.1109/TKDE.2005.66.

[19] Bianchi F., Redmond S.J., Narayanan M.R., Cerutti S., Celler B.G., Lovell N.H. Falls event detection using triaxial accelerometry and barometric pressure measurement. In: In Proceedings of the Annual International Conference of the IEEE Engineering in Medicine and Biology Society; 3–6 September 2009; MN, USA; 2009. p. 6111–6114. DOI: 10.1109/IEMBS.2009.5334922.

[20] Qiang L., Stankovic J.A., Hanson M.A., Barth A.T., Lach J., Gang Z. Accurate, fast fall detection using gyroscopes and accelerometer-derived posture information. In: In Proceedings of the Sixth International Workshop on Wearable and Implantable Body Sensor Networks; 3–5 June 2009; Berkeley, CA, USA; 2009. p. 138–143. DOI: 10.1109/BSN.2009.46.

[21] Dadashi F., Mariani B., Rochat S., Büla C., Santos-Eggimann B., Aminian K. Gait and foot clearance parameters obtained using shoe-worn inertial sensors in a large-population sample of older adults. Sensors. 2014;14(1):443–457. DOI: 10.3390/s140100443.

[22] Pogorelc B., Gams M. Detecting gait-related health problems of the elderly using multidimensional dynamic time warping approach with semantic attributes. Multimed. Tools Appl. 2013;66:95–114. DOI: 10.1007/s11042-013-1473-1.

[23] Sposaro, F., Tyson, G. iFall: an android application for fall monitoring and response. In: Proceedings of the Annual International Conference of the IEEE on Engineering in Medicine and Biology Society (EMBC); 3–6 September 2009; Minneapolis, MN, USA. IEEE; 2009. p. 6119–6122. DOI: 10.1109/IEMBS.2009.5334912.

[24] Dai J., Bai X., Yang Z., Shen Z., Xuan D. Mobile phone-based pervasive fall detection. Pers. Ubiquitous Comput. 2010;14(7):633–643. DOI: 10.1007/s00779-010-0292-x.

[25] Yavuz G., Kocak M., Ergun G., Alemdar H., Yalcin H., Incel, O.D., et al. A smartphone based fall detector with online location support. In: In Proceedings of the International Workshop on Sensing for App Phones; 2 November 2010; Zurich, Switzerland; 2010. p. 31–35.

[26] Zhao Z., Chen Y., Liu J. Fall detecting and alarming based on mobile phone. In: In Proceedings of the 7th International Conference on Ubiquitous Intelligence & Computing and 7th International Conference on Autonomic & Trusted Computing (UIC/ATC); 26–29 October 2010; Shanxi, China; 2010. p. 494–497. DOI: 10.1109/UIC-ATC.2010.44.

[27] Fahmi P., Viet V., Deok-Jai C. Semi-supervised fall detection algorithm using fall indicators in smartphone. In: In Proceedings of the 6th International Conference on Ubiquitous Information Management and Communication; 20–22 February 2012; Kuala Lumpur, Malaysia. 2012. DOI: 10.1145/2184751.2184890.

[28] He Y., Li Y. Physical activity recognition utilizing the built-in kinematic sensors of a smartphone. Int. J. Distrib. Sens. Netw. 2013; 2013, p. 1–10. DOI: 10.1155/2013/481580.

[29] Majumder A.J.A., Rahman F., Zerin I., Ebel W., Jr., Ahamed S.I. iPrevention: towards a novel real-time smartphone-based fall prevention system. In: In Proceedings of the 28th Annual ACM Symposium on Applied Computing; 18–22 March 2013; Coimbra, Portugal; 2013. p. 513–518. DOI: 10.1145/2480362.2480462.

[30] Dai J., Bai X., Yang Z., Shen Z., Xuan D. PerFallD: a pervasive fall detection system using mobile phones. In: In Proceedings of the 8th IEEE International Conference on

Pervasive Computing and Communications Workshops (PERCOM Workshops); 29 March–2 April 2010; Mannheim, Germany. IEEE; 2010. p. 292–297. DOI: 10.1109/ PERCOMW.2010.5470652.

[31] Lee R.Y., Carlisle A.J. Detection of falls using accelerometers and mobile phone technology. Age Ageing. 2011;40(6):690–696. DOI: 10.1093/ageing/afr050.

[32] Cao Y., Yang Y., Liu W. E-FallD: A fall detection system using android-based smart-phone. In: In Proceedings of the 9th International Conference on Fuzzy Systems and Knowledge Discovery (FSKD); 29–31 May 2012; Sichuan, China. IEEE; 2012. p. 1509–1513. DOI: 10.1109/FSKD.2012.6234271.

[33] Fang S.-H., Liang Y.-C., Chiu K.-M. Developing a mobile phone-based fall detection system on android platform. In: In Proceedings of the Computing, Communications and Applications Conference (ComComAp); 11–13 January 2012; Hong Kong, China. IEEE; 2012. p. 143–146. DOI: 10.1109/ComComAp.2012.6154019.

[34] Viet V.Q., Lee G., Choi D. Fall detection based on movement and smart phone tech-nology. In: In Proceedings of the IEEE RIVF International Conference on Computing and Communication Technologies, Research, Innovation, and Vision for the Future (RIVF); 27 February–1 March 2012; Ho Chi Minh City, Vietnam. IEEE; 2012. p. 1–4. DOI: 10.1109/rivf.2012.6169847.

[35] Mehner S., Klauck R., Koenig H. Location-independent fall detection with smartphone. In: In Proceedings of the 6th International Conference on PErvasive Technologies Related to Assistive Environments; 28–31 May 2013; Rhodes, Greece. 2013. DOI: 10.1145/2504335.2504346.

[36] Koshmak G.A., Linden M., Loutfi A. Evaluation of the android-based fall detection system with physiological data monitoring. In: In Proceedings of the 35th Annual International Conference of the IEEE on Engineering in Medicine and Biology Society (EMBC); 3–7 July 2013; Osaka, Japan. IEEE; 2013. p. 1164–1168. DOI: 10.1109/EMBC. 2013.6609713.

[37] Kau L.J., CHen C.S. A smart phone-based pocket fall accident detection, positioning, and rescue system. IEEE J. Biomed. Health Inform. 2014;19(1):44–56. DOI: 10.1109/JBHI. 2014.2328593.

[38] Suryadevara V.K., Rizkalla M. Smartphone based fall detection and logic testing application using android SDK. J. Biomed. Sci. Eng. 2015;8(9):616–624. DOI: 10.4236/ jbise.2015.89057.

[39] Viet V., Choi D.J. Fall detection with smart phone sensor. In: In Proceedings of the 3rd International Conference on Internet (ICONI); 15–19 December 2011; Sepang, Malaysia; 2011. p. 27-31.

[40] Shi Y., Shi Y., Wang X. Fall detection on mobile phones using features from a five-phase model. In: In Proceedings of the 9th International Conference on Ubiquitous Intelli-gence & Computing and 9th International Conference on Autonomic & Trusted

Computing (UIC/ATC); 4–7 September 2012; Fukuoka, Japan. IEEE; 2012. p. 951–956. DOI: 10.1109/UIC-ATC.2012.100.

[41] Zhao Z., Chen Y., Wang S., Chen Z. FallAlarm: smart phone based fall detecting and positioning system. Procedia Comput. Sci. 2012;10:617–624. DOI: FallAlarm: Smart Phone Based Fall Detecting and Positioning System.

[42] Kansiz A.O., Guvensan M.A., Turkmen H.I. Selection of time-domain features for fall detection based on supervised learning. In: In Proceedings of the World Congress on Engineering and Computer Science; 23–25 October 2013; San Francisco, CA, USA; 2013.

[43] Medrano C., Plaza I., Igual R., Sánchez Á., Castro M. The effect of personalization on smartphone-based fall detectors. Sensor. 2016;16(1):E117. DOI: 10.3390/s16010117.

[44] Abbate S., Avvenuti M., Bonatesta F., Cola G., Corsini P., Vecchio A. A smartphone-based fall detection system. Pervasive Mobile Comput. 2012;8(6):883–899. DOI: 10.1016/j.pmcj.2012.08.003.

[45] Habib M., Mohktar M., Kamaruzzaman S., Lim K., Pin T., Ibrahim F. Smartphone-based solutions for fall detection and prevention: challenges and open issues. Sensors. 2014;14(4):7181–7208. DOI: 10.3390/s140407181.

[46] Goetz C.G., Stebbins G.T., Wolff D., DeLeeuw W., Bronte-Stewart H., Elble R., et al. Testing objective measures of motor impairment in early Parkinson's disease: feasibility study of an at-home testing device. Mov. Disord. 2009;24(4):551–556. DOI: 10.1002/mds.22379.

[47] Dijkstra B., Kamsma Y.P., Zijlstra W. Detection of gait and postures using a miniaturized triaxial accelerometer-based system: accuracy in patients with mild to moderate Parkinson's disease. Arch. Phys. Med. Rehabil. 2010;91(8):1272–1277. DOI: 10.1016/j.apmr.2010.05.004.

[48] Moore S.T., MacDougall H.G., Ondo W.G. Ambulatory monitoring of freezing of gait in Parkinson's disease. J Neurosci Methods. 2008;167(2):340–348.

[49] Bächlin M., Roggen D., Plotnik M., Hausdorff J.M., Giladi N., Tröster G. Online detection of freezing of gait in Parkinson's disease patients: a performance characterization. In: Proceedings of the 4th International Conference on Body; Brussels, Belgium; 2009. p. 693–698. DOI: 10.4108/ICST.BODYNETS2009.5852.

[50] Salarian A., Russmann H., Vingerhoets F.J.G., Burkhard P.R., Aminian K. Ambulatory monitoring of physical activities in patients with Parkinson's disease. IEEE Trans. Biomed. Eng. 2007;54(12):2296–2299. DOI: 10.1109/TBME.2007.896591.

[51] Mazilu S., Blanke U., Hardegge M., Tröster G., Gazit E., Dorfman M., et al. GaitAssist: a wearable assistant for gait training and rehabilitation in Parkinson's disease. 2014 IEEE International Conference on Pervasive Computing and Communications Workshops (PERCOM Workshops); 24–28 March 2014; Budapest. IEEE; 2014. p. 135–137. DOI: 10.1109/PerComW.2014.6815179.

[52] Cancela J., Pansera M., Arredondo M.T., Estrada J.J., Pastorino M., Pastor-Sanz L. A comprehensive motor symptom monitoring and management system: the bradykinesia case. In: In Proceeding of the 32nd Annual Conference of the IEEE Engineering; 31 Aug 2010–4 Sept 2010; Buenos Aires. IEEE; 2010. p. 1008–1011.

[53] Barth J., Klucken J., Kugler P., Kammerer T., Steidl R., Winkler J., et al. Biometric and mobile gait analysis for early diagnosis and therapy monitoring in Parkinson's disease. In: In Proceedings of the 33rd Annual Conference of the IEEE Engineering in Medicine and Biology Society; 30 Aug 2011–3 Sept 2011; Boston, MA, USA. IEEE; 2011. p. 868–871. DOI: 10.1109/IEMBS.2011.6090226.

[54] Klucken J., Barth J., Kugler P., Schlachetzki J., Henze T., Marxreiter F., et al. Unbiased and mobile gait analysis detects motor impairment in Parkinson's disease. PLoS One. 2013;8(2):e56956. DOI: 10.1371/journal.pone.0056956.

[55] Zwartjes D.G.M., Heida T., van Vugt J.P.P., Geelen J.A.G., Veltink P.H. Ambulatory monitoring of activities and motor symptoms in Parkinson's disease. IEEE Trans. Biomed. Eng. 2010;57(11):2778–2786. DOI: 10.1109/TBME.2010.2049573.

[56] Tzallas A.T., Tsipouras M.G., Rigas G., Tsalikakis D.G., Karvounis E.C., Chondrogiorgi M. PERFORM: a system for monitoring, assessment and management of patients with Parkinson's disease. Sensor. 2014;14(11):21329–21357. DOI: 10.3390/s141121329.

[57] Arora S., Venkataraman V., Donohue S., Biglan K.M., Dorsey E.R., Little M.A. High accuracy discrimination of Parkinson's disease participants from healthy controls using smartphones. In: 2014 IEEE International Conference on Acoustics, Speech and Signal Processing (ICASSP); 4–9 May 2014; Florence. IEEE; 2014. p. 3641–3644. DOI: 10.1109/ICASSP.2014.6854280.

[58] Pepa L., Ciabattoni L., Verdini F., Capecci M., Ceravolo M.G. Smartphone based fuzzy logic freezing of gait detection in Parkinson's disease. In: 2014 IEEE/ASME 10th International Conference on Mechatronic and Embedded Systems and Applications (MESA); 10–12 Sept 2014; Senigallia. IEEE; 2014. p. 1–6. DOI: 10.1109/MESA.2014.6935630.

[59] Kim H., Lee H.J., Lee W., Kwon S., Kim S.K., Jeon H.S., et al. Unconstrained detection of freezing of Gait in Parkinson's disease patients using smartphone. In: 2015 37th Annual International Conference of the IEEE Engineering in Medicine and Biology Society (EMBC); 25–29 Aug. 2015; Milan. IEEE; 2015. p. 3751–3754. DOI: 10.1109/EMBC.2015.7319209.

[60] KostikisN., Hristu-Varsakelis D., Arnaoutoglou M., Kotsavasiloglou C. A smartphone-based tool for assessing Parkinsonian hand tremor. IEEE Trans. Biomed. Eng. 2015;19(6):1835–1842. DOI: 10.1109/JBHI.2015.2471093.

[61] Pan D., Dhall R., Lieberman A., Petitti D.B. A mobile cloud-based Parkinson's disease assessment system for home-based monitoring. JMIR Mhealth Uhealth. 2015;3(1):e29. DOI: 10.2196/mhealth.3956.

[62] iRhythm. Available from: http://www.irhythmtech.com/ [Accessed: Mar. 2016].

[63] Corventis [Internet]. Available from: http://www.corventis.com/ [Accessed: Mar. 2016].

[64] Rosenberg M.A., Samuel M., Thosani A., Zimetbaum P.J. Use of a noninvasive continuous monitoring device in the management of atrial fibrillation: a pilot study. Pacing Clin. Electrophysiol. 2012;36(3):328–333. DOI: 10.1111/pace.12053.

[65] Turakhia M.P., Hoang D.D., Zimetbaum P., Miller J.D., Froelicher V.F., Kumar U.N., et al. Diagnostic utility of a novel leadless arrhythmia monitoring device. Am. J. Cardiol. 2013;112(4):520–524. DOI: 10.1016/j.amjcard.2013.04.017.

[66] Engel J.M., Chakravarthy N., Katra R.P., Mazar S., Libbus I., Chavan A. Estimation of patient compliance in application of adherent mobile cardiac telemetry device. In: 2011 Annual International Conference of the IEEE Engineering in Medicine and Biology Society; 30 Aug 2011–3 Sept 2011; Boston, MA, USA. IEEE; 2011. p. 1536–1539. DOI: 10.1109/IEMBS.2011.6090448.

[67] Higgins S.L. A novel patch for heart rhythm monitoring: is the Holter monitor obsolete? Future Cardiol. 2013;9(3):325–333. DOI: 10.2217/fca.13.13.

[68] Verkruysse W., Svaasand L.O., Nelson J.S. Remote plethysmographic imaging using ambient light. Opt. Express. 2008;16(26):21434–21435.

[69] Lobodzinski S.S., Laks M.M. New devices for very long-term ECG monitoring. Cardiol. J. 2012;19(2):210–214.

[70] Imec. [Updated: Mar. 2016]. Available from: www2.imec.be.

[71] Poh M.Z., McDuff D.J., Picard R.W. Non-contact, automated cardiac pulse measurements using video imaging and blind source separation. Opt Express. 2010;18(10): 10762–10774. DOI: 10.1364/OE.18.010762.

[72] Poh M.Z., McDuff D.J., Picard R.W. Advancements in noncontact, multiparameter physiological measurements using a webcam. IEEE Trans. Biomed. Eng. 2011;58(1):7–11. DOI: 10.1109/TBME.2010.2086456.

[73] Zhao F., Li M., Qian Y., Tsien J.Z. Remote measurements of heart and respiration rates for telemedicine. PLoS One. 2013;8(10):e71384. DOI: 10.1371/journal.pone.0071384.

[74] Azumio. Instant Heart Rate [Internet]. Available from: http://www.azumio.com/apps/heart-rate/ [Accessed: Mar. 2016].

[75] Philips. VitalSigns Camera [Internet]. Available from: http://www.vitalsignscamera.com/ [Accessed: Mar. 2016].

[76] AliveCor. Available from: http://www.alivecor.com/home [Accessed: Mar. 2016].

[77] Zhao F., Li M., Tsien J.Z. Technology platforms for remote monitoring of vital signs in the new era of telemedicine. Expert Rev. Med. Devices. 2015;12(4):411–429. DOI: 10.1586/17434440.2015.1050957.

[78] Tensys Medical. TL-300 [Internet]. Available from: http://tensysmedical.com/us/products/.

[79] Eeftinck Schattenkerk D.W., van Lieshout J.J., van den Meiracker A.H., Wesseling K.R., Blanc S., Wieling W., et al. Nexfin noninvasive continuous blood pressure validated against Riva-Rocci/Korotkoff. Am. J. Hypertens. 2009;22(4):378–383. DOI: 10.1038/ajh. 2008.368.

[80] Garnier R.P., van der Spoel A.G., Sibarani-Ponsen R., Markhorst D.G., Boer C. Level of agreement between Nexfin non-invasive arterial pressure with invasive arterial pressure measurements in children. Br. J. Anaesth. 2012;109(4):609–615. DOI: 10.1093/bja/aes295.

[81] Saugel B., Meidert A.S., Hapfelmeier A., Eyer F., Schmid R.M., Huber W. Non- invasive continuous arterial pressure measurement based on radial artery tonometry in the intensive care unit: a method comparison study using the T- Line TL-200pro device. Br. J. Anaesth. 2013;111(2):185–190. DOI: 10.1093/bja/aet025.

[82] Leboulanger B., Guy R.H., Delgado-Charro M.B. Non-invasive monitoring of pheny-toin by reverse iontophoresis. Eur. J. Pharm. Sci. 2004;22(5):427–433.

[83] Tao D., Adler A. In Vivo Blood Characterization From Bioimpedance Spectroscopy of Blood Pooling . IEEE Trans. Instrum. Meas. 2009;58(11):3831-3838. DOI: 10.1109/TIM. 2009.2020836.

[84] Caduff A., Talary M.S., Mueller M., Dewarrat F., Klisic J., Donath M., et al. Non-invasive glucose monitoring in patients with Type 1 diabetes: a multisensor system combining sensors for dielectric and optical characterisation of skin. Biosens. Bioelectron. 2009;24(9):2778–2784. DOI: 10.1016/j.bios.2009.02.001.

[85] Tura A., Sbrignadello S., Cianciavicchia D., Pacini G., Ravazzani P. A low frequency electromagnetic sensor for indirect measurement of glucose concentration: in vitro experiments in different conductive solutions. Sensors. 2010;10(6):5346–5358. DOI: 10.3390/s100605346.

[86] Arnold M.A., Small G.W. Noninvasive glucose sensing. Anal. Chem. 2005;77(17):5429–5439.

[87] Vonlilienfeldtoal H., Weidenmuller M., Xhelaj A., Mantele W. A novel approach to non-invasive glucose measurement by mid-infrared spectroscopy: the combination of quantum cascade lasers (QCL) and photoacoustic detection. Vib. Spectrosc. 2005;38(1–2):209–215. DOI: 10.1016/j.vibspec.2005.02.025.

[88] Ellis D.I., Goodacre R. Metabolic fingerprinting in disease diagnosis: biomedical applications of infrared and Raman spectroscopy. Analyst. 2006;131(8):875–885.

[89] Larin K.V., Eledrisi M.S., Motamedi M., Esenaliev R.O. Noninvasive blood glucose monitoring with optical coherence tomography: a pilot study in human subjects. Diabetes Care. 2002;25(12):2263–2267.

[90] Malik B.H., Coté G.L. Real-time, closed-loop dual-wavelength optical polarimetry for glucose monitoring. J. Biomed. Opt. 2010;15(1):017002. DOI: 10.1117/1.3290819.

[91] Lee S., Nayak V., Dodds J., Pishko M., Smith N.B. Glucose measurements with sensors and ultrasound. Ultrasound Med. Biol. 2005;31(7):971–977.

[92] March W.F., Mueller A., Herbrechtsmeier P. Clinical trial of a noninvasive contact lens glucose sensor. Diabetes Technol. Ther. 2004;6(6):782–789.

[93] Alexeev V.L., Das S., Finegold D.N., Asher S.A. Photonic crystal glucose-sensing material for noninvasive monitoring of glucose in tear fluid. Clin. Chem. 2004;50(12): 2353–2360.

[94] Yao H., Shum A.J., Cowan M., Lähdesmäki I., Parviz B.A. A contact lens with embedded sensor for monitoring tear glucose level. Biosens. Bioelectron. 2011;26(7):3290–3296. DOI: 10.1016/j.bios.2010.12.042.

[95] Patel J.N., Gray B.L., Kaminska B., Gates B.D. Flexible three-dimensional electrochemical glucose sensor with improved sensitivity realized in hybrid polymer microelectromechanical systems technique. J. Diabetes Sci. Technol. 2011;5(5):1036–1043.

[96] Liao Y.T., Yao H., Lingley A., Parviz B., Otis B.P. A 3- \mu \hbox CMOS glucose sensor for wireless contact-lens tear glucose monitoring. IEEE J. Solid-St. Circ. 2012;47(1):335–344. DOI: 10.1109/JSSC.2011.2170633.

[97] Tacconi C., Mellone S., Chiari L. Smartphone-based applications for investigating falls and mobility. In: In Proceedings of the 5th International Conference on Pervasive Computing Technologies for Healthcare (PervasiveHealth); 23–26 May 2011; Dublin, Ireland; 2011. p. 258–261.

[98] Bai Y.W., Wu S.C., Tsai C.L. Design and implementation of a fall monitor system by using a 3-axis accelerometer in a smart phone. IEEE Trans. Consum. Electron. 2012;58(4):1269–1275. DOI: 10.1109/TCE.2012.6414995.

[99] Hsieh S.L., Su M.H., Liu L.F., Jiang W.W. A finite state machine-based fall detection mechanism on smartphones. In: In Proceedings of the 9th International Conference on Ubiquitous Intelligence & Computing and 9th International Conference on Autonomic & Trusted Computing (UIC/ATC); 4–7 September 2012; Fukuoka, Japan. IEEE; 2012. p. 735–739. DOI: 10.1109/UIC-ATC.2012.153.

[100] Bai Y.W., Wu S.C., Yu C.H. Recognition of direction of fall by smartphone. In: In Proceedings of the 26th Annual IEEE Canadian Conference on Electrical and Computer Engineering (CCECE); 5–8 May 2013; Regina, SK, Canada. IEEE; 2013. p. 1–6. DOI: 10.1109/CCECE.2013.6567781.

5

Moving towards Sustainable Electronic Health Applications

Sahr Wali, Karim Keshavjee and Catherine Demers

Abstract

Electronic healthcare applications, both web-based and mobile health (mHealth) provide new modalities for chronic disease. These tools allow patients to track their symptoms and help them manage their condition. The sustainability of these tools is often not considered during their development. To ensure these applications can be adopted and sustainable, where policy differs amongst states and provinces, we must present the benefits of our findings to highlight the justification for its development. For technology to be sustainable it has to utilize infrastructure that is secure, stable and to be agile so that it can be deployed quickly with minimal interruption to patients, family members and healthcare professionals.

Keywords: sustainability, self-care, eHealth, mHealth, technology, co-design

1. Introduction

Within the healthcare industry, innovation remains to be the leading force in the quest to balance health care quality and costcontainment [1]. Mobile health (mHealth) applications are one of the fastest growing segments in drive for innovation in the health care sector. With the rising use of mobile phones, mHealth applications (apps) provide individuals with a simple and accessible way to manage their health at the tip of their fingers [1].

Unfortunately, many mHealth interventions continue to be developed without the consideration of long term sustainability, which has left many apps with vast potential but nowhere to move forward. This is one of the growing problems with health app development, where in spite of the advances made with technology, apps fail to be used due to the methodological challenges associated with designing for sustainability [2]. In this chapter, we focus on address-ing the main issues app publishers face during the design process. We then outline the key components that should be included to assure the sustainability of an electronic health app.

We define the issues with innovation by three main components that include (1) end-user usability, (2) clinician and informal caregiver (spouse, children, friend) input and (3) impact of agencies outside development. Many electronic health apps fail to consider these major factors in its design, which in turn is often what limits the sustainability of its use. We believe that these three factors are essential as it evaluates the health apps design according to the user, their main members of care and finally the environment it is used. If the health app being designed does not simplify or improve the current model of care, there is no incentive for its use. Instead, the benefits associated with the app will be overshadowed by its complications or drawbacks.

This leads to our section in the chapter on designing for sustainability. We start by signify-ing the importance of putting the end-user first and then introduce the information system research framework that help identify user needs, design preferences and potential barriers to increase health app adoption. This is followed by the next stage of designing for sustainabil-ity, where we outline the steps to get all the potential players on board in support for the new innovation. We highlight the inevitable resistance to change that will occur, and explain the concept of 'behavioral intention' to use a technology and how this will help improve health app sustainability.

Finally, for the purpose of long-term sustainability, we expand on preparing for the expected and unexpected, by evaluating change management plans and regulations in place during health app design. Towards the end of the chapter, we develop a market and feasibility analy-sis framework for the adoption and scalability of the health app on a national scale. This allows us to ensure all key factors have been addressed; leaving the app design and efficacy to become unquestionable.

2. Issues with innovation

Over the past decade, there have been a number of advancements within the healthcare industry, yet there is still a strong resistance present towards the implementation of health innovation [3]. The lack of certainty in the interventions independent sustainability is one of the leading factors responsible for this resistance [4]. Electronic health apps may hold great promise for better health tracking [5], providing education [6], changing and enforcing health behaviors [7], and monitoring treatment adherence [8], however despite these benefits, they are still not being used [9]. This can be attributed due to nine key design barriers that are out-lined in Chindalo et al. literature review [9] (**Table 1**).

These barriers have created a stigma around stakeholders investing in health app develop-ment. Currently, the perceived return on investment (ROI) with health apps remains low, as the issues with innovation remain high. The beneficial impact of health apps may seem promising, but from a sustainability standpoint, they fail to address the underlying question that is 'will these benefits outweigh the cost of its development?'

Barrier	Explanation
1. Apps provide information conflicting from what is received from clinicians	Patients/end-users are less likely to use an app when it conflicts with information from their clinician. They will not feel confident in the content provided or its functionality
2. Language used too complex for end-user health literacy level	Patients/end-users often have lower levels of health literacy. They require technology to be adapted to their needs or the app will not be used sufficiently
3. Manual data input required	Treatment regimens are already perceived as complex by patients/end-users. Manual data input further complicates this process, as it is exhaustive and error-prone
4. Information provided has no value/meaningless data	If the app information has no beneficiary tie to the patient (e.g. cannot order diagnostic testing or prescribe medications) then the content becomes useless
5. Daily app use not required	Health apps aiming to help patients/end-users with their treatment regimen should be used daily and in accordance with their prescribed treatment. It the health app does not require daily use, this can reduce treatment adherence as the patient will not get into the habit of using it
6. Lack of incentives to use	Any source of change is viewed as burdensome, thus, if no incentive (cost savings or social approval) for a patient/end-user to utilize the tool is present, they are less likely to use it
7. Data collected not valued by clinician	If the data collected brings forward information important for the patient/end-users care, the clinician would be more likely to promote its use. However, if there is no functional value for the data, both clinicians and end-users/patients will not use the tool
8. No way for physicians to use data collected	Health apps may collect large amounts of data, but if they cannot visualize or analyze the meaning behind the data, it comes useless
9. No way to integrate app data into electronic medical record (EMR) for analysis or follow-up	If the data collected cannot be combined with previous medical information the context required for analysis will be lost, leaving the data to be meaningless

Table 1. Design barriers associated with decreased health app usage (adapted from [9]).

To ensure that resources being spent on an application are adequately being used and the above barriers are addressed, the needs, wants and expectations of the health apps primary stakeholders should be evaluated [10]. However, it is this lack of stakeholder consideration within app design that builds the three prime issues with innovation, which we describe below [1, 9].

1. Poor end-user usability: who are you designing for?

The overall hype of innovation, and mHealth solutions, has led developers into a cycle where app ideas centered on addressing patient challenges seem to forget about the patient once in development [11]. Consequently, this lack of end-user engagement has led health app usage to fall to 2% amongst patients at hospitals in the US [11]. The low percentage for health app usage may seem surprising, but when a tool does not suit the needs or capabilities of the end-user, the percentage becomes less surprising and more understandable.

Findings reveal that patients with chronic disease, such as heart failure and diabetes, have positive attitude towards using mobile technology if they are simple and effective [12].

However, the key issue here is that app developers seem to show greater motivation by the cleverness of the technology rather than the improvements in health outcomes, which often results in complicating the apps functionality [13]. Thus, in the eyes of the developer the app may seem effective, but they do not consider that the individual they are designing it for will not have the same understanding. As a result, apps will not meet user needs or capabilities, which in turn leads to the development of the first six barriers highlighted in **Table 1**. This poor product usability can be attributed due to the lack of end-user involvement or input during the development process [11]. Some would argue the most successful health apps are those that address real-life challenges in the context that the patient lives. Therefore, to assure the sustainability of a health application the question the developer must ask is not 'does it solve a problem', but rather 'does it help the patient directly'. If an application is in any way a burden, or adds more effort into their treatment, it will not be used.

2. **Lack of clinician and informal caregiver input: What are you designing it for and how will it improve clinical outcomes?**

The primary objective for a health application is to improve clinical outcomes and reduce the level of work required, clinicians and informal caregivers (spouse, children, friend) play a pivotal role in establishing the criteria for these improvements [14]. Clinicians provide the complete medical background surrounding patient care as well as clinical workflow operations, while informal caregivers allow developers to have a magnified look into the day-to day challenges that prevent adherence and worsen symptoms [3, 14]. Both key members of care contribute substantively in increasing adherence, improving self-care, quality of life and outcomes for patients [14]. However, the reality is, numerous apps are/ have been developed with either none or some clinician and/or caregiver feedback, but the inclusion of both are pivotal to assure sustainability.

As every tool must have an objective for its development, the use of clinician and caregiver input provides developers with the necessary content to build their objective around. The lack of clinician and caregiver feedback in current health apps limits app efficacy and is responsible for design barriers seven and eight in **Table 1**. Without the consideration of both the *physiological* and *social* factors provided by clinicians and caregivers, health apps will continue to be designed around the question 'does it a solve a problem', and developers will inevitably fall short in the effectiveness of their app design [10].

3. **Fail to consider impact of agencies outside development: does it effect current operations?**

Aside from the lack of usability considerations, other factors including, government regulations and organization operations, are also commonly neglected. The development and implementation of healthcare innovations is bounded by a set of regulations that must be followed [15]. These regulations are set in place as a standard to prevent public health risk and improve patient safety. In the United States, the Food and Drug Administration (FDA) issued a draft for the regulation of mobile medical applications [16]. However, as many of the standards currently in place are set to regulate medical devices, a large group of apps still do not fall within the categories for regulation. This leaves them to be generated without regulatory precaution or guidance, which in turn promotes the development of less effective and integrative health apps [17]. For example, one key element that would increase app use and sustainability would the use of data integration amongst EMRs and the respective health app. This would allow the data collected to be combined with current medical information, which would potentially improve clinical outcomes and future diagnosis [9]. However, as this is not a required component within health app development, it has become a barrier, instead of a benefit, for health app usage (**Table 1**).

Nevertheless, one area of regulation all health apps must adhere to involves privacy and security of personal health information. Ensuring that the introduction of a health app does not threaten the privacy of the data obtained is one of the pillars for a sustainable health intervention. However, as many health apps are very development-focused these pivotal components are not acknowledged early on. This results in complicating the design process and restraining development in the later stage [10]. Similarly, as many workflow operations may be changed with the introduction of an electronic health app, failing to consider the necessary requirements early in design process leads implementation to become more disruptive than beneficial [18]. An effective health app design would identify the key organizational barriers and resistance points that may occur prior to actual implementation. Thus, the problems associated with security and workflow operations are built upon the underlying issue that they are not considered until the start of implementation.

Furthermore, electronic health apps may have undeniable potential to improve health outcomes in a cost-effective manner, but the underlying issues with innovation are preventing their potential from being fully utilized [15]. Stakeholders may have different objectives for the outcome of a health app, but regardless, the app designer must still address their needs regarding usability, content, safety, clinical and cost-effectiveness accordingly. There is already a resistance for innovation in healthcare; therefore, to build a model for health app sustainability, we outline a series of frameworks to minimize the occurrence of these issues.

3. Designing for sustainability

Prior to designing an electronic health application or any innovative health tool, we must consider the who, what, where, when and how of the intervention. Who will be using it? What will it do? Where and when will it be used? Lastly, how will it work? These questions allow the designer of the tool to recognize its primary stakeholders, the risks and costs of innovation and whether it will work with current operations in place [10]. When designing for sustainability the goal should be to bridge a practical solution for a prominent issue. Therefore, addressing these common questions has framed our guideline for moving towards sustainable electronic health applications. In this section, we start by identifying the end-user and their needs, followed by an outline to creating a user-centered health app, and finally end with the steps required to gain support for app implementation.

3.1. Putting the end-user first

Whether older adults with heart failure or adolescents with diabetes will use a health application, identifying the end-user and their needs at the start of the design process is pivotal for the next steps towards development [19, 20]. Nevertheless, although the importance behind end-user evaluation has been signified, various studies confirm the lack of health apps available suiting their needs and capabilities [1, 21–23]. In the Delphi study, a literature review was conducted overviewing the determinants of innovation in health care organizations [24]. Their results indicated that many innovation studies failed to adjust their strategies according to feedback obtained, or that the data on the determinants was insignificant as it came from non-users [24]. In this case, the study highlights that it is not enough to simply obtain random feedback, but we must obtain useful input and apply it into the design [24].

Often times, the benefits of the end product overshadow the content required for adequate usability, leaving both the app developer and the end-user at a disadvantage. For example, by simplifying intervention processes and health education it is estimated that this will improve clinical outcomes. However, what is not considered is that the sustainability of these benefits will only be seen when the app is user-friendly and end-users can independently utilize it with confidence [25, 26]. To get to this stage, developers must recognize what components intended users need, so it becomes both easy to use and useful. Thus, to accomplish this, a user-centered framework has been developed which we summarize below.

3.1.1. Information system research (ISR) framework

As many electronic health interventions are designed according to the current healthcare system processes, this limits their impact potential compared to those that involve end-user input [27]. The ISR framework uses three research cycles, (1) relevance cycle, (2) design cycle and (3) rigor cycle, to identify user needs, design preferences as well as any barriers that will prevent the uptake or sustained use of the app [27, 28].

In the *Relevance Cycle*, developers or researchers seek out to understand the end-user in the context of their environment [19]. It is the environment that shapes the specificities behind the arising problems, the purpose of this cycle is to provide the requirements for the health app, as well as set of criteria for users to evaluate its functionality [28, 29]. Thus, to meet the goals of this cycle focus group style sessions with intended stakeholders and end-users are commonly used [27, 29]. By the end of this cycle, we should be able to answer the question, 'Does this app improve the user's environment, and how?' [28].

The heart of development occurs during the *Design Cycle*, as the content from the relevance cycle is used to build the health app and evaluate it accordingly [28]. This cycle continues in an iterative manner, where a series of designs will be generated and evaluated against the respective user requirements, until all key components are addressed. The design of the app can move relatively quickly, however, it is the continual evaluation and feedback for refinements that challenges developers [29]. Nevertheless, end-users often stop using apps that do not immediately engage them, so by repeatedly conducting prototype testing with key stakeholders, this increases the expected usability and sustainability of the end product.

Finally, the *Rigor Cycle* is the background check of the ISR framework [29]. It reviews and evaluates the current knowledge base present within the desired applications domain [27, 28]. This enhances the degree of innovation for the health apps design. In many cases, this cycle is conducted after the relevance cycle to increase the overall effectiveness of the apps design [27] (**Figure 1**).

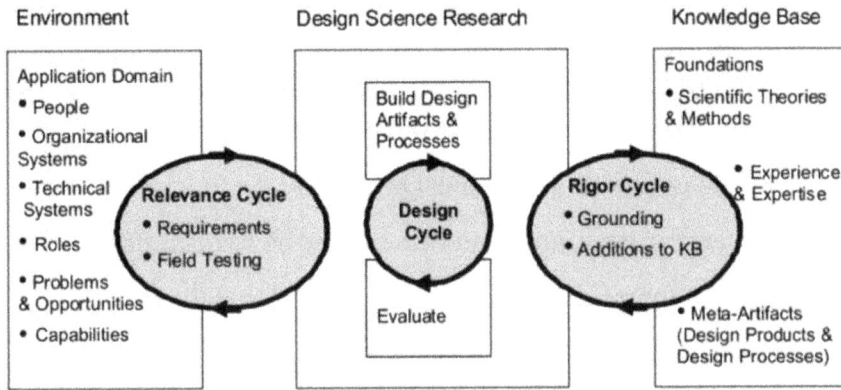

Figure 1. The ISR framework divided into three design science research cycles, (1) relevance cycle, (2) design cycle and (3) rigor cycle [28].

3.1.2. Creating a user-centered design: ISR and end-user co-design

The foundation of a user-centered design is centralized on three major components, (1) understanding how the device will be used, (2) curating information relevant to the end-user and (3) framing the tool in the user's environmental context and lifestyle [4]. The ISR framework allows developers to assess the needs of the end-user while evaluating current interventions in place [28]. However, the co-design method moves one step further by using a participatory approach where end-users and primary stakeholders work together on all aspects of the health apps development [30, 31]. By using the ISR framework in parallel with the co-design method, we believe this iterative process will lead towards a more effective user-centered end product over the long-term [29, 31].

Many electronic health app interventions fail to engage users in the design and usability stages [31]. In a systematic review of co-designed mHealth interventions, studies included patients in the development stages, but none assessed the intervention's effectiveness afterwards [31]. Conversely, in another study, users evaluated the interventions usability, but were not involved in its design [32]. The lack of fluidity between mHealth development and user input reduces end-user empowerment and overall app usability. The healthcare system is already burdened with various pre-mature innovation investments that have fallen short in its beneficial return. Therefore, from a sustainability standpoint, by using the ISR framework, this will allow all factors surrounding the end-user and the current knowledge base to be covered, whereas the co-design aspect will be pivotal to assure its usability.

3.2. How to get everyone on board

One of the greatest obstacles towards developing sustainable electronic health interventions involves getting primary stakeholders in support for its development and implementation [3]. This challenge has been shaped due to the three paradoxes of innovation [33]. First, the uptake of the dubious and rejection of the good. The explosion of electronic health apps created a consumer fad where a number 'breakthrough' apps left individuals in regret and stakeholders reluctant to invest again. Second, the wisdom and failings of democracy. Working with professional groups can be effective to ensure implementation of a new technology, however, solely relying on their cooperation results in killing the product before it is even complete. Third, health systems are not able to keep up. Innovation results in causing change in an organization, but this creates challenges that innovators are often not prepared for and results in causing more disruption than improvement [33].

In order to move past these challenges we must be address the following questions:

1. What evidence is there that it will improve outcomes and how will it effect current operations?

2. Will any additional support be needed before it can be introduced?

3. How should it be monitored during introduction?

The first question allows us to determine whether the electronic health app will be worth the investment. The second and third questions are key for its sustainability, as it recognizes components pivotal for a smooth implementation procedure [33]. Breaking down the barriers built by failed innovative interventions may be difficult, but it is beyond worthwhile to develop an effective health app. Answering these questions will be essential when developing a plan to obtain stakeholder support, thus we further discuss the specific steps to break down the resistance and prepare for the change below.

3.2.1. Battling the resistance to change

With any type of change there is an inevitable build-up of resistance that is formed. This resistance is derived from the fear of failure, similar to the first paradox of innovation; executives and end-users do not want to waste their time with another unbeneficial intervention [3, 33]. With this in mind, assimilating the idea of putting a new intervention into practice will be uphill road to climb. Nevertheless, two models described below help shape the key factors and steps involved towards achieving this goal.

3.2.1.1. Technology acceptance model (TAM)

The TAM was developed to drive the use of new technology and increase its acceptance by assessing the end-users *perceived ease of use (PEOU)* and *perceived usefulness (PU)* [33, 34]. This model suggests that by clarifying that a new source of innovation will reduce the amount of effort required (PEOU) and enhance performance it will be more likely to be accepted amongst end-users and other key stakeholders [35]. Thus, in the context of health care, executives, clinicians and patients will find an electronic health app more useful and user-friendly if they are familiar with the technology [3, 34].

With this in mind, when designing an electronic health app, developers must understand what the stakeholders needs, wants and expectations are. Once this is discovered, we can adequately highlight how the health app will benefit each of them specifically. Finally, when a foundation of acceptance for the app has been established, appropriate training protocols should be instilled to prevent any former resistance from re-establishing (**Figure 2**).

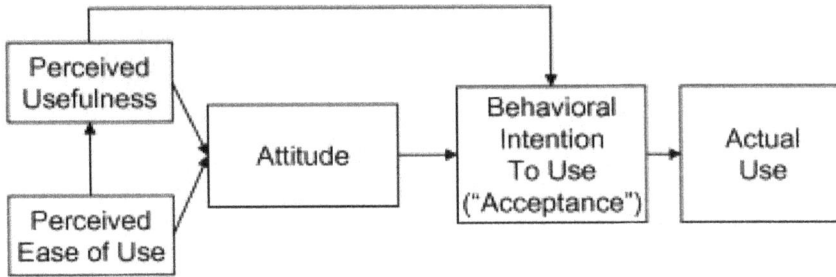

Figure 2. The technology acceptance model assessing the end-users perceived ease of use and perceived usefulness of technology to determine their behavioral intention and actual usage potential [34].

3.2.1.2. Diffusion of innovation (DOI) theory

The DOI theory is used to increase the adoption of technology [3]. This is one of the oldest theories, yet it remains to be continually used during innovative design. The DOI theory states that an organization will consider a technology to be innovative if it is perceived as new and relevant. It proposes that four main elements contribute to the diffusion of an idea, (1) the idea itself, (2) communication channels, (3) time and (4) a social system [36]. Similar to the TAM, the DOI theory suggests highlighting the perceived advantage and relevance of the innovations development. Therefore, in the context of electronic health apps, the benefit the of the app should be communicated amongst various influencers, and then stakeholder support must be established before the app can be readily adopted. As health apps must be widely adopted amongst all stakeholders and end-users before it can become self-sustaining, tackling this challenge will be key for the apps long-term success.

3.2.1.3. Presenting the benefits: results to support longevity

In both the TAM and the DOI theory, the key message to help obtain stakeholder support was to simply present why the app is beneficial for them. Why should they care about what we are developing? The real question developers should ask is, 'How will it help them?' This leads into one of the key components towards breaking down the barrier of stakeholder resistance and moving towards designing a sustainable health app. To adequately present the benefits of an application we must have the appropriate evidence to support our claim.

In many cases, a health app may be the first of its kind or an idea may be an advancement of a previous intervention. Regardless of whether a pilot study has been conducted to support the benefits of its use or its benefits have yet to be evaluated, the success of the product can be supported by answering the same question mentioned above, 'How will it help them'. We must outline what the problem currently is and why the development of this health app will help address it. It is not enough to state that a problem exists; it is the reasoning behind the solution that highlights the justification for its development.

Moreover, it is important to present the evidence supporting the benefits of the health app, but we must also present this support in the context of each stakeholder. Depending on the type of app being designed the stakeholders will differ, but to increase each claims value, we must understand the factors that will influence health app acceptance and evaluate them accordingly.

3.2.1.4. Testing health app acceptance: unified theory of acceptance and use of technology (UTAUT)

After assessing stakeholder needs and presenting the advantages associated with the health app, one of the next steps towards sustainability is to evaluate whether the proposed solution will be accepted amongst various users [37]. The UTAUT is a technology acceptance model commonly used to predict a user's behavioral intention to use a technology [37]. This model is based on four key components, [38].

1. **Performance expectancy:** providing an incentive to use a technology is key to ensure its acceptance. Performance expectancy is defined as the extent that the technology will benefit the end-user in completing a certain task. It is expected that increasing the health app's beneficial value, this will increase users behavioral intention. Therefore, to present these benefits, performance expectancy is constructed by four main evaluative criteria: (1) perceived usefulness: how much they will believe the technology will improve their performance, (2) extrinsic motivation: what other valued outcomes (money, fame) they will receive from its use, (3) job fit: how suitable technology is to increase performance and (4) relative advantage: benefit of new technology compared to what it will cost [39].

2. **Effort expectancy:** ease of use is a critical component of technology acceptance. Effort expectancy refers to how easy or difficult it is viewed to use the technology. Past technology acceptance models, such as TAM and DOI, have signified how applications that are simpler to use are more often accepted [40]. Thus, to reduce effort expectancy and increase acceptance rates, health apps should be less complex and instead easier to use [39].

3. **Social influence:** in many cases, the decision making process is influenced by specific individuals or the social norm. Social influence is the degree a user perceives that key individuals (family, friends) believe the use of the technology is important. This can be caused by informational influence where information from other people impact a decision or it can be normative influence where a user conforms their decision according to what is defined as 'acceptable' according to a certain group or situation. Regardless, social influence can be an ultimate determinate regarding the overall acceptance and usage of a health app [39].

4. **Facilitating conditions:** to ensure technology acceptance, users must feel its implementation is both feasible and realistic. Facilitating conditions is the degree individuals believe that existing organization and technical infrastructure is present to support its usage. These conditions can vary depending on a health app's objective, but regardless, they have a significant impact on its adoption and usage [40].

These four concepts have a direct influence on the behavioral intention to use a health app. Age, gender, experience and voluntariness are also associated with indirectly influencing behavioral intention and technology usage, as they moderate the four UTAUT component relationships. Thus, by incorporating the UTAUT within the health app design process, this will allow us to predict users' intention to adopt the app in an organizational context [38]. Nevertheless, as majority of health apps are focused on the users setting and the challenges they face, we recommend the usage of the more updated UTAUT2.

Compared to the original UTAUT, the extended UTAUT2 has shown to improve the variance in behavioral intention and technology use [38]. The UTAUT2 builds on the core UTAUT principles around extrinsic motivation, and adds three other components to improve the prediction of behavioral intention, which we describe below.

1. **Hedonic motivation:** hedonic motivation is defined as how enjoyable the technology is to use. It is used to analyze the emotional and psychological aspect of the technology, which is often overlooked by most evaluative models. The functionality of a health app will only go so far in influencing technology acceptance; it is the user experience that ultimately determines its long-term use and sustainability. Therefore, by evaluating the users internal satisfaction, this will result in improving technology usage [38, 39].

2. **Price value:** the price value determines whether the benefit of the technology is greater than its monetary cost. If the price value is high then individuals feel the benefit of use is greater than the cost of investment. However, this is not always the case and it is pivotal to assess this aspect of health app design to ensure its sustainability [38].

3. **Habit:** habit is the degree individuals automatically perform tasks due to learnt behaviors [38]. This construct was added to the UTAUT2 as it helps assess whether user-activity will be sustained. Often times, there is a fall out in health app usage due to the tasks becoming burdensome. Thus, if we were able to make these tasks more like a reflex than an extra step, this would reduce the effort required and improve technology acceptance (**Figure 3**).

With the addition of these factors to the UTAUT2, this helps tailor the health app evaluation to users in their context, which in turn helps improve its overall acceptance (**Table 2**). In many cases, it is these factors that prevent the sustainability of a health app. App publishers are focused on eliciting a behavior change or improving clinical outcomes, so they tend forget about the individual in their context. To reduce the resistance to change and move towards acceptance, it is the responsibility of the app publisher to ensure that the tool they are introducing is not only effective, but also it is 'fun', affordable, easy and relatable, or else it will simply not be used. Therefore, we believe by using the UTAUT2 principles during health app design, this will allow for the development of a more effective product, and will lead into a smoother transition phase during implementation.

3.2.2. Preparing for the expected and the unexpected

The implementation of any new source of innovation will come with many challenges that are both expected and unexpected, however, being prepared for both is what ensures optimal sustainability. We highlight below two of the major areas that result in impeding health app implementation, which is (1) regulations and (2) change management. Both are essential to incorporate during the design plan of a health app, we describe the detailed steps we recommend to tackle both areas effectively.

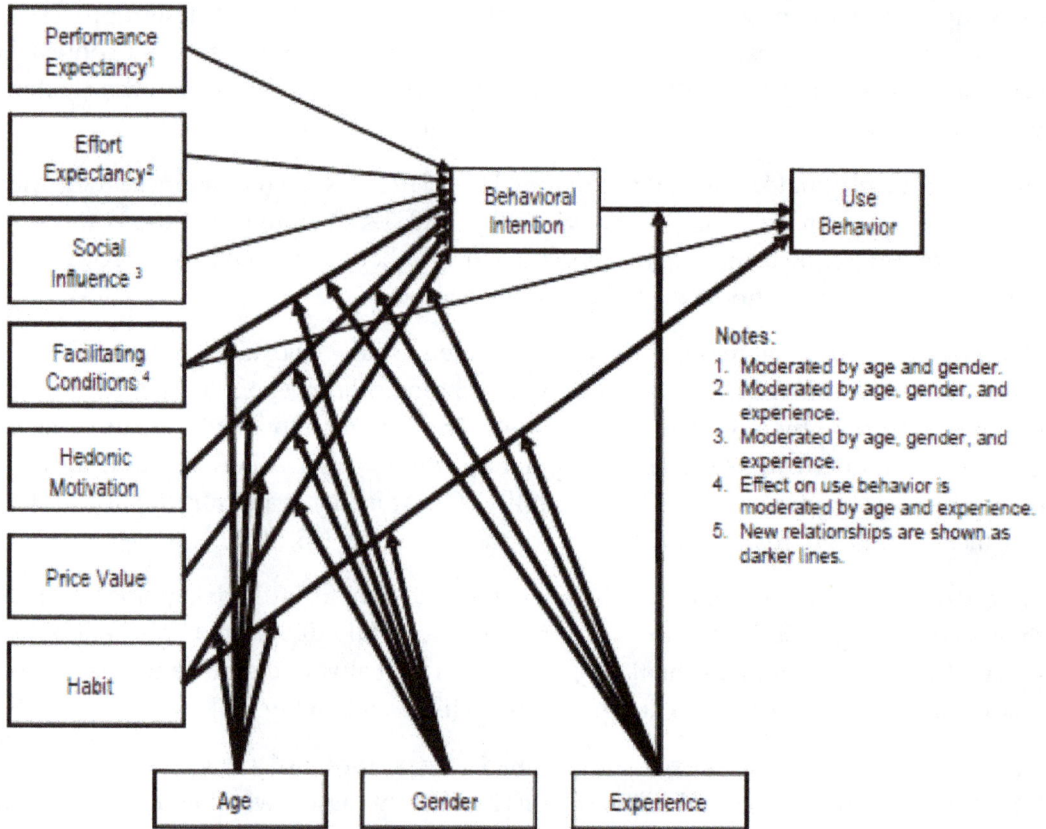

Figure 3. The UTAUT2 model with addition of hedonic motivation motivation, price value and habit to determine behavioral intention and technology use. All factors contribute in influencing behavioral intention to use except for 'facilitating conditions' and 'habit' which directing effect use behavior [38].

3.2.2.1. What regulations?

When implementing any new intervention into the health care industry there are a series of regulations that must be reviewed [15]. The FDA and Health Canada have issued a set of restrictions when developing an electronic application used as a medical device; however, most health apps do not fall under this category [17]. Nevertheless, one aspect of regulation all health apps must oblige to involves privacy and security. As many health apps are mobile phone based, this creates a challenging situation where more data can be obtained but data privacy is not secure. Policymakers are still in the works of establishing specific criteria required for patient safety, however we have listed a series of components that should be included within the health apps design to protect data integrity and prevent any unexpected threats.

(1) Data Sharing and Consent Management—Who can share my data

   All data shared must have consent, as well as meet the Health Insurance Portability and Accountability Act (HIPAA) standards for data sharing [17].

(2) Access Control and Authentication—Who can access data

To assure that only the approved individuals can access the data, an authentication procedure should be implemented. With most health data, data encryption and a respective login passcode are usually required.

(3) Confidentiality and Anonymity—Who knows it's my data

Depending on the level of consent and the data obtained, most personal data should remain confidential and possibly anonymous if used for public-health purposes [17].

Higher degrees of data security protocols can be implemented into health app designs, however, we believe that by incorporating these three aspects of privacy and security, this will make the app more desirable for both its end-users and its respective stakeholders during development. Ultimately, being prepared with the proper security measures gives stakeholders the confidence in the product, and will ease the process of change management.

			1	2	3	4	5
Performance expectancy	PE1	I find the health app useful in my daily life					
	PE2	Using the health app increases my chances of achieving things that are important to me					
	PE3	Using the health app helps me accomplish things more quickly					
	PE4	Using the health app increases my productivity					
Effort expectancy	EE1	Learning how to use the health app is easy for me.					
	EE2	My interaction with the health app is clear and understandable					
	EE3	I find the health app easy to use					
	EE4	It is easy for me to become skillful at using the health app					
Social influence	SI1	People who are important to me think that I should use the health app					
	SI2	People who influence my behavior think that I should use the health app					
	SI3	People whose opinions that I value prefer that I use the game					
Facilitating conditions	FC1	I have the resources necessary to use the health app					
	FC2	I have the knowledge necessary to use the health app					
	FC3	The health app is compatible with other technologies I use					
	FC4	I can get help from others when I have difficulties using the health app					

			1	2	3	4	5
Hedonistic motivation	HM1	Using the health app is fun					
	HM2	Using the health app is enjoyable					
	HM3	Using the health app is very entertaining					
Price value	PV1	The health app is reasonably priced					
	PV2	The health app is a good value for the money					
	PV3	At the current price, the health app provides a good value					
Habit	HT1	The use of the health app has become a habit for me					
	HT2	I am addicted to using the health app					
	HT3	I must use the health app					
	HT4	Using the health app has become natural to me					
Behavioral intention	BI1	I intend to continue using the health app in the future					
	BI2	I will always try to use the health app in my daily life					
	BI3	I plan to continue to use the health app frequently					

Table 2. UTAUT2 questionnaire used to evaluate health app acceptance amongst end-users.

3.2.2.2. Change management is key for smooth sailing

With the introduction of any new intervention this will result in causing changes in work-flow that in some cases may be disruptive. These challenges are expected, but to assure the implementation process runs smoothly, a set of change management plans can be pre-developed [41]. To develop a proper strategy, we must consider three primary levels of change management.

(1) Individual change management: how people experience the change and what their needs are to successfully make the transition.

(2) Organizational/initiative change management: what are the primary groups that will directly be impacted and what changes will need to be completed respectively.

(3) Enterprise change management capability: this is the overall organizational approach to managing change. It usually involves executive discussion, and reflects the organizations capability to allow and embrace change. This level is key as top-down support has a direct relationship on how a change will be perceived at the lower levels.

All three levels of change management can be addressed through the three-phase change management process (**Figure 4**) [41]. Phase 1, prepare for the change, we must determine who will be impacted by the change and what level of support we will need to smoothly move forward. During this phase, it will be key to understand all the challenges that will be in play, as

Phase 1 – Preparing for Change

| Define your change management strategy |
| Prepare your change management team |
| Develop your sponsorship model |

Phase 2 – Managing Change

| Develop change management plans |
| Take action and implement plans |

Phase 3 – Reinforcing Change

| Collect and analyze feedback |
| Diagnose gaps and manage resistance |
| Implement corrective actions and celebrate successes |

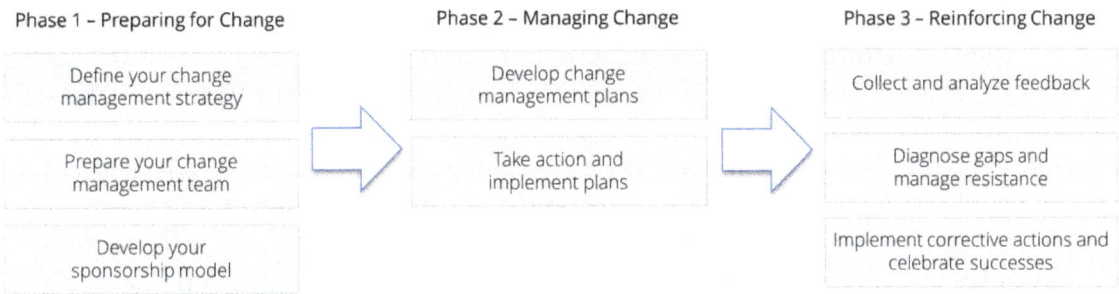

Figure 4. The change management process indicated by three phases (1) preparing for change, (2) managing change and (3) reinforcing change [41].

we will need instill that the perceived usefulness will remain to be stronger. Phase 2, manage the change, focuses on supporting the individuals impacted by the change. With respect to the implementation of health apps, this phase would be heavily focused on the end-users and what additional training that may be required to increase its perceived ease of use and prevent resistance from re-establishing. Phase 3, reinforcing change, evaluates the current status of the intervention to identify any issues and address them accordingly. This phase is key for the long-term sustainability of the health app as it ensures the change is maintained and provides evidence to support its benefits [41]. By following this three-phase change management plan, the health app design process will move more efficiently and will lead to a higher adoption rate.

4. Ensuring adoption and scalability

Moving from end-user usability and primary stakeholder needs, app publishers must also consider the underlying factors for national adoption. State or province specific regulations, needs, and resources available are likely to differ across a country. Thus, for optimal scalability, technology should be agile enough to utilize the infrastructure that is in place without causing disruption.

For instance, in Canada, policies regarding home-care differ between provinces, leaving some provinces with funding and others with none. When introducing a health app with similar objectives to home-care, developers must consider how the app can be used independently and concurrently, without losing its value. To ensure long-term adoption and scalability, the ideal health app should be designed to seamlessly coincide with the current practices that are in place. We describe below what evaluative steps we recommend to maximize national health app potential.

4.1. Long-term sustainability: where will it work?

We have described components should be included to please various stakeholders and ensure a smooth transition process. However, true sustainability stems from its capability to be seamlessly used in multiple settings. To accomplish this, we must conduct a market analysis to understand what interventions and regulations are currently in place, followed by a feasibility assessment to determine if those factors will jeopardize its implementation on a national scale [2, 42].

Depending on the health app being developed, different factors contributing to the market will be evaluated. However, before evaluating any components, the objective of the health app must be distinguished. This will narrow the scope of market factors that we will need to consider. We will then need to determine whether the health app will be an improvement of a current intervention or if it will stand alone in its functionality. Once this has been decided, we can readily evaluate what market factors are at play by answering a set of questions as outlined in **Figure 5**. Moving forward, depending on the con-current usage of the health app the steps may differ. Nonetheless, both ends of the evaluation will move in the same direction towards evaluating app feasibility, by determining what regulations/policies are in place, how cost-effective the app will be and most importantly if there is any funding available to support its implementation (**Figure 5**). This evaluative framework regarding the market forces and feasibility will determine whether the app will be sustainable across national regulations, or if it requires substantial changes in its design construct.

In the health app industry, it is common for enthusiasm regarding innovation to overshadow the drive to tackle sustainability, let alone feasibility. In this chapter, we focused on the high-lighting the importance beyond designing sustainable electronic health applications. We started by addressing what barriers regarding sustainability were present and outlined what steps were needed to avoid them. The importance of identifying the needs, wants and expectations of the health apps primary stakeholders were also signified, as we understand that it is not only

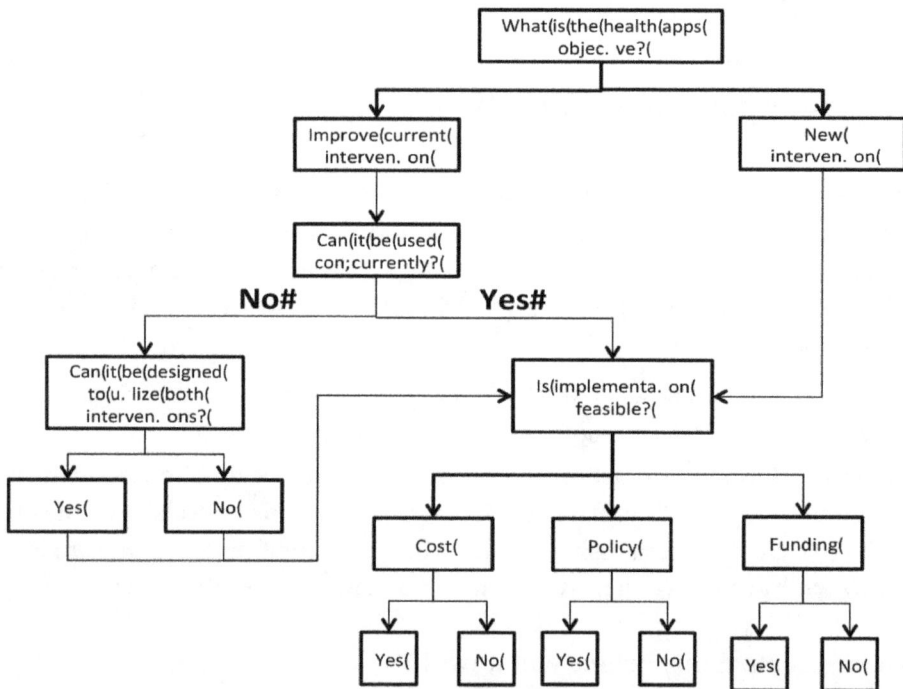

Figure 5. Market evaluation and feasibility analysis framework to help determine national sustainability of the intervention. The analysis begins by highlighting the health apps objective and determining whether it will improve current processes or introduce a new one. This leads to evaluating how the health app will function with current practices in place and if it will be suitable moving forward. In this framework, each block represents a form of analysis that is conducted, which leads to the final block that assesses overall feasibility and/or potential health app re-design/modifications needed.

important from a usability standpoint, but it shapes whether it will be sustainable across the country. Designing for sustainability may be a tiresome process, but if executed properly, the end results will bring more value than anticipated.

Author details

Sahr Wali[1], Karim Keshavjee[2] and Catherine Demers[1*]

*Address all correspondence to: demers@hhsc.ca

1 McMaster University, Hamilton, Canada

2 InfoClin Inc, Toronto, Canada

References

[1] Research2guidance. App Developer Economics 2015. 2015. Available from: http://research-2guidance.com/r2g/r2g--App-Developer-Economics-2015.pdf [Accessed: November 27, 2017]

[2] Proctor E, Luke D, Calhoun A, McMillen C, Brownson R, McCrary S, Padek M. Sustainability of evidence-based healthcare: Research agenda, methodological advances, and infrastructure support. Implementation Science. 2015;**10**(88):1-13. DOI: 10.1186/s13012-015-0274-5

[3] Thakur R, Hsu SHY, Fontenot G. Innovation in healthcare: Issues and future trends. Journal of Business Research. 2012;**65**:562-569

[4] Marshall D, Demers C, O'Brien B, Guyatt G. Economic evaluation. In: Dicenso A, Guyatt G, Ciliska D, editors. Evidence-Based Nursing: A Guide to Clinical Practice. St Louis: Elsevier Mosby; 2005. pp. 298-317

[5] Abril EP. Tracking myself: Assessing the contribution of mobile technologies for self-trackers of weight, diet, or exercise. Journal of Health Communication. 2016;**21**(6):638-646

[6] Hartin PJ, Nugent CD, McClean SI, Cleland I, Tschanz JT, Clark CJ, Norton MC. The empowering role of mobile apps in behavior change interventions: The gray matters randomized controlled trial. JMIR mHealth uHealth. 2016;**4**(3):e93

[7] Carter MC, Burley VJ, Nykjaer C, Cade JE. Adherence to a smartphone application for weight loss compared to website and paper diary: Pilot randomized controlled trial. Journal of Medical Internet Research. 2013;**15**(4):e32

[8] Cook KA, Modena BD, Simon RA. Improvement in asthma control using a minimally burdensome and proactive smartphone application. The Journal of Allergy and Clinical Immunology. In Practice. 2016;**4**(4):730-737

[9]   Chindalo P, Keshavjee K, Karim A, Brahmbhatt R, Saha N. Health apps by design: A refer-ence architecture for mobile engagement. International Journal of Handheld Computing Research. 2016;7(2):34-43

[10] Omachonu VK. Innovation in healthcare delivery systems: A conceptual framework. Public Sector Innovation Journal. 2010;15(1):1-20

[11] Patient Empowerment Network. Designing with the patient in mind. 2016. Retrieved from: https://powerfulpatients.org/2016/01/26/designing-with-the-patient-in-mind/

[12] Kuerbis A, Mulliken A, Muench F, Moore AA, Gardner D. Older adults and mobile tech-nology: Factors that enhance and inhibit utilization in the context of behavioral health. Mental Health and Addiction Research. 2017;2(2):1-11

[13] Patient Empowerment Network. Are we ready for mobile health. 2016. Retrieved from: https://powerfulpatients.org/2016/01/04/are-we-ready-for-mobile-health/

[14] Kotz D, Gunter CA, Kumar S, Weiner JP. Privacy and security in mobile health: A research agenda. IEEE Computer. 2016;49(6):22-30

[15] Faulkner A, Kent J. Innovation and regulation in human implant technologies: Developing comparative approaches. Social Science & Medicine. 2001;53(7):895-913

[16] Hollis C, Moriss R, Martin J, Amani S, Cotton R, Denis M, Lewis S. Technological innova-tions in mental healthcare: Harnessing the digital revolution. British Journal of Psychiatry. 2015;206(4):263-265

[17] Barton AJ. The regulation of mobile health applications. BMC Medicine. 2012;10(46):1-4

[18] Avgar AC, Litwin AS, Pronovost PJ. Drivers and barriers in health IT adoption. Applied Clinical Informatics. 2012;3:488-500

[19] Aidemark J, Asskenas L, Nygardh A, Stromberg A. User involvement in the co-design of self-care support systems for heart failure patients. Procedia Computer Science. 2015;64: 118-124

[20] McCurdie T, Taneva S, Casselman M, Yeung M, McDaniel C, Ho W, Cafazzo J. mHealth consumer apps: The case for user-centered design. Horizons: Technology and Design. 2012;46:49-56

[21] Brahmbhatt R, Niakan S, Saha N, Tewari A, Pirani A, Keshavjee N, Mugambi D, Alavi N, Keshavjee K. Diabetes mHealth apps: Can they be effective. Studies in Health Technology and Informatics. 2017;234:49-53

[22] Martinez-Perez B, Torre-Diez I, Lopez-Coronado M, Herreros-Gonzalex J. Mobile apps in cardiology: Review. JMIR mhealth uhealth. 2013;1(2):e15

[23] Creber RMM, Maurer MS, Reading M, Hiraldo G, Hickey KT, Iribarren S. Review and analysis of existing mobile phone apps to support heart failure symptom monitoring and self-care management using the mobile application rating scale (MARS). JMIR mHealth uHealth. 2016;4(2):e74

[24] Fleuren M, Wiefferink K, Paulussen T. Determinants of innovation within health care organizations: Literature review and Delphi study. International Journal for Quality in Health Care. 2004;**16**(2):107-123

[25] Gandhi S, Chen S, Hong L, Sun K, Gong E, Li C, Yang LL, Schwalm JD. Effect of mobile health interventions on secondary prevention of cardiovascular disease: Systematic review and meta-analysis. Canadian Journal of Cardiology. 2017;**33**:210-231

[26] Bonoto BC, de Araujo VE, de Lemos LL, Godman B, Bennie M, Diniz LM, Junior AA. Efficacy of mobile apps to support the care of patients with analysis of randomized controlled trials. JMIR mHealth uHealth. 2017;**5**(3):e4

[27] Schnall R, Rojas M, Bakken S, Brown W, Carballo-Dieguez A, Carry M, Gelaude D, Patterson Mosley D, Travers J. A user-centered model for designing consumer mobile health (mHealth) applications (apps). Journal of Biomedical Informatics. 2016;**60**:243-251

[28] Hevner ARA. Three cycle view of design science research. Scandinavian Journal of Information Systems. 2007;**19**(2):87-92

[29] Cronholm S, Gobel H. Evaluation of the information systems research framework: Empirical evidence from a design science research project. The Electronic Journal Information Systems Evaluation. 2016;**19**(3):158-168

[30] Donetto S, Pierri P, Tsianakas V, Robert G. Experience-based co-design and healthcare improvement: Realising participatory design in the public sector. International Journal for All Aspects of Design. 2015;**18**(2):227-248

[31] Eyles H, Jull A, Dobson R, Firestone R, Whittaker R, Te Morenga L, Goodwin D, Ni Mhurch C. Co-design of mhealth delivered interventions: A systematic review to assess key methods and processes. Current Nutrition Report. 2016;**5**(30):160-167

[32] Lloyd T, Buck H, Foy A, Black S, Pinter A, Pogash R, Eismann B, Balaban E, Chan J, Kunselman A, Smyth J, Boehmer J. The Penn state heart assistant: A pilot study of a web-based intervention to improve self-care of heart failure patients. Health Informatics Journal. 2017:1-12. Web

[33] Dixon-Woods M, Amalberti R, Goodman S, Bergman B, Glasziou P. Problems and promises of innovation: Why healthcare needs to rethink its love/hate relationship with the new. BMJ Quality and Safety. 2011;**20**(1):47-51

[34] Davis FD. Perceived usefulness, perceived ease of use, and user acceptance of information technology. MIS Quarterly. 1989;**13**(3):319-340

[35] Holden RJ, Karsh BT. The technology acceptance model: Its past and its future in health care. Journal of Biomedical Informatics. 2010;**43**(1):159-172

[36] Rogers EM. Diffusion of Innovations. 5th ed. New York, NY: Free Press; August 2003. pp. xv-xxi

[37] Venkatesh V, Morris MG, Davis GB, Davis FD. User acceptance of information technology: Toward a unified view. MIS Quarterly. 2003;**27**(3):425-478

[38] Venkatesh V, Thong JYL, Xu X. Consumer acceptance and use of information technology: Extending the unified theory of acceptance and use of technology. MIS Quarterly. 2012;**36**(1):157-178

[39] Huang CY, Kao YS. UTAUT2 based predictions of factors influencing the technology acceptance of phablets by DNP. Mathematical Problems in Engineering. 2015;**2015**:1-23

[40] Chang A. UTAUT and UTAUT2: A review and agenda for future research. The Winners. 2012; **13**(2):106-114

[41] Prosci. What is change management. 2018. Retrieved from: https://www.prosci.com/change-management/what-is-change-management

[42] Swerissen H, Crisp BR. The sustainability of health promotion interventions for different levels of social organization. Health Promotion International. 2004;**19**(1):123-130

6

Mobile Cloud-Based Blood Pressure Healthcare for Education

Chin-Feng Lin, Shere-Er Wang, Yen-Chiao Lu,
Chung-I Lin, Chung-Cheng Chang, Tim Yeh,
Candice Lee, Jeffson Huang, Chic-Erh Weng,
Sue-Hsien Chen, Bing-Leung Sun,
Chao-Sheng Wang, Shiue-Li Cheng, Shiou-Yu Li and
Lan-Yu Wu

Abstract

Mercury, pneumatic, and electronic sphygmomanometers were widely used for traditional blood pressure (BP) measurement. Cloud BP database, and mobile information and communication technology (MICT) do not integrate to these BP measurement methods. Pen and papers were employed to record BP values for nurses and physicians, and recording errors are possible to occur. In the chapter, the cloud-based BP platform solution and advanced wireless hospital BP measurement technologies were studied. These cloud-based BT measurement technologies were used as teaching aids to train students of electrical and nursing fields for mobile BP healthcare and health promotion education, and hence interdisciplinary teaching and learning were conducted. The teachers include professors of electrical and nursing fields, physicians, hospital nurses, and the engineer and health management experts of Microlife. The interdisciplinary teaching and learning of mobile BP healthcare and health promotion for smart aging were conducted in the Department of Nursing Division, Chang Cung Memorial Hospital, Keelung Branch, Department of Nursing Ching Kuo Institute of Management and Health, School of Nursing Chung Shan Medical University, and Department of Electrical Engineering, National Taiwan Ocean University. The students of electrical and nursing fields participated for joint interdisciplinary learning. The concepts of interdisciplinary mobile BP healthcare learning and teaching involve nursing and technology, healthy aging, BP health care for smart aging, telenursing, BP care for smart aging, community/home telecare, and MICT. The objective of teaching and learning is training the design and making electrical engineers to understand BP healthcare and health promotion, and nurses to understand mobile BP healthcare and health promotion system for smart aging.

Keywords: BP healthcare, smart aging, cloud-based BP measurement technologies, jointly interdisciplinary learning and teaching, mobile information and communication technology

1. Introduction

In this chapter, computers, Internet access, mobile computing, Web page systems, short messaging services, multimedia messaging services, and e-mails were examined with respect to students of medical, nursing, and health science disciplines [1]. The advanced technologies help health science students to access healthcare information and adopt effective methods to develop their skills. Mobile information and communication technology (MICT) has been used in the learning and teaching process of health and medicine science education, and has enabled learning and access to health education knowledge anywhere and at any time [2]. Mazzola et al. [3] demonstrated how physical activity, nutrition, and training through a combination of processes and mobile technologies are related to overweight teenagers and obesity in behavioral education. The People for Ecosystem-based Governance in Assessing Sustainable development of Ocean and coast (PEGASO) scenarios [3] include motion sensors to detect physical activity, GPS location service, and the smartphone acts as a communication gateway for these sensors with feedback functions and information. The awareness and self-management of obesity risks are important to motivate teenagers to engage in affective learning and trigger a behavioral change. Smartphone applications were exploited to improve participants' health-related quality of life and healthcare utilization for rheumatic diseases self-management [4]. Disease-associated self-management strategies can be designed using mobile health (mHealth) technologies. Azevedo et al. [4] reviewed several aims, platforms, and characteristics of smartphone applications for self-management of rheumatic diseases.

mHealth is a "medical and public health practice supported by mobile devices, such as mobile phones, patient monitoring devices, personal digital assistants, and other wireless devices" [5], and is recognized by the World Health Organization. Advanced mobile Web-based and Internet technologies have transformed current healthcare models with regard to monitoring of physical activity or encouraging physiological changes that stimulate positive health behaviors. Zhang et al. [6] illustrated how to extend a mobile Web-based app with multimedia features for psychiatry education in Singapore, and found out through a survey that MICT helped them save a significant amount of time in clinical activities. MICT must ensure that the physiological signals provided within are accurate and credible. Healthy behaviors (e.g., sports lifestyle, healthy eating habits, and blood pressure (BP) monitoring) help in reducing fatal health risk, disability, healthcare use and health-related costs [7]. Weight management, physical activity, smoking cessation, self-management of diabetes mellitus, and hypertension care using MICT were demonstrated [8]. MICT-supported health behavior interventions are designed to prevent or manage illness and lead to fundamental changes in health practices, thereby, providing an opportunity to stimulate and sustain healthy behaviors [6, 7]. Chan et al. [9] described that problem-based learning using multimedia, such as video clips, Web sites, images, or photos, was implemented in the health sciences learning process, and students could use their mobile Internet technology to access the knowledge and enhance their process of learning using laptops, tablets, and smartphone mobile devices on a cloud-based learning platform. Problem identification, problem description, problem exploration, applicability, and integration strategies were recommended in the problem-based learning approach [10].

Elliott et al. [11] implemented a mobile electronic health records (EHR) system for medical education. The functionality, connectivity, ease of use, and usage challenges of the developed EHR system in the hospital environment were investigated for learning. Davies et al. [12] developed a mobile learning model using a personal digital assistant (PDA) loaded with medical resources for undergraduate medical students in the clinical environment. MICT was used to provide new learning methods with respect to problem identification and solving skills. ISO/IEEE 11073 and Health Level 7(HL7) V2.6 protocols were used to develop and evaluate self-management mobile Personal Health Record mobile health application for Android 4.0.3 by the Continua Health Alliance for continuous self-management of chronic disease patients [13]. It has the potential to promote new treatment and medical opportunities as well as to reduce medical costs and time for an aging society. It monitors their vital signs using mobile network technology (MNT); thereby, ensuring better healthcare. The user interface, applications, seamless transmission protocol, personal health record, and database managers were demonstrated for the application.

Wu et al. [14] proposed a cellular and iridium network-based blood pressure and body temperature remote measurement platform for mobile healthcare education. The overview of mobile telemedicine research fields was provided by Lin [15, 16]. In previous studies [17–21], 802.11n and ultra-wideband wireless telemedicine transmission schemes, multicode code division multiple access (CDMA) cellular mobile telemedicine transmission mechanism, and multi-satellites wideband CDMA and orthogonal frequency division multiplexing (OFDM) transport architectures were proposed. In this article, a cloud-based mobile blood pressure (BP) healthcare education program for smart aging is investigated.

2. Teaching methodology and concept

Our teaching team included professors from electrical and nursing fields, as well as physicians, the engineers, and health management experts for Microlife. Cloud-based and mobile BP healthcare knowledge was the focus of studies for students in electrical and nursing fields. The could-based and mobile BP platform of Microlife was used in the healthcare program for interdisciplinary learning. The tele-BP healthcare for smart aging course was offered through the Department of Electrical Engineering, National Taiwan Ocean University, and the School of Nursing Chung Shan Medical University, during February 2014 and June 2014. Fourteen students in the electrical field and 19 nursing students participated for joint interdisciplinary learning. The distance between National Taiwan Ocean University and Chung Shan Medical

University is 180 km. Facebook videoconferences were used for team discussions associated with problem-based learning and problem solving. The BP healthcare for smart aging course was offered through the Department of Electrical Engineering, National Taiwan Ocean University, and the Department of Nursing, Ching Kuo Institute of Management and Health, during September 2014 and January 2015. Thirteen students in the electrical field and 34 nursing students participated for joint interdisciplinary learning. In the learning teams, students in the electrical field provided the MICT know-how, and nursing students contributed user experience and healthcare knowledge. The course outline of tele-BP healthcare for smart aging is as follows:

• Nursing and technology

• Healthy aging

• BP healthcare for smart aging

• Telenursing

Video materials were recorded and uploaded to the course Web site for students enrolled in the course so that they could download the information to study anytime and anywhere.

Nursing and technology video material [22]: Lu discussed the relationship between nursing and technology, technology's effects on nursing, the connection between nurse's experiences with technology and new technology design, advanced nursing processes, future trends in nursing education, and future trends in the development of nursing technologies.

Healthy aging video material [23]: Lu defined aging and discussed the aging process, changes in bodily functions, longevity, elderly food intake and arrangements, elderly movement, and approaches to caring for the elderly, as well as definitions of healthy aging, aging attitudes, and planning.

BP healthcare for smart aging video material [24]: Lin discussed health and medical, issues, medical care for smart aging, cardiovascular disease, BP definition, the principles of BP changes, classifications of hypertension, techniques and times for measuring BP, and principles and operational modes regarding mercury, pneumatic, and electronic sphygmomanometers. Other topics included risk factors, symptoms, and complications of hypertension, and preventive measures for the disease.

Telenursing video material [25]: Lu discussed the definitions of telehealth, telecare, telemedicine, and telenursing, community-based telecare, home-based telecare, and agency-based telecare, as well as the roles, opportunities, and challenges of telecare nurses.

The course outline of BP healthcare for smart aging is as follows:

• BP care for smart aging

• Community/home telecare

• MICT

BP care for smart aging digital material [26]: Wang discussed the significance of low and high BP, the factors influencing BP, the significance of BP tracking, the risk of brain/cardiovascular disease associated with BP, and the challenge of telecare.

Community/home telecare digital material [27]: Wang discussed community-based telecare in Taiwan, the project model for telecare, physiological signal monitoring, locations and energy services for smart aging, health counseling and interpersonal assistance for smart aging, and design considerations for products for smart aging.

MICT digital material [28]: Lin discussed the definition and history of communication technology, definition and history of the Internet, introduction to multimedia communications and communications and network infrastructure in Taiwan, mobile communications and networks, the architecture of telecare, and the definition and history of telemedicine.

3. Experiment-based and visit-based learning

In the experiment-based learning process, interdisciplinary students can understand the principle and technology of mobile BP healthcare solutions for smart aging. **Figure 1** shows several BP measurements for the same personal, taken in different situations. The systolic BP values for lying, sitting, standing, and walking are 122, 123, 128, and 136 mmHg, respectively. The diastolic BP values are 62, 70, 75, and 90 mmHg, respectively. We observed the range of the systolic and diastolic BP values by taking measurements in several situations. The maximum measurement value of BP is reported for walking, and the minimum measurement value is reported for lying.

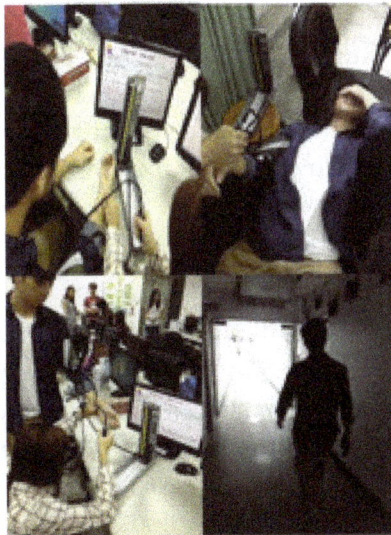

Figure 1. Several BP measurements for the same personal taken in different situations.

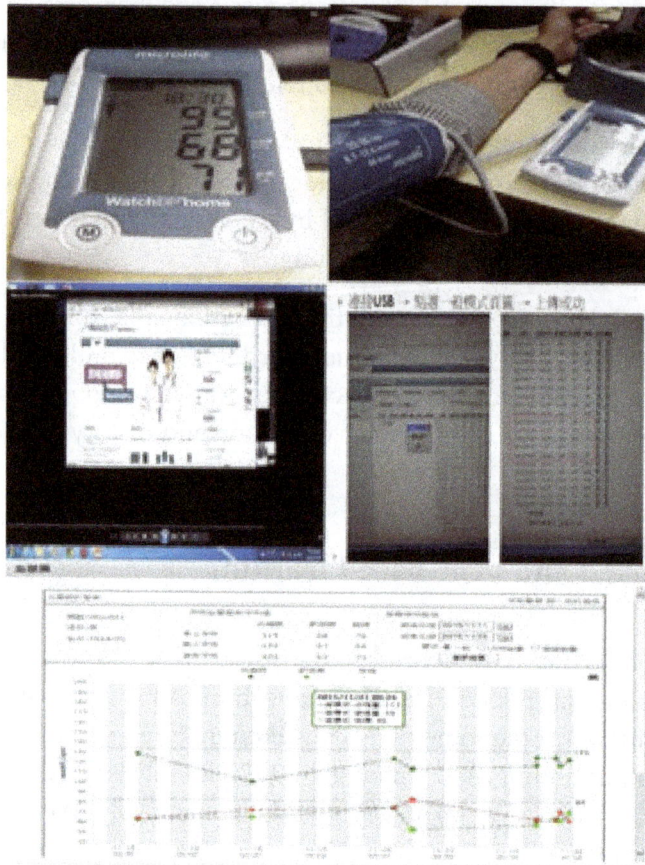

Figure 2. The cloud-based BP platform solution developed by Microlife [29]. Values are presented.

As shown in **Figure 2**, the cloud-based BP platform solution developed by Microlife was adopted in the course to train students in mobile BP healthcare [29]. The BP measurement times were before sleep and after getting up, and the times were recorded with a USB-based sphygmomanometer that can store 256 BP measurement times, as well as the values for pulse, diastolic, and systolic BP. These values can be uploaded to the cloud-based mobile BP platform from the USB-based sphygmomanometer using a USB transmission interface. In the cloud-based BP platform, the BP measurement time and pulse, diastolic, and systolic BP values are recorded, and the trend and changes of pulse, diastolic, and systolic BP are noted.

We can also obtain the sleep habits of the cloud-based BP platform users. The joint interdisciplinary learning process for cloud-based BP healthcare solutions in the courses of tele-BP healthcare and BP healthcare for smart aging is shown in **Figure 3**. The third-generation (3G) mobile cellular network was used to connect notebooks to the cloud-based BP platform at anytime and anywhere. Observation, interdisciplinary cooperation, reverse thinking and feedback, innovative design, and an applied science and technology learning methodology were utilized. Cloud-based BP healthcare solutions for smart aging were learned, using integration, innovation, design, and thinking skills. The interdisciplinary students posed and answered the following questions:

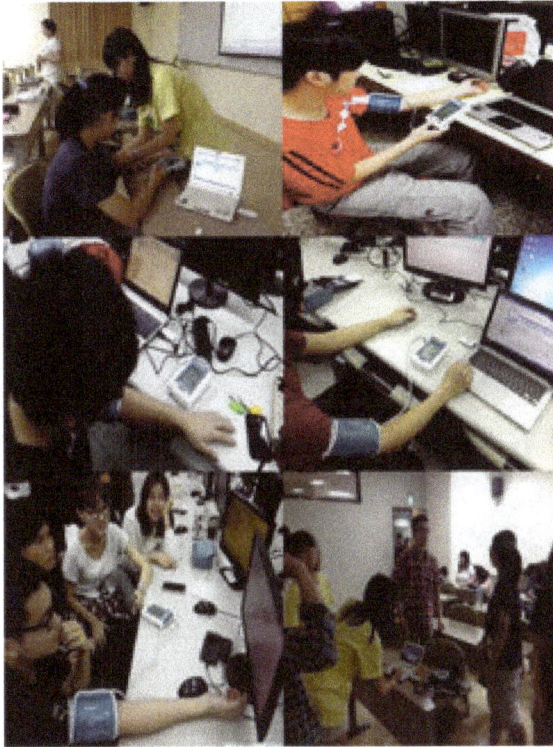

Figure 3. The joint interdisciplinary learning process for cloud-based BP healthcare solutions in the courses of tele-BP healthcare and BP healthcare for smart aging.

What healthcare services are available?

What kinds of smart aging groups are available?

Why are these kinds of smart aging groups suitable?

How are these kinds of smart aging groups used?

What kinds of carers and operators are needed?

What kinds of sensors and control devices are used?

What are the kinds of MICT devices, HMI, and network needs?

What are the functions of the cloud database?

What are the costs to be paid?

Who are the payers?

What are the self-management strategies of lifestyle and the treatment concept in mobile BP healthcare education for smart aging using MICT?

What are the advantages and disadvantages?

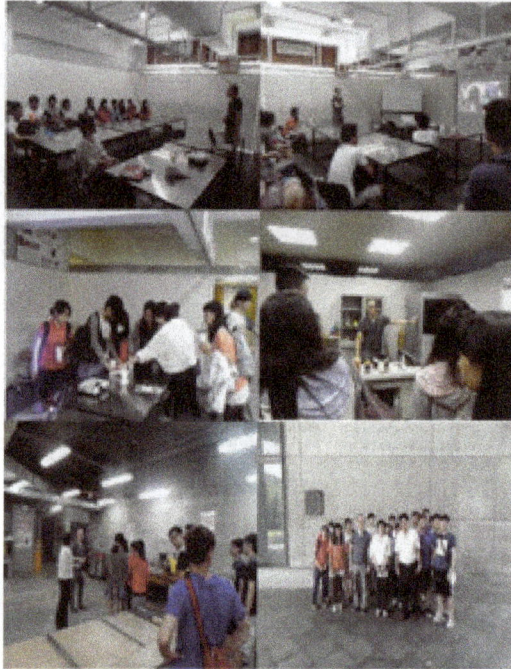

Figure 4. The interdisciplinary course outline of tele-BP healthcare for smart aging included a visit to the Department of Industrial Design, Shih Chien University, in July 2, 2014.

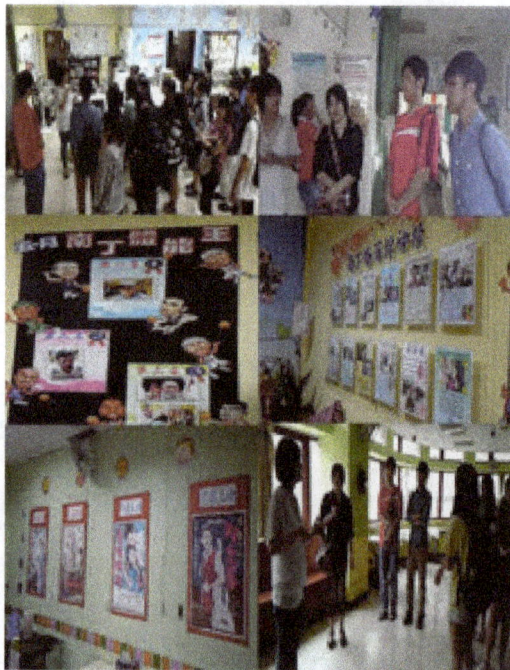

Figure 5. The interdisciplinary course outline of tele-BP healthcare for smart aging also included a visit to the Nightingale Nursing home for Smart Aging, Taichung, in June 2014.

The interdisciplinary course outline of tele-BP healthcare for smart aging included a visit to the Department of Industrial Design, Shih Chien University, in July 2, 2014, as shown in **Figure 4**. Prof. Z.C. Wang presented the principle and technology of industrial design of nursing and a 3D printer. The course outline also included a visit to the Nightingale Nursing home for Smart Aging, Taichung, in June 2014, as shown in **Figure 5**. Students studied the life behaviors, diet, entertainment, and movement habits in the care center. In addition, the interdisciplinary course outline of BP healthcare for smart aging included a visit to a hospice and iodine 131 wards at Chang Cung Memorial Hospital, Keelung Branch, in November 2014, as shown in **Figure 6**, for an overview of the hospice practices. A video phone was used in an iodine 131 ward to provide real-time interaction between patients inside the ward and doctors, nurses, family members, and friends outside the ward. The video phone technology ameliorated the sense of helpless and anxiety felt by patients in the isolation iodine 131 ward. In addition, the cloud-based, wireless sphygmomanometers used in the Chang Cung Memorial Hospital, Keelung Branch, were observed. The medical record number, BP measurement time, and pulse, diastolic, and systolic BP values transmitted in real time to the cloud-based hospital care platform using the wireless transmission technology. Thus, the interdisciplinary students studied mobile BP healthcare for smart aging through visit-based learning.

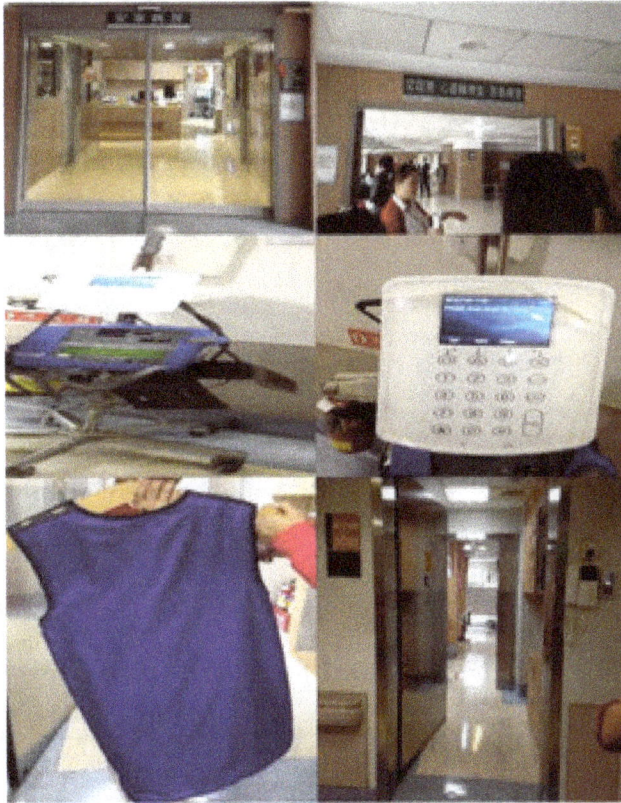

Figure 6. The interdisciplinary course outline of BP healthcare for smart aging included a visit to a hospice and iodine 131 wards at Chang Cung Memorial Hospital, Keelung Branch, in November 2014.

According to the teaching and learning experience, as well as the visit-based experience described in the above explanation, the learning tool was developed for mobile hypertension education, as shown in **Figure 7**. The development learning tools included the proximal display software, a notebook, tablet, or personal computer with the Microsoft operating system, and a 3G mobile modem. The C# program was used to develop the proximal display software. The adaptive screen with large font solutions for smart aging, cloud-based BP measurement solution of Microlife, cloud-based BP measurement solution of Sunshine Instrument [30], SKYPE videoconference solution [31], and Messenger Plus videoconference recording solution [32] were all integrated with each other. Cloud-based sphygmomanometer and electrocardiography instruments are approved by Food and Drug Administration (FDA), and Taiwan FDA medical equipment, respectively. The videoconference and videoconference recording solutions can be used for team discussions relating to problem-based learning and problem solving. The mobile hypertension care process was studied as regards nursing students, and the proximal display software technology and the principle of MICT were studied as regards electrical students.

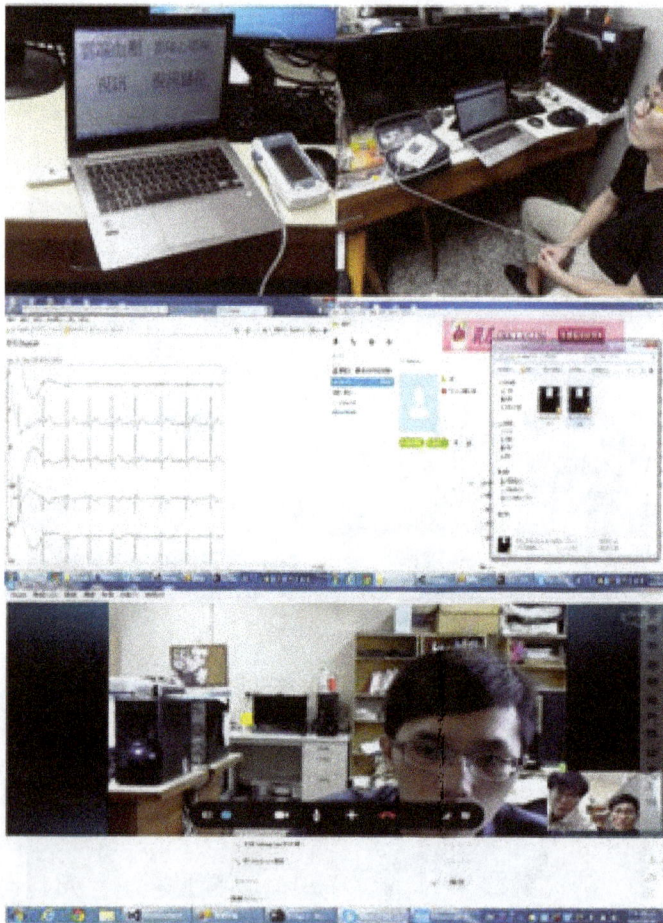

Figure 7. The learning tool was developed for mobile hypertension education.

A learning tool developed by Microlife Corporation for 3G mobile agent and cloud-based multiuser real-time BP measurement system is shown in **Figure 8**. The 3G mobile agent and cloud-based multiuser real-time BP measurement system includes radiofrequency identification (RFID) cards, a Bluetooth-based sphygmomanometer, 3G gateway with Bluetooth network, 3G mobile modem, auto login sensor, and tablet. Each user has an RFID card, such as an Easycard, or a student card, to identify the user number. The Bluetooth-based sphygmomanometer is in a shutdown state. When the RFID-based student card senses the Bluetooth-based sphygmomanometer, the device is turned on, and the BP is measured. Real-time BP values are transmitted to the 3G gateway via the Bluetooth network, and a 3G mobile modem is used for transmission of these values to a cloud-based BP platform. When the RFID-based student card senses auto login, the auto login sensor uses the 3G mobile modem to login into the cloud-based BP monitoring Web page, and the real-time BP values in the Web page are displayed on the tablet. Each user can access BP reports on the cloud-based Web page at any instance from any global location.

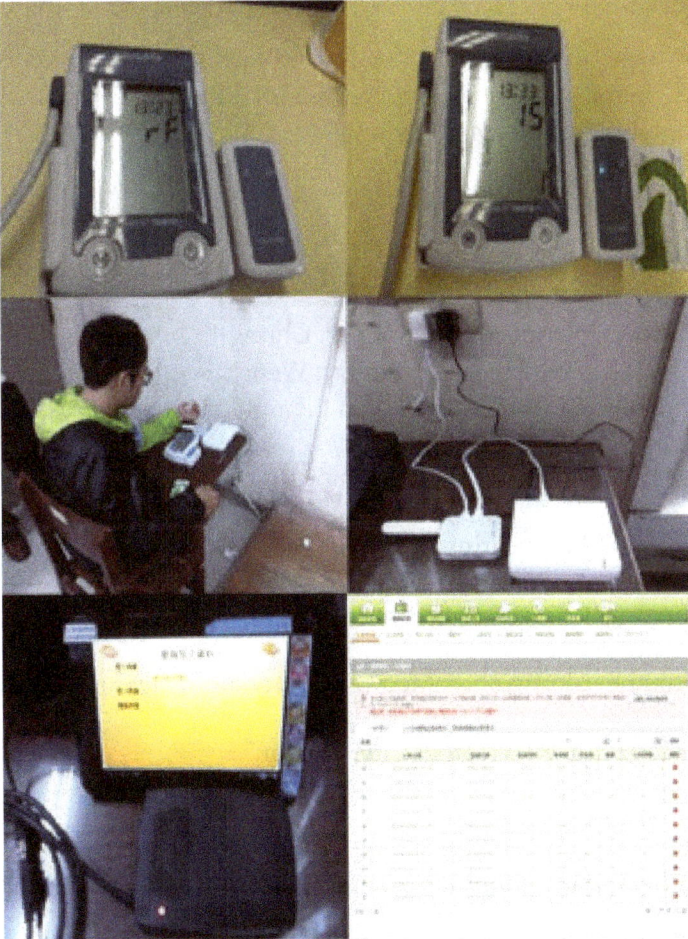

Figure 8. A learning tool developed by Microlife Corporation for 3G mobile agent and cloud-based multiuser real time BP measurement system.

4. Conclusion

For students in electrical and nursing fields, mobile BP smart aging healthcare is a challenging area of joint interdisciplinary learning. A new educational model and innovative teaching methodology using a cloud-based mobile BP healthcare solution for BP healthcare smart aging education were proposed. Problem-based learning and a solving process, experiment-based learning, and visit-based learning were adopted. Facebook videoconferencing was used for team discussions of the problem-based learning and solving process among students in electrical and nursing fields. The cloud-based BP platform solution developed by Microlife was adopted in the course to train the students in mobile BP healthcare. This is a good learning and teaching program for mobile BP healthcare solutions for smart aging, and it is a beneficial contribution to the mobile BP healthcare industry of smart aging.

Acknowledgements

The author acknowledges the support of the Union Teaching of the Ministry of Education for Smart Aging, the Union Teaching of the Ministry of Education for Medical Electronics in Taiwan, and the valuable comments of the reviewers.

Author details

Chin-Feng Lin[1]*, Shere-Er Wang[2], Yen-Chiao Lu[3], Chung-I Lin[4], Chung-Cheng Chang[1], Tim Yeh[5], Candice Lee[5], Jeffson Huang[5], Chic-Erh Weng[6], Sue-Hsien Chen[6], Bing-Leung Sun[7], Chao-Sheng Wang[1], Shiue-Li Cheng[1], Shiou-Yu Li[1] and Lan-Yu Wu[1]

*Address all correspondence to: lcf1024@mail.ntou.edu.tw

1 Department of Electrical Engineering, National Taiwan Ocean University, Keelung, Taiwan

2 Department of Nursing, Ching Kuo Institute of Management and Health, Keelung, Taiwan

3 Department of Nursing, Chung Shan Medical University, Taichung, Taiwan

4 Health Center of Gongliao, New Taipei City, Taiwan

5 Microlife, Taipei, Taiwan

6 Department of Nursing Division, Chang Cung Memorial Hospital, Keelung Branch, Keelung, Taiwan

7 Department of Applied Information and Multimedia, Ching Kuo Institute of Management and Health, Keelung, Taiwan

References

[1] Ducut E, Fontelo AP. Mobile devices in health education: current use and practice. J Comput High Educ. 2008; 20:59–68. DOI:10.1007/s12528-008-9003-2

[2] Juanes JA, Ruisoto P. Computer applications in health science education. J Med Syst. 2015; 39:97. DOI:10.1007/s10916-015-0283-6

[3] Mazzola M, Arslan P, Cândea G, et al. Integrated architecture for next-generation m-Health services (education, monitoring and prevention) in teenagers. In: Duffy VG, editor. Digital human modeling. Applications in health, safety, ergonomics and risk management . Springer; Germany. 2014, p. 403–414.

[4] Azevedo AP, Sousa HM, Monteiro JF, et al. Future perspectives of smartphone applications for rheumatic diseases self-management. Rheumatol Int. 2015; 35:419–431. DOI:10.1007/s00296-014-3117-9

[5] Martinez-Perez B, Torre-Diez I, Lopez-Coronado M. Mobile health applications for the most prevalent conditions by the world health organization: review and analysis. J Med Internet Res. 2013; 15(6):e120. DOI:10.2196/jmir.2600

[6] Zhang MWB, Tsang T, Cheow E, et al. Enabling Psychiatrists to be mobile phone app developers: insights into app development methodologies. JMIR mHealth uHealth. 2014; 2(4):e53. DOI:10.2196/mhealth.3425

[7] Burke LE, Ma J, Azar KMJ, et al. Current science on consumer use of mobile health for cardiovascular disease prevention a scientific statement from the American Heart Association. Circulation. 2015; 132:1157–1213. DOI:10.1161/CIR.0000000000000232

[8] Brennan PF. Telehealth: bringing health care to the point of living. Med Care. 1999; 37:115–116.

[9] Chan LK, Bridges S, Doherty I, et al. How do health sciences students use their mobile devices in problem-based learning? In: Bridges S, et al., editors. Educational technologies in medical and health sciences education, advances in medical education 5, ch 6. Springer; 2016, p. 99–116. DOI:10.1007/978-3-319-08275-2_6

[10] Kamin CS, O'Sullivan PS, Deterding R, et al. A comparison of critical thinking in groups of third year medical students in text, video and virtual PBL case modalities. Acad Med. 2003; 78:204–211.

[11] Elliott K, Judd T, McColl G, et al. Utilising mobile electronic health records in clinical education, In: Bridges S, et al., editors. Educational technologies in medical and health sciences education, advances in medical education 5, ch 9. Springer; 2016, p. 159–179. DOI: 10.1007/978-3-319-08275-2_9

[12] Davies BS, Rafique J, Vincent TR, et al. Mobile medical education (MoMEd) – how mobile information resources contribute to learning for undergraduate clinical

students – a mixed methods study. BMC Med Educ. 2012; 12:1. DOI: 10.1186/1472-6920-12-1

[13] Park HS, Cho1 H, Kim HS. Development of a multi-agent m-health application based on various protocols for chronic disease self-management. J Med Syst. 2016; 40:36. DOI: 10.1007/s10916-015-0401-5

[14] Wu SM, Lin CF, Liu CC, et al. Cellular and iridium network based blood pressure measurement scheme for mobile healthcare education. In: Clary TS, editors. Horizons in computer science research. 13. Nova Science Publishers. USA.

[15] Lin CF. Mobile telemedicine: a survey study. J Med Syst. 2012; 36(2):511–520. DOI: 10.1007/s10916-010-9496-x

[16] Lin CF. An advance wireless multimedia communication application: mobile teleme-dicine. WSEAS Trans Commun. 2012; 9(3):206–215.

[17] Lin CF, Hung SI, Chiang IH. An 802.11n WLAN transmission scheme for wireless telemedicine applications. Proc Inst Mech Eng H. 2010; 224(10):1201–1208. DOI: 10.1177/0954411911434246

[18] Lin CF, Li CY. A DS UWB transmission system for wireless telemedicine. WSEAS Trans Syst. 2008; 7(7):578–588.

[19] Lin CF, Chang WT, Lee HW, et al. Downlink power control in multi-code CDMA mobile medicine system. Med Biol Eng Comput. 2006; 44:437–444. DOI:10.1007/s11517-009-0458-8

[20] Lin CF, Chang KT. A power assignment mechanism in Ka band OFDM-based multi-satellites mobile telemedicine. J Med Biol Eng. 2008; 28(1):17–22.

[21] Lin CF, Chen JY, Shiu RH, et al. A Ka band WCDMA-based LEO transport architecture in mobile telemedicine, In: Martinez L, Gomez C, editors. Telemedicine in the 21st century. Nova Science Publishers; USA. 2008, p. 187–201.

[22] Lu YC. Nursing and technology video material, 2014.

[23] Lu YC. Healthy aging video material, 2014.

[24] Lin CI. BP health care for smart aging video material, 2013.

[25] Lu YC. Telenursing video material, 2012.

[26] Wang SE. BP care for smart aging, 2014.

[27] Wang SE. Community/home telecare digital material, 2014.

[28] Lin CF. MICT digital material, 2014.

[29] WatchBP, Cloud-based Blood Pressure Healthcare System, Available from: https://cloud.watchbp.com.tw/

[30] CMATE, Cloud-based ECG Healthcare System, Available from: http://www.ecg.com.tw/ecg/

[31] SKYPE, Video Conference Software, Available from: http://www.skype.com/zh-Hant/home/

[32] Messenger Plus, Video Conference Record Software, Available from: http://www.msgplus.net/

7

Use of Artificial Intelligence in Healthcare Delivery

Sandeep Reddy

Abstract

In recent years, there has been an amplified focus on the use of artificial intelligence (AI) in various domains to resolve complex issues. Likewise, the adoption of artificial intelligence (AI) in healthcare is growing while radically changing the face of healthcare delivery. AI is being employed in a myriad of settings including hospitals, clinical laboratories, and research facilities. AI approaches employing machines to sense and comprehend data like humans has opened up previously unavailable or unrecognised opportunities for clinical practitioners and health service organisations. Some examples include utilising AI approaches to analyse unstructured data such as photos, videos, physician notes to enable clinical decision making; use of intelligence interfaces to enhance patient engagement and compliance with treatment; and predictive modelling to manage patient flow and hospital capacity/resource allocation. Yet, there is an incomplete understanding of AI and even confusion as to what it is? Also, it is not completely clear what the implications are in using AI generally and in particular for clinicians? This chapter aims to cover these topics and also introduce the reader to the concept of AI, the theories behind AI programming and the various applications of AI in the medical domain.

Keywords: artificial intelligence, healthcare delivery, medicine, machine learning, deep learning, intelligent agent and neural networks

1. Introduction

There has been an immense amount of discussion in recent years about the advent of artificial intelligence (AI) and the implication of its application in various domains. However, the concept of AI is not new and can be traced back to Ramon Llull's theory of a reasoning machine in 1300 CE and even Aristotle's syllogisms in 300 BC [1, 2]. However, it is only since the 1950s, clearer definitions and practical applications have been formulated [3, 4]. While there was a lull in the development of AI in the 70s and 80s because of loss of interest and funding, there has been in the most recent period a dramatic revival in the research and development of AI programs. Countries like China have prioritised AI development by investing billions of dollars into AI industrial hubs [5]. Other nations and global corporations have also invested into AI programming and creation of innovative AI applications [6–8]. Building on this trend, institutions are now increasingly paying attention to application of AI in healthcare. AI is being used to improve the efficiency in delivery of healthcare and address previously intractable health problems [1, 9, 10]. The hundreds of AI-based healthcare applications being introduced into the market in recent years is a testimonial to this focus. Commentators have discussed how application of AI in healthcare is at the early stages and there is yet more to come [1, 4, 6]. However, is AI just hype and are entities investing into a bubble? To get an answer, we first need to understand what AI is and its approaches and tools. This chapter covers these issues and how they specifically apply to healthcare and what is next for the use of AI in healthcare?

2. Development and application of AI

2.1. Definition

So, what is AI? Because of the complexity involved in developing synthetic intelligence that is comparable to human intelligence, there are varying interpretations of what AI is and what goes into developing AI. Some authors even frown upon the term 'AI' and prefer the term 'Computational Intelligence' [11]. However, if we consider what is the objective of AI and what resources go into achieving the objective, an acceptable definition encompassing these components can be fashioned. The end objective of AI is to create systems that think and act rationally like humans [2, 4, 12]. These systems can also be termed as 'intelligent agents' [2, 4]. If the goal of the system is to demonstrate intelligence and developing these systems requires computer programming, a formal definition of AI would read as *'a field of science concerned with the computational understanding of what is commonly called intelligent behaviour, and with the creation of intelligent agents that exhibit such behaviour'* [13]. Simpler definitions describe AI as 'machines assuming human like capabilities', 'extension of human intelligence through computers' and 'making computers do things which currently humans do' but a more accurate description would be 'the science of making intelligent machines' [1, 2, 4, 14].

2.2. Intelligent agent

AI theory can be best understood through the *intelligent agent* concept [11]. An intelligent agent incorporates the skills required to pass the Turing Test, which assesses whether a machine can think like a human? [2, 3]. So an intelligent agent should be skilled in perception, practical reasoning and have an ability to take action to achieve its goals. The agent utilises the environment, it operates within, to both receive input and take action (**Figure 1**). Some key inputs that feed into an agent and potentially, which it can draw itself are current observations about the environment, prior knowledge about the environment, past experiences

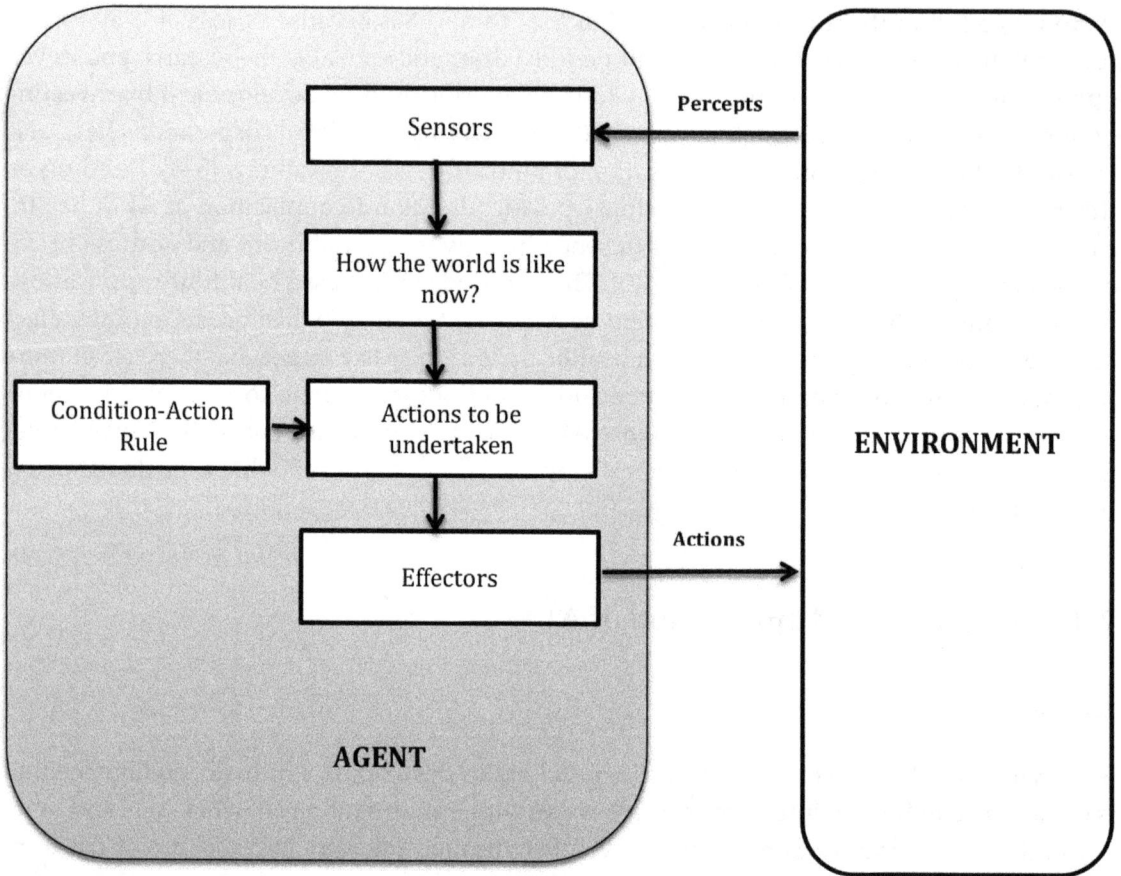

Figure 1. Concept of an intelligent agent.

that it can learn from and the objectives it needs to achieve. The agent perceives the environment through sensors and acts on the environment through effectors. When an intelligent agent is comprised of a computational core with physical actuators and sensors, it is termed a 'robot' [11]. When an agent is a program acting in a pure computational environment, it is an 'infobot' and when an advice providing program is coupled with a human expert, it is a 'decision support system'.

2.3. What makes up AI?

In the past, researchers aimed for AI to replicate human intelligence [2]. This approach is called 'Classical AI'. However, this was a limiting approach as it assumed human intelligence is the only form of intelligence. This approach also assumes human intelligence is the most intelligence can be. Intelligence mainly comprises of learning and reasoning [3, 13]. Constructing intelligence does not have to be defined by the limitations human intelligence poses. An apt analogy to discuss here is flight. While bird flight may be a source of inspiration for constructing aeroplanes, the aeroplane structure is not replicating the anatomic structure of a bird. So in constructing AI, it is more important to incorporate the vital characteristics of intelligence than merely replicate human intelligence.

Learning is an essential characteristic of intelligence [2, 4, 11]. Learning involves acquiring new knowledge, developing new skills through instruction or practise and knowledge representation and experimentation. If AI comprises learning, it has to demonstrate all the aforementioned features. A very common process through which AI systems achieve learning objectives is by *Machine Learning*. Machine learning is the modelling of different aspects of the learning process by computers [15]. Key goals of machine learning are for algorithms[1] to self-learn and improve through experience. The algorithms for machine learning typically fall into two categories: supervised and unsupervised categories [16]. Supervised learning involves an algorithm working with labelled training data. Categorisation of data and programming of the relationship between input and output data occurs in supervised learning. On the other hand, unsupervised learning allows the algorithm to identify a hidden pattern in a stack of data. Here the algorithm is run to check what patterns can be identified in the data and what outcomes may occur?

Reasoning and knowledge representation are the other aspects of AI [11]. In AI, reasoning involves manipulation of data to produce actions. Unlike traditional programming, the emphasis in AI is on what is to be computed rather than how it is to be computed? Structuring of this computation happens through design-time reasoning, offline computation and online computation. Earlier forms of AI involved algorithms based on the step-by-step reasoning model used to address predicated problems [2]. However, these models were not useful for uncertain situations or when there was incomplete information. AI reasoning models have now evolved to respond to these situations by drawing upon concepts from probability and economic theories. To resolve problems-certain or uncertain, AI systems require widespread knowledge about the relevant environment and then be able to represent this knowledge in a computable form [11]. For this to occur, AI uses a *Representation and Reasoning System* (RRS). An RRS is comprised of a programming language to communicate with a computer, a method to allocate meaning to the language and after input a process to figure out the answers. Knowledge is represented in different forms, but the most widely used method is Frames [2]. Frames are files in the computer where information is stored in slots. To enable AI knowledge representation and reasoning, programming languages and computational resources are two important properties. Different programming languages are used in AI, but the most popular are low-level programming languages such as Lisp, Python, C++ and Fortran. In the past, stand-alone computers and their limited processing power had restricted the advancement of AI. In recent years, AI reasoning and knowledge representation has immensely benefited from the rapid technological advances in computing power and wireless technology. These advances have helped in the deployment of sophisticated algorithms designed to resolve problems that could not have been addressed by AI applications in the past.

2.4. AI tools

AI systems employ several tools to automate problem-solving tasks. These tools are based on AI principles, some of which were discussed in the previous sections. The tools are used to

---

[1]In computer science, an algorithm is an explicit description of how to solve a class of problems? [2–4].

create AI applications to resolves issues across various disciplines and industries. Some commonly utilised tools are discussed in this section.

Search in AI system mirrors real-life problem solving but draws upon computing power to resolve the problems [17]. Search problems are classified based on the amount of information that is available to the search process. This information may relate to the whole of the problem area or a specific component of the problem. AI through an independent search planning process analyses multiple options and identifies an optimal solution. AI adopts a faster and better process to search and optimisation than conventional techniques [17, 18]. The search process that separates AI from conventional techniques is its process remembers past results, learns and refines its performance in relation to past searches, plans its path forward and answers search queries akin to human intelligence. One such example of AI search and optimisation tool is *Evolutionary Computation*. Evolutionary Computation is the umbrella term for algorithms based on natural evolutionary processes that incorporate mechanisms of natural selection and survival of the fittest principle [1, 10]. Foremost of the evolutionary computation algorithms are the *Genetic Algorithms*. Genetic Algorithms are a category of stochastic search and optimisation algorithms based on Darwin's natural biological evolution. These algorithms use a population-based search process to create random solutions for the problem at hand. These solutions are termed chromosomes. The chromosomes are comprised of random values derived from various control values. The variations in the values are utilised for the search process. The population of chromosomes is then assessed for an objective function. This population of solutions then evolves from one generation to another to arrive at an acceptable solution. The ideal solutions are retained and the mediocre ones disposed of. Through a process of repetition, improvements and generation of new solutions would occur.

In their quest to replicate biological intelligence, AI researchers inspired by the biological nervous system have developed *Artificial Neural Networks (ANNs)* [1, 19]. Artificial Neural Networks attempt to simulate nerve cell (neurons) networks of the brain. This approach of copying biological neuronal networks to function independently differs from conventional computing process that primarily seeks to support human brain computation. A very simple base algorithm structure (see **Figure 2**) lies behind the artificial neural networks but it can be adapted to a range of problems. The artificial neurons, which are computer processors, are interconnected with each other and are capable of performing parallel computations for data processing and knowledge representation [19]. These neural networks are capable of learning from historical examples, examining non-linear data, and managing imprecise information. ANNs are categorised into two main categories: *Feedforward Neural Networks* and *Recurrent Neural Networks*. In feedforward network the signal passes in only one direction and in recurrent neural networks, feedback and short-term memories of previous inputs are enabled. In both categories, application of deep learning, which is a class of machine learning that uses a cascade of multiple layers of non-linear processing units, enhances the problem-solving capabilities of the neural networks. So we have deep feedforward and deep recurrent neural networks increasingly being used to resolve real-world problems through language modelling, analysis of unstructured data and strategy formulation.

Hidden

Input

Output

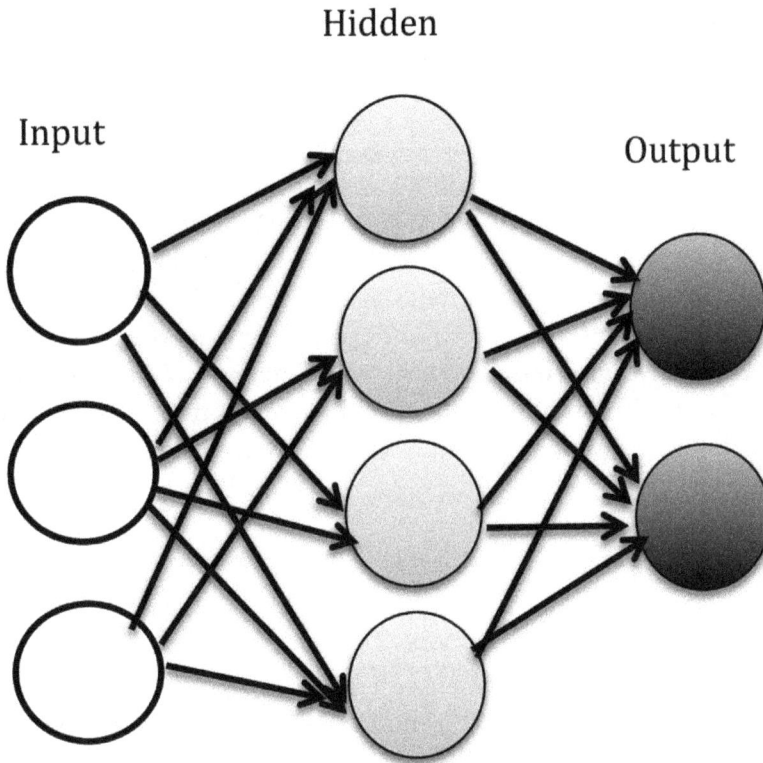

Figure 2. Schematic representation of an artificial neural network.

Logic is important to reasoning, which in turn is a key component of intelligence. Classical logic is based on the assumption that only two truth-values (false and true) exist [2]. This assumption is called *bivalence*. On the other hand, *Fuzzy Logic* reflects real world phenomenon, where everything is a matter of degree [1, 2, 10]. A fuzzy logic can be viewed as a fuzzy extension of a multi-valued logic i.e. instead of recognising everything is black and white, it recognises there are shades of grey. Fuzzy logic uses continuous set membership from 0 to 1 in opposition to Boolean logic, which relies on sharp distinctions such as 0 for false and 1 for true. Fuzzy applications utilise a structure of series of 'if-then' rules for modelling. This approach by fuzzy logic permits ambiguity and can be used in AI systems for indeterminate reasoning.

Another important AI technique is *Natural Language Processing*. Natural language processing (NLP) is concerned with the use of software programming to understand and manipulate natural language text or speech for practical purposes [20]. With NLP, the process of language analysis is decomposed into various stages mirroring theoretical linguistic distinctions as outlined by syntax, semantics and pragmatics [4, 20]. NLP enables machines to read and understand human language. NLP can also be utilised to gather and analyse unstructured data such as free text. In recent years, progress in NLP specifically in the field of syntax has led to development of effective grammar characterisation and chart parsing. Development of numerous conceptual tools has led to formation of systems and interface subsystems to use for experiments. Part-of-speech identification and word sense disambiguation have become standard processes in NLP. Other current applications of NLP include information retrieval, machine translation and text mining.

Use of *Hybrid Artificial Intelligent Systems* (HAIS), which are a combination of AI techniques, is becoming popular because of its capabilities to address real world complex problems that individual AI techniques cannot address [21]. By combining different AI learning and adaptation techniques, HAIS overcomes the limitations associated with a particular technique. HAIS may involve a combination of agents and multi-agent systems, fuzzy systems, artificial neural networks, optimisation models and so forth. By combining symbolic and sub-symbolic techniques, complex issues involving indistinctness, ambiguity and vagueness can be resolved by HAIS. The synergy in HAIS also allows it to adjust to common sense, mine knowledge from raw data, use human like reasoning, and learn to adapt to a changing environment.

3. AI in healthcare

AI lends itself to healthcare delivery very well. In fact, in the recent years there has been an exponential increase in the use of AI in clinical environments [1, 6, 21–24]. With modern Medicine facing a significant challenge of acquiring, analysing and applying structured and unstructured data to treat or manage diseases, AI systems with their data-mining and pattern recognition capabilities come in handy. Medical AI is mainly concerned with the development of AI programs that help with the prediction, diagnosis and treatment or management of diseases. In contrast to non-AI medical software application, which relies on pure statistical analysis and probabilistic approaches, medical AI applications utilise symbolic models of diseases and analyse their relationship to patient signs and symptoms [1, 25–27]. For example, diagnostic AI applications gather and synthesise clinical data and compare information with predefined categories such as diseases to help with diagnosis and treatment. Medical AI applications have not just been used to support diagnosis but also treatment protocol development, drug development and patient monitoring too [1].

3.1. History of use of AI in healthcare

Discussion of the use of AI in medicine coincides with the advent AI in the modern era. This is not surprising as AI systems initially intend to replicate the functioning of the human brain [2]. In 1970, William B Schwartz, a physician interested in the use of computing science in medicine, published an influential paper in the *New England Journal of Medicine* titled '*Medicine and the computer: the promise and problems of change*' [28]. In the paper he argued '*Computing science will probably exert its major effects by augmenting and, in some cases, largely replacing the intellectual functions of the physician*'. By the 1970s there was a realisation that conventional computing techniques were unsuitable for solving complex medical phenomenon [2, 4]. A more sophisticated computational model that simulated human cognitive processes, that is AI models, was required for clinical problem solving. Early efforts to apply AI in medicine consisted of setting up rules-based systems to help with medical reasoning. However, serious

clinical problems are too complex to lend them to simple rules-based problem solving techniques. Problem solving in medicine then progressed to construction of computer programs based on models of diseases. It was not just with the field of general medicine, that AI was being explored to assist with problem solving. In 1976, the Scottish surgeon Gunn used computational analysis to diagnose acute abdominal pain [1]. This was achieved through clinical audits of structured case notes through computers, whereby diagnosis through this route proved to be about 10% more accurate than the conventional route. By the 1980s, AI research communities were well established across the world but especially in learning centres in the US [1, 2, 4, 13]. This development helped in expansion of the use of novel and innovative AI approaches to medical diagnoses. Much of this push was because medicine was an ideal testing ground for these AI applications. A significant number of AI applications in medicine at this stage were based on the *expert system* methodology [1, 25, 29–31]. By the end of the 1990s, research in medical AI had started to use new techniques like machine learning and artificial neural networks to aid clinical decision-making. The next section explores current application of AI in various aspects of healthcare.

3.2. Application of AI techniques in healthcare

The wide acceptance of AI in healthcare relates to the complexities of modern medicine, which involves acquisition and analysis of the copious amount of information and the limitation of clinicians to address these needs with just human intelligence. Medical AI applications with their advanced computing ability are overcoming this limitation and are using several techniques to assist clinicians in medical care.

AI is being used for all the three classical medical tasks: diagnosis, prognosis and therapy but mostly in the area of medical diagnosis [9, 32]. Generally, the medical diagnosis cycle (**Figure 3**) involves observation and examination of the patient, collection of patient data, interpretation of the data using the clinician's knowledge and experience and then formulation of a diagnosis and a therapeutic plan by the physician. If we can compare the medical diagnostic cycle (**Figure 3**) to the concept of an intelligent agent system, the physician is the intelligent agent, the patient data is the input and the diagnosis is the output. There are several methods, through which AI systems can replicate this diagnostic cycle and assist clinicians with medical diagnosis. One such approach is the use of *Expert Systems*. Expert systems are based on rules clearly outlining the steps involved in progressing from inputs to outputs [2]. The progression occurs through the construction of a number of IF-THEN type rules. These rules are constructed with the help of subject experts like clinicians who have interest and experience in the particular domain. The success of the expert system relies on the explicit representation of the knowledge area in the form of rules. The core of the expert system is the inference engine, which transforms the inputs into actionable outputs.

Commonly, the application of the expert system approach in medical software programming is seen in *Clinical Decision Support Systems* (CDSS). Simply put, CDSS are software programs that enable clinicians to make clinician decisions [33, 34]. CDSS provides customised assessment or advice based on analysis of patient data sets. An early version of CDSS was the MYCIN program developed in the 1970s. MYCIN was a CDSS focusing on the management

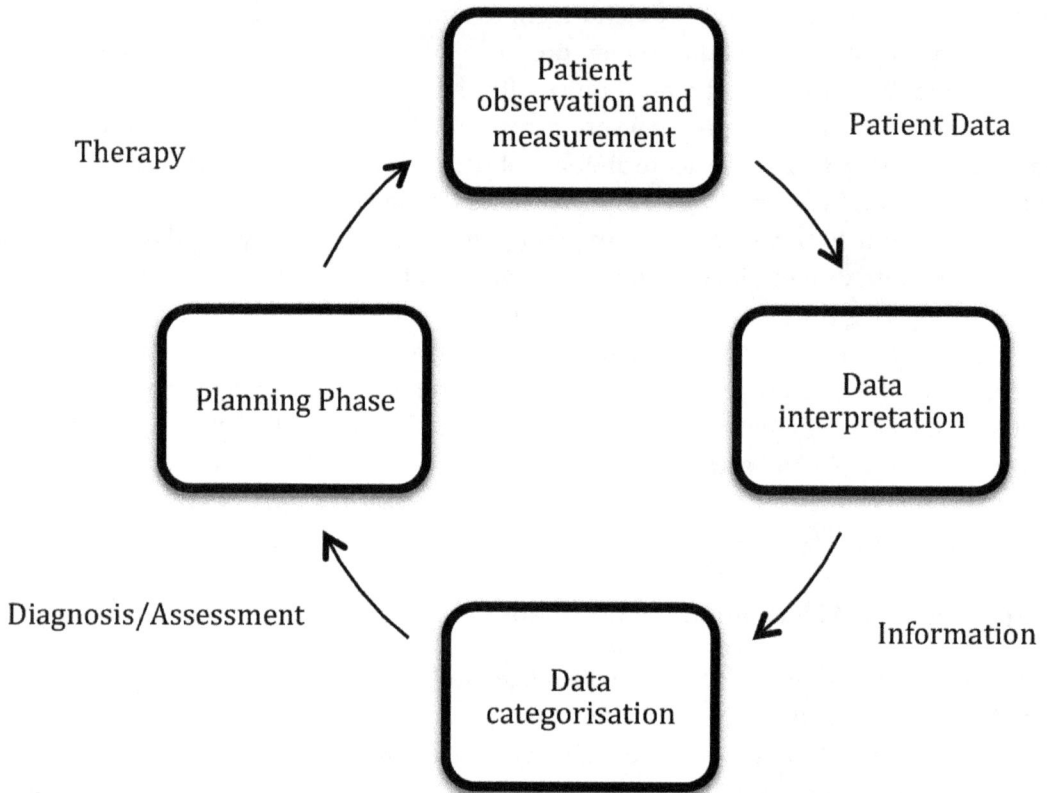

Figure 3. Medical diagnostic-therapeutic cycle.

of infectious disease patients. Infectious disease knowledge was represented in the form of production rules, which are conditional statements as to how observations can be inferred appropriately. However, MYCIN had less emphasis on diagnosis and more on the management of patients with infectious diseases. In a later evaluation of the MYCIN system, it was found it compared favourably with the advice provided by infectious disease experts. MYCIN paved the way for the development of knowledge-based systems and the commercialisation of rule-base approaches in medicine and other fields. Another CDSS that was initially developed around the same time period as MYCIN but continues to be used is the QMR system [35]. The QMR system utilises a customised algorithm modelled on the clinical reasoning of one single University of Pittsburgh internist. Hence the system was initially called INTERNIST-I. By considering historical and physical findings, QMR system generates the differential diagnosis. Utilising a large database that categorises disease findings into 'evoking strengths', 'importance' and 'frequencies' domains, the system generates the differential diagnosis. Heuristic rules drove the system to produce a list of ranked diagnoses founded on disease knowledge domains in-built into the system. Where the system was unable to make a determined diagnosis it probed the user with further questions or provided advice about further tests until a determination of the condition was made. While MYCIN and QMR systems offered diagnostic support, other forms of CDSS can provide alerts and reminders and advice about patient treatment and management. These systems operate by creating predictive models and multi-dimensional patient view through aggregation of data from multiple sources including knowledge and patient information databases. As treatment and management of diseases have evolved, CDSS architecture is now utilising multi-agent systems [26]. Each of the multiple agents performs distinct tasks and operations in various capacities or different locations but transmit data to a central repository so aggregated data can be used for knowledge discovery.

Unlike experts systems where a serial or sequential data processing approach is utilised, ANN processing utilises a parallel form of data processing analogous to the brain [19]. In ANNs, the processing elements, otherwise called as neurons, process data simultaneously while communicating with each other. The processing elements are arranged in layers and the layers, in turn, are connected to each other. The links between the processing elements are associated with a numerical weight. The memory and adaptation of ANNs are adjusted by changing the weights, which leads to the amplification of the effects of afferent connection to each processing element. As a result of this architecture, ANNs can be trained to learn from experience, analyse non-linear data and manage inexact information. These abilities have led to ANN techniques being one of the most popularly utilised AI techniques in medicine [1]. ANNs in addition to medical diagnosis have been used for radiology and histopathology analysis. In radiology, gamma camera, CT, ultrasound and MRI all create digital images, which can be manipulated by ANNs and used as inputs. The digitised inputs are then transmitted through the hidden and output layers to produce desired outputs (see **Figure 2**). Using the Backpropagation approach, a learning algorithm, ANNs have successfully identified orthopaedic trauma from radiographs [36]. When ANNs and radiologists interpret the same radiological images separately, research has identified good diagnostic agreement [1, 36]. ANNs have also been used for analysis of cytological and histological specimens too [1, 25]. For example, ANNs has been used to screen abnormal cells from slide images for haematology and cervical cytology. Further, ANNs have also been used to interpret ECGs and EEGs through waveform analysis. For this to occur, a multi-layered neural network is trained with waveform data from both people with the disease and without [1]. Evaluation of the waveform interpretations by ANNs has identified excellent pattern approximation and classification abilities and comparable in interpretation to clinicians.

Data Mining acts as the foundation for machine learning. Data mining is the process for identifying previously unknown patterns and trends in large databases and then utilising the same to create predictive models [37, 38]. Data mining involves multiple iterative steps (**Figure 4**) that includes retrieval of data sets from data warehouses or operational databases, cleaning of data to remove discrepancies, analysis of data sets to identify patterns that represent relationships amongst the data, validation of the patterns with new data sets and culminating in knowledge extraction [39]. Use of data mining has become hugely popular in healthcare largely because of the generation of data too voluminous and complex to be processed by conventional computational techniques. The potential application of data mining in healthcare can be huge but practically data mining has been used in evaluating the effectiveness of medical treatments, analyse epidemiological data to identify disease outbreaks and act as an early warning system, analyse hospital records to identify acute medical conditions and help with interventions, quality assessment of medical interventions and predicting survival

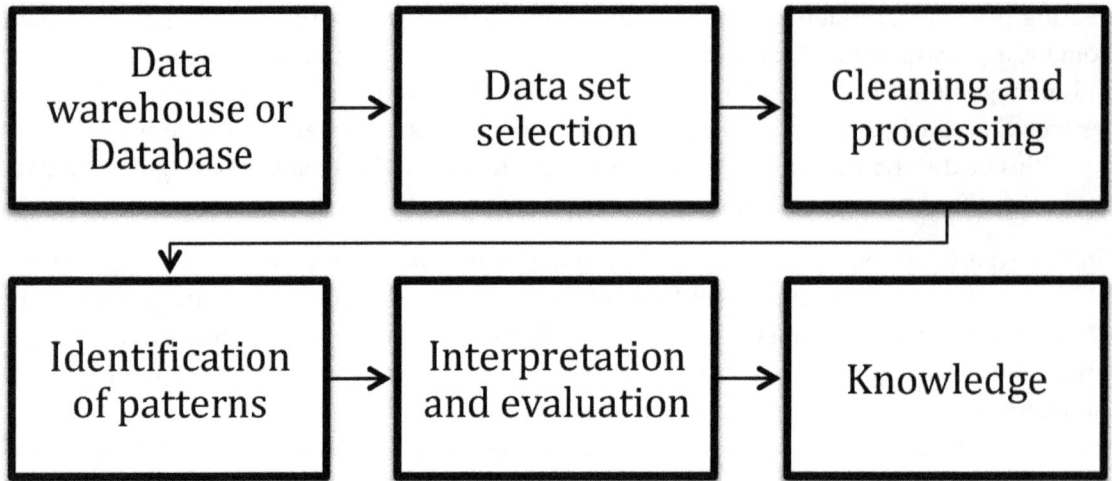

Figure 4. Data mining process. Adapted from Huang et al. [39].

time for chronic disease and cancer patients [8, 38–40]. Data mining medical data faces two main issues: heterogeneity of data sometimes with incomplete recording or filing of data and complexity of the requested outputs [27]. Fuzzy logic, which we discussed in an earlier section, with its proficiency to represent assorted data, strength in adapting to change in the user environment and its distinctive expressiveness can support data mining in addressing these issues. Thus data mining utilising fuzzy logic has been used for a range of situations in healthcare including prediction of the prognosis of cancer and assessing the satisfaction of clinicians for patient information management systems.

There are an estimated 5 billion mobile phone subscriptions in the world [41]. Many mobile phones now have memories and processing power equivalent to the capacity of mini-computers [42]. So it is natural to see mobile communication devices being harnessed to deliver healthcare. The use of wireless communication devices to support delivery of healthcare is called *Mobile Health* or in a popular terminology: *mHealth* [41]. Mobile health applications are being used in many areas of healthcare delivery including education and awareness, point-of-care support and diagnostics, patient monitoring, disease surveillance, emergency medical response and patient information management [41, 43–46]. The rapid development in mHealth has coincided with the increase in AI research and development of AI techniques. Consequently, there has been an increased application of AI techniques in mHealth. The move has worked well as characteristics of an intelligent agent system lend themselves to the objectives of mHealth. The intelligent agent perceives the environment and autonomously acts upon it. In case of multi-agent systems, the agents can communicate between themselves, dynamically manage data and resource and handle the complexity of solutions through decomposition, modelling and reorganisation of relationships. These abilities mean agent-based mobile applications can be used for remote monitoring of patients especially elderly and chronic disease patients, support clinical decision-making and provide remote training for health workers. The application of AI has not been restricted to mobile communication devices but has been extended to other smart devices. When these smart devices are connected to each other to create a cyber-physical smart pervasive network, it is termed as the *Internet of Things* (IoT) [47, 48]. IoT is being used across for many purposes including prediction of natural disasters, water scarcity monitoring and intelligent transport systems but in health care, the concept is being used to design smart homes to assist senior citizens to accomplish their daily living activities while preserving their privacy and to remotely monitor their health conditions and medicine intake [48]. An IoT powered by AI and set up to address the healthcare need of senior and incapacitated patients is called as *Ambient Assisted Living* (AAL) [49]. As the main aim of AAL is to extend the independent living of elderly individuals in their homes, automation, security, control and communication are key aspects of AAL modular architecture. The system also includes sensors, actuators and cameras to collect different types of data about the individual and home. The constituent system sets up a smart home environment where activities and the health condition of the resident are not only tracked but also predicted [50].

In addition to the examples discussed above, AI techniques have been successfully used in other areas of medicine. Genetic algorithm techniques have been used to predict outcomes in acutely ill and cancer patients, to analyse mammograms and MRI images and fuzzy logic techniques have been used in diagnosing various cancers, characterise ultrasound and CT scan images and predict survival in cancer patients and administer medication and anaesthetics [1, 6].

Of all the AI applications that have been developed over the past many decades, IBM's Watson is one of the well-recognised applications. IBM Watson is a cognitive computing technology that groups together the competencies of reading, reasoning and learning to reply to questions or investigate original connections [40]. IBM Watson aggregates huge volumes of structured and unstructured data from multiple sources into a single repository called Watson corpus. IBM incorporates machine learning and NLP techniques to process and analyse data to undertake problem solving. The technology of IBM Watson has been extended to the medical domain to assist medical scientists and clinicians in improving patient care [31, 51–53]. Some of the published examples of the use of IBM Watson in health care include automated problem list generation from electronic medical records, drug target identification and drug repurposing, interpretation of genetic testing results, oncological decision making support, and to support the roll-out of government healthcare programs.

3.3. Future trends and application of AI in healthcare

As more AI research is undertaken and AI systems become more trained and consequently intelligent, it is foreseeable that these agents replace some of, if not all, the human elements of clinical care [6]. While leaving the communication of serious matters and final decision making to human clinicians, AI systems can take responsibility for routine and less risky diagnostic and treatment processes. The intention here is not to replace human clinicians but enable a streamlined high-quality healthcare delivery process.

Of all the promising medical AI novelties that are being explored, robotics driven by AI will have an important role in the medical automation process. Robots embody AI and give it a form, while AI algorithms/programming provide intelligence to the robots [2]. Robotic assistants have already been employed to conduct surgeries, deliver medication and monitor hospital patients but the most promising area for their use is in elderly care [31]. Mobile robotic assistants are already being used to assist the elderly people in their day-to-day activities either in their home or in aged care settings [51]. The robotic assistants mainly undertake tasks that remind them of their routine activities including medication intake or guidance in their environments. With advances in AI and robotics, the employment of robotic assistants in elderly care is only bound to grow.

While the conventional thinking is that robots act as a vessel for a silicon-based artificial brain, there is emergence of a school of thought that imagines the use of biological brains in robots [2]. With advances in science now allowing the culture of biological neurons, the potential use of a biological brain in a robotic frame through which it can sense the world and move around is not inconceivable. This *Cyborg* model presents a true blurring of the boundaries between human and artificial intelligence and the imaginable development of a hybrid human-artificial intelligence health worker that can revolutionise healthcare delivery.

3.4. Challenges

While the application of AI in delivery of healthcare has very promising potential, challenges-both technical and ethical exist. AI research is largely led and driven by computer scientists without medical training and it has been commented that this has led to a very technologically focused and problem oriented approach in the application of AI in healthcare delivery [24]. Contemporary healthcare delivery models are very dependent on human reasoning, patient-clinician communication and establishing professional relationships with patients to ensure compliance. These aspects are something AI cannot replace easily. Use of robotic assistants in healthcare has raised issues about the mechanisation of care in vulnerable situations where human interaction and intervention is probably more appealing [6]. There is also the reluctance of clinicians in adopting AI technologies that they envisage will eventually replace them. Yet there is no qualm in them using technologies that automate and speed up laboratory diagnostic process [1]. This has led to some suggesting a model of co-habitation [6]. This is a model that accommodates both the AI and human elements in healthcare delivery and anticipates the inevitable automatisation of significant components of medical processes while preserving the human aspects of clinical care like communication, procedures and decision-making.

4. Conclusion

Healthcare delivery has over years become complex and challenging. A large part of the complexity in delivering healthcare is because of the voluminous data that is generated in the process of healthcare, which has to be interpreted in an intelligent fashion. AI systems with their problem solving approach can address this need. Their intelligent architecture, which incorporates learning and reasoning and ability to act autonomously without requiring constant human attention, is alluring. Thus the medical domain has provided a fertile ground for AI researchers to test their techniques and in many instances; AI applications have successfully solved problems with outcomes comparable to that of human clinicians. As healthcare delivery becomes more expensive, stakeholders will increasingly look to solutions that can replace the expensive elements in patient care and AI solutions will be sought after in these situations. However, cold technology cannot totally replace the human elements in patient care and a model that incorporates both technological innovations and human care has to be investigated.

Notice

The chapter was submitted to a double blind review and it is in line with COPE Ethical Guidelines.

Author details

Sandeep Reddy

Address all correspondence to: sandeep.reddy@deakin.edu.au

School of Medicine, Faculty of Health, Deakin University, Australia

References

[1] Ramesh AN, Kambhampati C, Monson JRT, Drew PJ. Artificial intelligence in medicine. Annals of the Royal College of Surgeons of England. 2004;**86**(5):334-338

[2] Warwick K. Artificial Intelligence: The Basics. Abingdon: Routledge; 2012

[3] Simmons AB, Chappell SG. Artificial intelligence—Definition and practice. IEEE Journal of Oceanic Engineering. 1988;**13**(2):14-42

[4] Kok JN, Boers EJW, Kosters WA, Van Der Putten P, Poel M. Artificial Intelligence: Definition, Trends, Techniques, and Cases. Oxford, UK: Encyclopedia of Life Support Systems; 2013

[5] Cyranoski D. 'China enters the battle for AI talent'. Nature [Online]. 2018. Available from: https://www.nature.com/articles/d41586-018-00604-6 [Accessed: Jan 12, 2018]

[6] Diprose W, Buist N. Artificial intelligence in medicine: Humans need not apply? The New Zealand Medical Journal. 2016;**129**(1434):73-76

[7] Baker S. Final Jeopardy: The Story of Watson, the Computer That Will Transform Our World. New York: Houghton Mifflin Harcourt Publishing Company, Mariner Books; 2012

[8] Chen HCH, Zeng D. AI for global disease surveillance. IEEE Intelligent Systems. 2009;**24**(6):66-82

[9] Szolovitz P. Artificial intelligence in medical diagnosis. Annals of Internal Medicine. 1988;**108**(1):80

[10] Gambhir S, Malik SK, Kumar Y. Role of soft computing approaches in healthcare domain: A mini review. Journal of Medical Systems. 2016;**40**(12):2-20

[11] Poole DL, Mackworth A, Goebel RG. Computational intelligence and knowledge. In: Computational Intelligence: A Logical Approach. New York: Oxford University Press; no. Ci. 1998. pp. 1-22

[12] Poole DL, Mackworth AK. Artificial Intelligence: Foundations of Computational Agents. 2nd ed. Cambridge, UK: Cambridge University Press; 2017

[13] Shapiro SC. Encyclopedia of Artificial Intelligence. 2nd ed. New York: Wiley-Interscience; 1992

[14] Szolovits P, Stephen PG. Medicine Flowchart—How Can We Emulate Diagnosis? Categorical and Probabilistic Reasoning in Medical Diagnosis; Artificial Intelligence. 1978;**11**:115-144

[15] Bell J. Machine learning. In: Machine Learning: Hands-on for Developers and Technical Professionals. Indianapolis, USA: John Wiley & Sons; 2015

[16] Michalski RS, Carbonell JG, Mitchell TM. An overview of machine learning. In: Michalski RS, Carbonell JG, Mitchell TM, editors. Machine Learning: An Artificial Intelligence Approach. Palo Alto: Springer; 1983. p. 23

[17] Chandel A, Sood M. Searching and optimization techniques in artificial intelligence: A comparative study and complexity analysis. International Journal of Advanced Research in Computer Engineering & Technology. 2014;**3**(3):866-871

[18] Badar A, Umre BS, Junghare AS. Study of artificial intelligence optimization techniques applied to active power loss minimization. IOSR Journal of Electrical and Electronics Engineering. 2014;**2014**(1989):39-45

[19] Priddy KL, Keller PE. Artificial Neural Networks: An Introduction. Bellingham: SPIE Press; 2005

[20] Spyns P. Natural language processing in medicine: An overview. Methods of Information in Medicine. 1996;**35**(4-5):285-301

[21] Abraham A. Hybrid artificial intelligent systems. In: Corchado E, Corchado J, Abraham A, editors. Innovations in Hybrid Intelligent Systems—Advances in Soft Computing. Berlin: Springer Berlin Heidelberg; 2007

[22] Kim E-Y. Patient will see you now: The future of medicine is in your hands. Healthcare Informatics Research. 2015;**21**(4):321-323

[23] Mishra S, Takke A, Auti S, Suryavanshi S, Oza M. Role of artificial intelligence in health care. BioChemistry: An Indian Journal. 2017;**11**(5):1-14

[24] Coiera EW. Artificial intelligence in medicine: The challenges ahead. Journal of the American Medical Informatics Association. 1996;**3**(6):363-366

[25] Scott R. Artificial intelligence: its use in medical diagnosis. Journal of Nuclear Medicine. 1993;**34**(3):510-514

[26] Wimmer H, Yoon VY, Sugumaran V. A multi-agent system to support evidence based medicine and clinical decision making via data sharing and data privacy. Decision Support Systems. 2016;**88**:51-66

[27] Koh HC, Tan G. Data mining applications in healthcare. Journal of Healthcare Information Management. 2005;**19**(2):64-72

[28] Schwartz WB. Medicine and the computer: The promise and problems of change. The New England Journal of Medicine. 1970;**283**(23):1257-1264

[29] Sim I, Gorman P, Greenes RA, Haynes RB, Kaplan B, Lehmann H, Tang PC. Clinical decision support systems for the practice of evidence-based medicine. Journal of the American Medical Informatics Association. 2001;**8**(6):527-534

[30] Khanna S, Sattar A, Hansen D. Advances in artificial intelligence research in health. The Australasian Medical Journal. 2012;**5**(9):475-477

[31] Topol E. The Patient Will See You Now: The Future of Medicine Is in Your Hands. New York: Basic Books; 2015

[32] Farrugia A, Al-Jumeily D, Al-Jumaily M, Hussain A, Lamb D. Medical diagnosis: Are artificial intelligence systems able to diagnose the underlying causes of specific headaches? In: Proceedings of 2013 6th International Conference on Developments in eSystems Engineering (DeSE); 2013. pp. 376-382

[33] Littenberg B, MacLean C, Gagnon M. Clinical decision support system. US Pat. App. 11/640,103; 2006. pp. 1-10

[34] Pusic M, Ansermino JM. Clinical decision support systems. The British Columbia Medical Journal. 2004;**46**:236-239

[35] Miller RA, McNeil MA, Challinor SM, Masarie FE Jr, Myers JD. INTERNIST-1: An experimental computer-based diagnostic consultant for general internal medicine. The New England Journal of Medicine. 1982;**307**:468-476

[36] Olczak J, Fahlberg N, Maki A, Razavian AS, Jilert A, Stark A, Sköldenberg O, Gordon M. Artificial intelligence for analyzing orthopedic trauma radiographs: Deep learning algorithms—Are they on par with humans for diagnosing fractures? Acta Orthopaedica. 2017;**88**(6):581-586

[37] Milovic B, Milovic M. Prediction and decision making in health care using data mining. International Journal of Public Health Science. 2012;**1**(2):69-76

[38] Zhang Y, Guo SL, Han LN, Li TL. Application and exploration of big data mining in clinical medicine. Chinese Medical Journal. 2016;**129**(6):731-738

[39] Huang MJ, Chen MY, Lee SC. Integrating data mining with case-based reasoning for chronic diseases prognosis and diagnosis. Expert Systems with Applications. 2007;**32**(3):856-867

[40] Kelly JE III, Hamm S. Smart Machines: IBM's Watson and the Era of Cognitive Computing. New York: Columbia University Press; 2013

[41] Barton AJ. The regulation of mobile health applications. BMC Medicine. 2012;**10**:2-5

[42] Dagon D, Martin T, Starner T. Mobile phones as computing devices: The viruses are coming! IEEE Pervasive Computing. 2004;**3**(4):11-15

[43] Mohammadzadeh N, Safdari R. Patient monitoring in mobile health: Opportunities and challenges. Medieval Archaeology. 2014;**68**(1):57

[44] Alnosayan N, Lee E, Alluhaidan A, Chatterjee S, Houston-Feenstra L, Kagoda M, Dysinger W. MyHeart: An intelligent mhealth home monitoring system supporting heart failure self-care. In: 2014 IEEE 16th International Conference on e-Health Networking, Application & Services (HealthCom); 2015. pp. 311-316

[45] Minutolo A, Sannino G, Esposito M, De Pietro G. A rule-based mHealth system for cardiac monitoring. In: Proceedings of 2010 IEEE EMBS Conference on Biomedical Engineering and Sciences (IECBES); 2010. pp. 144-149

[46] Boulos MNK, Wheeler S, Tavares C, Jones R. How smartphones are changing the face of mobile and participatory healthcare: An overview, with example from eCAA-LYX. Biomedical Engineering Online. 2011;**10**:1-14

[47] Islam SMR, Kwak D, Kabir H, Hossain M, Kwak K-S. The Internet of things for health care: A comprehensive survey. IEEE Access. 2015;**3**:678-708

[48] Da Xu L, He W, Li S. Internet of things in industries: A survey. IEEE Transactions on Industrial Informatics. 2014;**10**(4):2233-2243

[49] Costa R, Carneiro D, Novais P, Lima L, Machado J, Marques A, Neves J. Ambient assisted living. Applied Soft Computing. 2008;**51**:86-94

[50] Amiribesheli M, Benmansour A, Bouchachia A. A review of smart homes in healthcare. Journal of Ambient Intelligence and Humanized Computing. 2015;**6**(4):495-517

[51] Pollack ME, Engberg S, Matthews JT, Dunbar-jacob J, Mccarthy CE, Thrun S. Pearl: A mobile robotic assistant for the elderly. Architecture. 2002;**2002**:85-91

[52] Chen Y, Argentinis E, Weber G. IBM Watson: How cognitive computing can be applied to big data challenges in life sciences research. Clinical Therapeutics. 2016;**38**(4):688-701

[53] Devarakonda M, Tsou C-H. Automated problem list generation from electronic medical records in IBM Watson. In: 29th AAAI Conference on Artificial Intelligence (AAAI) 2015 and the 27th Innovative Applications of Artificial Intelligence Conference, IAAI 2015; vol. 5; 2015. pp. 3942-3947

8

Empowering Diabetes Patient with Mobile Health Technologies

Matjaž Krošel, Lana Švegl, Luka Vidmar and
Dejan Dinevski

Abstract

Chronic diseases, especially diabetes mellitus, are huge public health burden. Therefore, new health care models for sharing the responsibility for care among health care
providers and patients themselves are needed. The concept of empowerment promotes patient's active involvement and control over their own health. It can be achieved
through education, self-management, and shared decision making. All these aspects can
be covered by mobile health technologies, the so-called mHealth. This term comprises
mobile phones, patient monitoring devices, tablets, personal digital assistants, other
wireless devices, and numerous apps. Many challenges of diabetics can be addressed
by mHealth, including glycemic control, nutrition control, physical activity, high blood
pressure, medication adherence, obesity, education, diabetic retinopathy screening,
diabetic foot screening, and psychosocial care. However, mHealth plays only minor role
in diabetes management, despite numerous apps on the market. Namely, these apps
have many shortcomings and the majority of them does not include important
functions. Moreover, these apps lack the perceived additional benefit by the user and
the ease of use, important factors for acceptance of mHealth. Studies of diabetes apps
regarding usability and accessibility have shown moderate results. Beside improvements of apps usability, the future of diabetes mHealth lies probably in personalized
education and self-management with the help of decision support systems. At the same
time, work on artificial pancreas is in progress and smartphone could be used as user
interface.

Keywords: mobile health, diabetes, empowerment, smartphone, chronic disease management

1. Introduction

Aging and chronic conditions represent a huge burden on the health care budgets. Moreover, in the future this burden will only increase [1]. At the same time, the patients require a better service, while there are fewer health care professionals and lesser resources. The states currently act mainly in two dimensions. On the one hand, they are strengthening their efforts on prevention. They develop or update existing programs, which promote healthy and active life styles. On the other hand, they are transforming the existing health care. Namely, the health care systems as we know them were developed to treat the acute diseases. However, the chronic diseases spent more than 70% of the health care budgets [2, 3]. The prevention programs can prolong the healthy period of each individual, but some chronic diseases, such as diabetes, cannot eliminate. Therefore, there is a need for transformation of the existing health care whose goals are better health results, better quality of service and quality of patient life, and economic feasibility. This transformation is as follows [2]:

- from the health care model centered on acute medical care to the model adopted to the needs of chronic patients,

- from reactive model to proactive model to cure, care for and prevent based on risk factors,

- from passive patients to a model with a patient in the center, actively managing his disease,

- from a fragmented model with lack of coordination to a model enabling continuity of care, and

- from activities primarily in acute hospitals to activities in more suitable environments, such as homes.

The key enablers for such transformation are patient empowerment, use of information and communications technology (ICT), integrated care, and adopted business models.

This chapter explores the concept of empowerment of diabetes patients by presenting current and future possibilities of mobile health technology.

2. Diabetes mellitus

Number of diabetes patients around the world has reached 415 million and it is predicted to climb up to 642 million by the year 2040. Diabetes can also be linked to around 5 million deaths each year and it is associated with high financial burden, since health spending on diabetes accounts for around 12% of total health expenditure worldwide. The costs include increase use of health services as well as loss of productivity or disability and are estimated to range from 673 billion USD to 1197 billion USD [4]. With such troubling predictions, we are obligated to look for new methods to facilitate patient care. Introduction of new methods should be done with the understanding that more than 95% of diabetes care is done by the patients themselves [5]. This is just one of several reasons why diabetes patients are excellent candidates for managing their disease with the help of mobile health technologies (mHealth) and why this may improve many aspects of personal and public health.

Diabetes is medically defined by the following criteria: patient fasting plasma glucose level ≥126 mg/dl (7.0 mmol/l) or HbA1c (glycated hemoglobin) ≥6.5% or patient plasma glucose level 2-h after OGTT (oral glucose tolerance test) ≥200 mg/dl (11.1 mmol/l) or patient random plasma glucose level ≥200 mg/dl (11.1 mmol/l) [6]. After the diagnosis, diabetes patients need to endure life-long management of their disease, which include medications and significant lifestyle changes. Disease progress should be monitored with the help of health care professionals in order to ensure prevention and quick diagnosis of long-term complications of hyperglycemia. Most commonly seen diabetes complications are retinopathy with a potential loss of vision, nephropathy that can result in renal failure, peripheral neuropathy leading to foot ulcers, Charcot foot and amputation, autonomic neuropathy that can causes gastrointestinal, genito-urinary, and cardiovascular symptoms. The patients with a chronically elevated glucose level have high incidence of atherosclerotic vascular changes, which cause development of peripheral arterial disease, cerebrovascular, and cardiovascular complications [6, 7]. Number of complications can be reduced, if patients maintain good glycemic control. Every patient who reduces HbA1c level for 1% decreases the risk of microvascular complication for 37% and the risk for diabetes related deaths for 21% [8].

3. Adherence to treatment

World Health Organization defines adherence as an extent to which a person's behavior: taking medication, following a diet, and/or executing lifestyle changes, corresponds with agreed recommendations from a health care provider [9]. One of the key challenges in diabetes management is a lack of adherence to medication regime and lack of lifestyle changes. Adherence to oral hypoglycemic agents is between 36 and 93% for the first 9–24 months of treatment and adherence to insulin treatment for type 2 diabetes patients is between 62 and 64%. Patients even less complain when it comes to dietary and other lifestyle recommendations [10, 11]. Regardless of the type of treatment, it was proven that introduction of self-monitoring of blood glucose level is associated with better glycemic control [12], but there are still around 29% patients treated with insulin, 65% patients treated with oral hypoglycemic agents, and 80% patients treated with dietary restriction, who do not practice self-monitoring or they do it less than once a month [13]. Poor adherence is also a public health issue. For every 10% increase in adherence, there is 8.6% decrease in annual health care cost. Furthermore, there is evidently a link between number of hospitalizations and adherence to medication therapy, which is reduced by 23.3% when adherence had increased from 50 to 100%. Even more evident reduction of 46.2% is seen in number of emergency department visits. Both events, i.e., number of hospitalization and emergency department visits are associated with lower costs [14, 15]. When dealing with nonadherence, it is valuable to consider various reasons why this phenomenon occurs. It can be attributed to demographic factors, psychological factors, social factors, medical system factors, disease and treatment characteristic, but mostly it is a result of combinations of multiple factors [11, 16]. For example, glycemic control and treatment outcomes are less promising among racial minorities, men and people with depression or anxiety disorders [17, 18]. Those differences emphasize the importance of individualized and patient-centered care.

4. Concept of empowerment

Patient empowerment is a paradigm of transferring the responsibility of patient's health care in the hands of patients. Such paradigm is in contradiction with the traditional health care where the care was in the hands of the medical staff.

Compliance and adherence are concepts that arise from an idea of patient submitting and agreeing with health professional, who acts as an authority, whereas empowerment promotes patient active involvement and control over their own health [19].

The empowerment can be achieved through education, self-management, and shared decision making.

To obtain satisfactory outcome, there is more to be done than just encourage patients to self-manage their chronic disease. Patients need to be educated about their disease, motivated, provided with patient-centered care, which means that self-management plan needs to be tailored to fit patient priorities, goals, resources, culture, and lifestyle [19].

The education typically occurs at the clinic by the doctor and/or nurse. At Stanford School of Medicine, a Chronic Disease Self-Management Program (CDSMP) [20] was developed which empowers patients through a series of workshops in community settings. Its success is evident in Denmark, which decided to implement it in its health care. As a result, Danish patients are the most empowered [21]. This program was also used in EU project EMPOWER [22].

While face-to-face patient education has positive effects, not much work has been done to evaluate the effect of virtual education. Moreover, patient knowledge is a necessary, but not a sufficient factor for change in the self-care behavior [23]. Patients require self-management support. It can be achieved through face-to-face interaction, through self- and telemonitoring and virtually [24–27].

Collaborative decision making represents collaboration and exchange of knowledge among patients, formal and informal care givers. Because it currently occurs in face-to-face meetings in most cases, there is no evidence for the effects of virtual collaborative decision making.

The goal of such efforts is to shape individuals that make rational health care decisions regarding their health and wellness, are less depended on health care service and contribute to more cost-effective use of health care resources [28].

Finally, in the diabetes treatment, notions of compliance and adherence were replaced with the concept of patient empowerment [29]. With Diabetes Empowerment Scale, significant correlation between level of empowerment and better medication adherence, extensive diabetes knowledge, improved general diet and exercise, blood glucose control, and foot care, can be established [30]. In diabetes management, mobile health technologies are already offering different means for introduction of the concept of empowerment into patients' everyday life.

5. Use of information communication technologies (ICT) for patients with chronic diseases

Patients with chronic diseases need to monitor and record several biometric health parameters. For this purpose, in current health care system, they mainly note observations on a paper, although most devices in use enable storage of such biometric measurements. While there are issues with reading noted values from the papers or even with losing the papers, there are issues with transferring the stored data on the devices to general practitioners (GPs) or specialists. Moreover, the doctors would appreciate to monitor more parameters that are relevant for a holistic care.

On the market, there are devices that can automatically measure and transfer the measurements to the smartphones and dedicated servers: Fitbit wristlets measure user activity and sleep periods [31]; BitBite measures user nutrition habits [32]; iHealth [33], VitaDock [34], VPD [35], and Abbott [36] products measure temperature, blood pressure, pulse, blood oxygen saturation, and glucose level. The current trend is geared toward wearables and gadgets that help diagnose very specific diseases, such as peripheral neuropathy [37] and retinopathy [38], toward gadgets that can measure several parameters [39] and toward integration of functionalities from gadgets to smartphone applications, such as in Google Fit [40] and in Moves [41]. These applications perform comparably well as standalone devices [42].

Furthermore, there are numerous smartphone applications, working with manual data input or data from previously mentioned devices, that assist users in managing their health [43, 44] or diabetes in particular [45, 46]. Such applications do not only display the status of health parameters, but also provide personalized recommendations based on the input data. They mostly encourage users to change their behavior [47].

However, wearable devices and smartphone applications are only facilitators and not drivers of patient empowerment. The design of engagement strategies is more important for successful use and potential health benefits of these devices than the features of technology [48].

Several pilots have been conducted, suggesting positive effects on health and diabetes care, and a need for 24/7 support [49–51]. However, in use, there are mainly only solutions that enable patients to informatively monitor their health status. Solutions that would be used as a part of the general health care service are in the stage of pilots and are only very rarely deployed as part of the standard practice.

6. Why mobile health?

Mobile health is defined as a use of mobile communication devices, which include mobile phones, patient monitoring devices, tablets, personal digital assistants, and other wireless devices for health services, and information [52]. Currently, growing use of those devices can be seen in practically every part of the world. Number of mobile phone owners in the United States has reached 92% of a population and even number of smartphone owners has grown to 68%, while 45% of people own a tablet computer. Desktop or laptop computers were bought by 73% of Americans [53]. Surprisingly, similar rise in mobile technology use is also recorded among people in developing countries, where average share of people with mobile phones is around 83% [54]. With a vast majority of world population having an access to some type of mobile technology, this can certainly become a widely used to deliver deferent health care solutions to people. Role of mHealth is very broad and includes education and rising awareness, remote data collection, remote monitoring, communication with health care workers, support with diagnostic and treatment, and tracking diseases and epidemic outbreaks [55]. Most of these tasks are already performed by various mHealth applications for diabetes self-management.

7. Features of diabetes apps

There are different classifications of diabetes app features and in this section we present some of them.

Review of accessible diabetes applications has shown that they mostly focus on blood glucose monitoring, medications, physical exercise, and diet management, while they also include other features such as education, communication, weight or BMI and blood pressure tracking, integration with public health records, decision support systems, and social networking. Blood glucose monitoring is available in all reviewed applications, while other features are more rarely present. Educational tools are brought to use in just 18% of applications and only around 30% of applications offer means to monitor weight, blood pressure, and physical exercise [56]. Still, among all medical conditions, diabetes with weight control represents the most addressed medical issue by mHealth applications in mHealth research [57].

In a recent systematic review, 53% of apps offered documentation function (recording and displaying data), 17.8% analysis function (the possibility to analyze the recorded data and to graphically display the results), 11.4% reminder function (reminds the user of its periodic, predefined medication), 34.5% of apps offered an information function (inform about the illness). Data forwarding/communication function (opportunity to send the recorded data) was present in 31.1% of apps. Surprisingly, only 8.8% of the diabetes apps provided an advisory function (use of the recorded data to create individualized advice) or any other kind of therapeutic support. Besides, the previously described functions, 14.5% of the apps included suggestions for recipes suitable for the needs of diabetics. The majority of apps, i.e., 54.1% were limited to only one function, while there were only 28.2% with two and 17.7% with three and more functions [58]. In another classification, features of apps were grouped into three classes on the basis of prevalence. In class A, there were insulin and medication management, communication and patient monitoring by primary care providers, diet management, and physical activity. Class B included weight management, blood pressure management, and connection to personal health record (PHR). In class C, there were education, social media, and alerts. Class A comprised four major features and class B had significantly higher prevalence than class C [59].

mHealth research platform *Few Touch Application* (FTA) was developed to support management of diabetes. Applications and studies based on FTA allow automatic monitoring of blood glucose information, receiving short message service information about type 1 diabetes, mobile diary for type 2 diabetes, sharing diaries with doctor or nurse, mobile diary for type 1 diabetes, a food picture data, transfer of physical activity data on mobile phone, nutrition advices, context sensitivity, and modeling of blood glucose. Performance of each of the 10 FTA-based apps was analyzed and the conclusion was that all FTA apps are beneficial [60].

In the next sections, we will present 11 problems of diabetes disease that can be addressed by mHealth.

7.1. Glycemic control

Monitoring of blood glucose level is a base function of all available mHealth diabetes applications, because even without technology interventions self-monitoring of blood glucose (SMBG) is still an integral component of daily diabetes management, especially for insulin-treated patients [56, 61]. Unstructured SMBG is not recommended and does not produce the same results as structured SMBG, which links to behavioral changes, optimization of therapy, and improved clinical outcome. An example of such structured SMBG is a 7-point glucose profile, where blood glucose is measured every day of the week preprandially, postprandially, and at bedtime [62]. A pilot of such structured SMBG demonstrated a reduction in HbA1c levels up to 1.2% in 12 months [63]. To help patients in keeping up with structured SMBG, mHealth offers personal goal setting and various types of reminders [64]. Most commercially available devices for glucose monitoring enable patients to store and follow their blood glucose pattern. For this, patients need to transfer measurements to a computer through an USB cable or to a mobile phone with a direct connection through Bluetooth or Wi-Fi. Even more accurate glucose profile can be obtained with a use of continuous glucose monitor [61]. Regardless of a type of a mHealth intervention used, there is evidence in its positive impacts on reduction of HbA1c values by a mean of 0.5% over 6 months [65]. However, a review of 24 papers has shown that the effectiveness of mHealth interventions (blood glucose reading and transmission to server) measured in HbA1c value was inconsistent for both types of diabetes [66].

7.2. Nutrition control

For education, most of the technologies used for nutrition therapy rely on videoconferencing, while for food tracking and food selection various mobile apps [47]. Distinct features are being formed among behavior mHealth modalities. Food intake can be recorded to determine the quantity of calories consumed each day and the targeted quantity of calories automatically adjusted, based on patient's daily physical activities [67]. More widely adopted are different nutrition databases containing a rage of food items, including different brands and restaurant food, and real-time calculations of consumed calories. Similarly, there exists also a possibility to scan the barcode of brand names to see the nutrient content [47]. Growing number of possibilities provide a new generation of mHealth devices also known as wearables. For example, in diet self-management wrist monitors and electronic utensils can be used to track the amount and speed of bites, but such devices are practically not used yet [68]. Furthermore, mHealth may enable calories calculations with recognition of food from photography in free-living conditions. Even more promising are mobile applications that suggest appropriate meal based on preprandial blood glucose reading, which can facilitate patients' educated decision making [64].

7.3. Physical activity

Sixty nine percent of diabetes patients describe their exercise practices as nonexistent or less than recommended level [69]. It is recommended that adult patient with diabetes perform at least 150 min of moderate-intensity aerobic physical activity per week, spread over at least 3 days and with no more than two consecutive days without exercise [70]. For patients to monitor the extent of their daily physical activity, mHealth offers solutions in a form of body-worn activity monitors. Most easily accessible are pedometers, but besides number of steps taken they do not measure other forms of physical activity [64]. Meanwhile, accelerometers with a combination of gyroscope can record wider range of movements and accuracy of recordings is not dependent on person's body position [71]. When tested, people with access to fully automated system performed on average for 2 h and 18 min per week more of physical activity than people without it [72]. Wearable sensors still need to be complemented with education, planning, and feedback tools to successfully promote physical activity. Effectiveness of mHealth intervention was shown in improved daily number of steps, which was done by setting an achievable goal, providing real-time feedback about the amount of burned calories, and showing recorded progress. This raised the number of steps by 22% in 8 weeks [73].

It was observed that insufficient number of currently evaluable mHealth applications incorporate evidence-based behavior change techniques. This is especially true for techniques, such as relapse prevention, teaching to use props, time management, and agreement to form behavior contract [74].

7.4. Weight loss

Obesity should be diagnosed according to body mass index (BMI). BMI classes are normal weight (18.5–24.9 kg/m^2), overweight (25–29.9 kg/m^2), obesity class I (30–34.9 kg/m^2), obesity class II (35–39.9 kg/m^2), and obesity class III (≥40 kg/m^2). For Southeast Asians and Asian Indians, lower BMI cut-points may be appropriate. Lifestyle modifications including behavioral changes, reduced calorie diets, and appropriately prescribed physical activity should be implemented as the cornerstone of obesity management [75]. Weight loss can be achieved with 500–750 kcal/day reduction that means intake of 1200–1800 kcal/day depending on sex and baseline body weight [76]. Raised BMI, i.e., above 25 kg/m², is seen in more than 75% of diabetes patients [77]. Patients with high BMI and diabetes are significantly more likely to have poor glycemic control [78]. Overweight individuals with diabetes are encouraged to lose at least 5–10% of their weight, because this importantly reduces most cardiovascular risk factors, but it is worth mentioning that lager weight loss (10–15%) has even greater benefits [79]. Reviewed mHealth applications offer means to help achieve this recommendation by monitoring and facilitating physical activity (41% of the applications) and by improving users' diet (68% of the applications) [56]. An evaluation of 137 diabetes apps showed, that only 39% of them offered weight tracking [59]. Self-monitoring of weight and of body composition by using weight scales can now be accomplished wirelessly with mHealth apps or computer applications. This minimizes the burden on the user, while it also minimizes the error in data transcription. Tracked weight and fat mass can be graphically analyzed by the patient or health care practitioner [47].

SMS interventions were investigated to promote change in diet and physical activity. Small and short randomized controlled trials proved significant weight loss, while larger and longer studies showed no statistical significance [80].

Researchers investigated dietary self-monitoring-based electronic interventions using personal digital assistants (PDAs), electronic portable devices that share some of the features of mobile phones. PDA in the study was equipped with dietary and exercise software with and without feedback message. Patients were enrolled in three groups: PDA alone, PDA with feedback (feedback algorithm that provided daily messages tailored to their entries and provided positive reinforcement and guidance for goal attainment), and paper diary/record. All participants had statistically significant weight loss, but PDA group combined with feedback had the highest proportion of participants achieving greater than 5% weight loss in six months [81].

Studies incorporating podcasts compared to podcasts that included prompting by mobile app and interaction with study counselors and other participants on Twitter, did not show enhanced weight loss in the latter group [82].

Interventions delivered by smartphone app, website, or paper diary were also compared. App incorporated goal settings, self-monitoring of diet and activity, and feedback via weekly text message. The website group used commercially available slimming website. Trial retention, adherence, and achieved weight loss were significantly higher in the smartphone app group [80].

7.5. Blood pressure control

Elevated blood pressure is a common condition coexisting with diabetes and it is a clear independent risk factor for the cardiovascular complications. To reduce the risk, blood pressure should be routinely monitored and maintained at a targeted level. Recommended systolic pressure for diabetes patient is <140 mmHg and diastolic pressure <90 mmHg. Home-monitoring is greatly encouraged, because it is a way to exclude white coat hypertension and because research suggested better correlation between at home measurements and cardiovascular risk than office measurements [83]. Among reviewed diabetes applications, 23% of them currently offer means of self-monitoring of blood pressure [56]. Monitoring blood pressure with the help of mHealth program may detect hypertension patterns that would otherwise gone unreported [22]. Fully automatized blood pressure readings, which are immediately stored in mHealth device and send to a health care provider, enabled to 51% of diabetes patient to reach the targeted blood pressure level. This is a significant improvement compared to 37.5% of general diabetes population that succeed in lowering their blood pressure. Such improvement was achieved also due to by inclusion of daily reminders, alerts in a case of concern-reassign measurement and linkage to patient support system [84]. Home-monitoring alone does not produce the same results, proving telemedicine equal, but not more effective than standard approach, so this needs to be taken into consideration for future mHealth design [85].

7.6. Medication adherence

Previously, already discussed lack of adherence to pharmacological intervention in diabetes patients is an issue addressed by approximately 76% of reviewed mHealth applications [56]. One of the commonly reported barriers is patient forgetfulness, when it comes to medication intake regime. Mobile health technologies can offer different solution to this problem. Daily automatic electronic or text-message reminders may improve medication intake [86]. Those reminders can be upgraded by the use of real-time medication monitoring, which is possible with a use of electronic medication dispenser that records date and time of each opening. Consequentially, alert is only send in a case of forgotten medication dose. A trail confirmed that a baseline adherence of around 62% improved to 79.5% adherence after 1 year of use. Long-term effectiveness of this mHealth method peaked at 80.4% medication adherence, whereas control group adherence remained in a range of 68.4%. Majority of patients that used real-time medication monitoring also agreed that this method supported higher awareness of their medication use and reported positive experience with receiving SMS reminders [87, 88]. Considerable amount of patient, who tested real-time monitoring devices, were glad that physician knew if they took their medication and were reassured by technology supported communication [89].

7.7. Education

Diabetes education is a key element in patient care. To reassure adequate results, effective education strategies can be found in National Standards for Diabetes Self-Management Education and are worth applying to mHealth methods [90]. Even limited amount of education can result in improved weight control and potentially reduced cardiovascular risk [91]. Initial comparisons between in person diabetes education and education administrated through telemedicine already demonstrated a feasibility and equal effectiveness of technology supported methods [92]. Most diabetes self-management applications do not integrate educational information. When available, such information is often generic and is not personalized to the individual patient. This is more prominent in commercial applications [56]. Education and personalized feedback are still underdeveloped features, included in less than one third of reviewed mHealth applications. Only 20% of reviewed applications had an education module, and only 26% of these met the criteria for personalized education or feedback. Task of personalizing rapidly growing number of information is challenging, but it may be largely beneficial for diabetes patient [59]. Most widely used mHealth method for diabetes education is SMS. Meta-analysis of current findings has shown that mobile SMS education can improve glycemic control. The glycemic control is even better if diabetes education is done by a combination of SMS and internet methods, i.e., 86% effect in comparison with 44% that is achieved by SMS alone [93]. Positive results of e-mail and SMS education can also be seen in improved quality of life [94].

Numerous applications are available helping healthy people or people with risk factors to assess their risk for developing diabetes type 2 in the future. Only a few of these apps disclose the name of the risk calculator used for assessing the risk of diabetes, therefore the quality of their calculations is questionable [95].

7.8. Diabetic retinopathy screening

Diabetic retinopathy represents most frequent cause of newly occurring adult blindness. Incidence of diabetic retinopathy is highly depended on duration of diabetes itself. Among population with type 2 diabetes cumulative incidence after 4 years is estimated to be 26%, 38.1–41.0% after 6 years and 66% after 10 years [96]. Comprehensive eye examination should be performed after diabetes diagnosis and repeated every 2 years, if there are no visible changes, or annually, if initial retinopathy changes are already present [97]. To keep up with this requirement even with patient in remote and isolated areas, low cost smartphone-based intelligent system integrated with microscopic lens was developed and tested. System detects retinal abnormalities by a method of comparison with medical image database. Early testing has promisingly shown more than 87% accuracy rate in retinal disease detection [98].

7.9. Diabetic foot screening

Diabetic foot is a main cause for nontraumatic lower limb amputation and precedes 85% of the cases. Approximately 15% of diabetes patients will develop diabetic foot ulcers in their lifetime [99]. It is recommended for all diabetes patients to perform annual extensive foot examination to identify risk factors predictive of foot ulcers. Patient should be screened for signs of peripheral neuropathy and peripheral vascular disease, simultaneously paying attention to identify other risk factors such as foot deformities, past foot ulcers, visual impairment, and cigarette smoking [97]. Currently, researched mHealth method to facilitate foot care is using high quality photography to diagnose foot ulcers and preulcerative lesions. Trained professional can diagnose visible diabetic foot changes in valid and reliable manner, which implies methods usability as a monitoring tool in home environment [100]. Originally developed was a method for wound area measurement. The wound margins are recognized with the help of smartphone. First, the wound contour is copied on the foil. The area is then measured with smartphone app and compared with previous measurements [101].

7.10. Psychosocial care

Patients with diabetes should regularly be assessed for their psychosocial well-being. Care should include assessment of their attitudes about the illness and prognosis, mood changes, satisfaction with quality of life, financial, social and emotional conditions, and possible psychiatric disorders (depression, distress, anxiety, eating disorders, dementia). Screening is recommended for depression and cognitive impairment for older than 65 [76].

Telemedicine study researching depression and glycemic control in elderly showed a weak relationship between depression and HbA1C, but depression did not prospectively predict change in glycemic control [102]. In another study, web-based depression treatment for diabetics using cognitive behavior therapy was effective in reducing depressive symptoms, diabetes-specific emotional distress, while it had no benefit on glycemic control [103].

Telephone-based cognitive assessment (TBCA) was previously performed by conventional telephone. Because of better understanding of cognitive impairment, there is a possibility of more accurate TBCA. It needs more complex features of telephone which are easily achieved with the use of smartphones [104].

7.11. Personal health record (PHR)/electronic medical record (EMR) and social media integration

PHR is an internet-based set of tools that allows people to access and coordinate their lifelong health information and make appropriate parts of it available to those who need it [105]. Electronic medical record (EMR) is an electronic record with documents of patient's treatment in a clinic. Electronic health record (EHR) is a summary of individual's lifetime health status and care. Terms EMR and EHR are often used interchangeably [106].

Overall, 21% of commercial applications support synchronization of data with PHRs. Half of reviewed studies have integrated PHR with EMR and provide both patient and physician Web portal, whereas other included either a patient view or a clinician view of the EMR [56].

Social media integration is also emerging function of diabetes apps. It can help patients find similar users and communities in a dynamic fashion. But the majority of apps only provides links to their groups in well-known social networking sites such as Facebook and Twitter or maybe provides an account to a forum [59].

8. Usability, accessibility, and acceptability of diabetes apps

In a study of feasibility and acceptability of PDA-based (personal digital assistant-based) dietary self-monitoring of diabetes patients at the time of advent of the first smartphone high percentage of participants reported that they found PDA-monitoring useful, that the app was easy to use and that feedback was easily understandable [107]. In another study with PDAs, several limitations were found that may have contributed to perceived frustration including usability, data loss/errors (especially mistyped numbers) and time constraint (time consuming and tedious handling) [108]. A new study revealed that the perceived additional benefit and the perceived ease of use had the strongest impact on acceptance of diabetes smartphone technology by patients 50 or older. Less important factors were previous experiences, health status, support, confidence in own technical knowledge, perceived data security, and fault tolerance. The target group of diabetes patients aged 50 or older is a rather heterogeneous one and their needs are highly heterogeneous due to differences in previous knowledge, age, type of diabetes, and therapy. For that reason, it is impossible to address the needs of all diabetes patients adequately with one diabetes app in order to gain an additional benefit. Therefore, the contents of a helpful diabetes app should be individually adaptable [109]. There is a lack of systems that can perform automated translation of behavioral data into specific actionable suggestions that promote healthier lifestyle without any human involvement. The first attempts were made to create personalized, contextualized, actionable suggestions automatically from self-tracked information [110].

Ten percent of all available apps in 2013 were evaluated within usability evaluation by three experts considering the special requirements of diabetes patients age 50 years or older. Four main criteria were evaluated, being "comprehensibility," "presentation," "usability," and "general characteristics." The main criteria, "comprehensibility," rated best. In particular, the elderly benefit from easy, understandable semantics and easy, comprehensible, and interpretable images and depictions. It can lower inhibition thresholds, especially during the first time of use. The same is true for the influence of "easily understandable feedback" and an "intuitive usability" (main criterion "usability"). However, these two subcriteria performed worse within evaluation. Test of accessibility features indicated a very good operability of the screen readers. The criterion "fault tolerance" rated worst. Especially, inexperienced (elderly) users often have difficulties with inputting data. Some errors are unrecoverable or even cause the application to shut down [58].

9. Type 1 diabetes mellitus

We have to say some words about type 1 diabetes mellitus. We described until now mobile health interventions irrespective of the diabetes type. Because type 2 diabetes is much more widespread, studies included mostly or exclusively type 2 diabetes patients.

Young people with type 1 diabetes have many ideas and can help improve services and their own health-related quality of life. However, their lifestyle and their use of Web and smartphones to cope the disease are not well researched [111].

A systematic review was carried out, focused on the ability of mobile health tools to grant patients with type 1 diabetes greater glycemic control. The tools investigated took a variety of forms and provided a number of different services to a diabetic patient. The indicator demonstrating the intervention to be successful was HbA1c and it was decreased in majority of studies, but not all values were statistically significant. In addition, prospective studies were predominantly used instead of randomized controlled trials [112].

Qualitative interviewing and exploring how young people with diabetes type 1 make use of technology in their lives and in relation to their condition and treatment, was made. On that basis, many suggestions to develop apps were found including issues such as alcohol and diabetes, hypoglycemia and diabetes, illness and diabetes, and Twitter use for diabetics. All listed suggestions were taken forward for prototyping, with alcohol and diabetes being developed as clinically approved app. There were also many other issues suggested, that were not prototyped [111].

In UK, a competition for teams including at least one young person with diabetes to develop an app, that might help this group of patients in preparation for their diabetes appointments, was conducted. After the development, other young people with diabetes were invited to choose, test and review new apps. The competition proved successful, showing the app designers and developers a need to develop a range of new functions [113].

Insulin calculator apps for patients with diabetes were scrutinized, because self-medication errors are recognized source of avoidable harm. Users are at risk of both catastrophic overdose and more subtle—suboptimal glucose control. In a research, considering input, only 59% calculators included clinical disclaimer and only 30% documented the calculation formula. 91% lacked numeric input validation, problems were also with calculation with missing values, ambiguous terminology, even with numeric precision. Considering output, 67% of calculators carries a risk of inappropriate output dose recommendation that either violated basic clinical assumptions or did not match a stated formula or correctly update in response to changing user input. It is advised, that health care professionals should exercise substantial caution in recommending unregulated dose calculators to patients and take care for proper education about possible threats [114].

10. Doctors' involvement

Little attention has been paid to physicians' intentions to adopt mobile diabetes monitoring technology. Japan study showed that overall quality (system quality, information quality, and service quality) assessment does affect doctors' intention to use this technology, but only indirectly through perceived value. Net benefits (both ubiquitous control and health improvement) seem to be also a strong driver in both a direct and indirect manner [115].

Combined smartphone-based logging of different health parameters (e.g., blood sugar logging, insulin dose logging, bread unit logging, activity logging) can of course help doctor (diabetologist) in solving glycemic control problems. With these data, diabetologist can make individualized recommendations for every patient [116].

11. Economic effectiveness

It was establish that standard, technology unsupported, diabetes interventions are cost-effective. Effective base therapy typically costs up to $50,000 per each quality adjusted life year gained [117]. Activities that focus on intensive lifestyle changes, universal opportunistic screening for undiagnosed type 2 diabetes, intensive glycemic control, annual screening for diabetic retinopathy were proven to cost ≤$25,000 per life year gained or per quality-adjusted life year, what categorizes them as very cost-effective [118]. If there is to be expected that mHealth interventions will be introduced in everyday diabetes patients' care, they need to show themselves to be more cost-effective than standard treatment. In other words, they should cost less than an amount that we are already willing to pay for diabetes treatment. Current diabetes cost-effectiveness studies are sparse, but promising. Findings of one such study demonstrated annual cost decrease by using mHealth glucose meter with a support of disease management call center that outweighed higher program costs by several-folds. Implementation of technology supported care meant $50 per patient per month higher expenses than standard care, however in a year's time it was possible to register $3384 cost decrease compared with an increase of $282 among those with previously established course of treatment [119]. Immediate cost reduction after implementation of telehealth is primarily due to the absence of transportation costs per patient visit to outpatient clinic and productivity savings, because of eliminated need for frequent work absences. More substantial medical savings can be seen with a long term use [120]. Furthermore, it is reasonable to predict lowering of medical cost with growing number of diabetes patient included in automated telephone-linked interventions. For illustration, delivery of mHealth solution to 10,000 patients instead of 1000 can reduce expenses from £444 per patient to £301 [121]. In other economic evaluations, new management methods were determine to be associated with higher cost per quality adjusted life year and not cost-effective addition to standard care. This economic model argues that even with 80% reduction in equipment cost and full utilization of the telehealth service the probability of cost-effectiveness would only reach 61% at the £30,000 threshold of willingness to pay [122]. Still, individual research results are too heterogeneous to enable extraction of significant meaning regarding a possible medical expenditure reduction with continuous use of mHealth solution [123].

12. Future trends

Clinical decision support systems are active knowledge systems using two or more items of patient's data to generate case specific advice. It is in majority of cases standalone technology or integrated in provider's information system and is used by doctors or other medical staff [124]. Many mobile decision support software apps for smartphones are now available for diabetes and are intended to assist patients to make decisions for themselves in real time without having to contact their health care provider. For many minute-to-minute decisions, the questions are not sufficiently significant to warrant contacting a health care provider and there is insufficient time to wait for a reply. Mobile decision support apps can be helpful to assist patients to identify data patterns and make it easier for them to come to an immediate decision on their own [52]. With the advent of minimally invasive subcutaneous continuous glucose monitoring increasing academic and industrial effort has been focused on the development of SC-SC (subcutaneous-subcutaneous) artificial pancreas systems, using continuous glucose monitoring coupled with continuous subcutaneous insulin infusion. Next step is use of mobile system as user interface which is controlled by the patient. The interface is based on patient's commercial mobile phone [125].

13. Conclusion

Use of mobile health technology for empowerment of patients with diabetes is an emerging way to improve their health and wellbeing. It can address almost every problem of diabetic patient. But approaches are diverse and every app has its own properties and functionalities. There are many apps on the market, but only few of them are adequately certified by health care authorities. Therefore, their quality is questionable. But many studies showed, mHealth is effective and even cost-effective, though more research is needed.

The future applications should be more personally oriented, improved regarding usability and accessibility, and based on accepted clinical guidelines.

Author details

Matjaž Krošel[1], Lana Švegl[1], Luka Vidmar[2] and Dejan Dinevski[1*]

*Address all correspondence to: dejan.dinevski@uni-mb.si

1 Faculty of Medicine, University of Maribor, Maribor, Slovenia

2 Telekom Slovenije d.d., Ljubljana, Slovenia

References

[1] O'Grady MJ, Capretta JC. Health-care cost projections for diabetes and other chronic diseases: the current context and potential enhancements. Partnership to Fight Chronic Disease. [Internet]. 2009. Available from: http://www.fightchronicdisease.org/sites/default/files/docs/PFCD_whitepaper5.21.09.pdf [Accessed: 2016-02-15]

[2] Pauws S, Schonenberg H, Maramis C, et al. ACT Programme. Deliverable: Evaluation Engine for Advancing Care Coordination and Telehealth Deployment. DG SANCO; [Internet]. 2013. Available from: http://www2.med.auth.gr/act/documents/del2.pdf [Accessed: 2016-02-15].

[3] Eriksson T. A Danish Chronic Care Model & Risk Stratification. EQuiP. [Internet]. 2007. Available from: http://equip2.dudal.com/dcmpage/national_pages/denmark/a_danish_chronic_care_model_risk_stratification/ [Accessed: 2016-02-15].

[4]   International Diabetes Federation. IDF diabetes Atlas. 7th ed. [Internet]. 2015. Available from: http://www.diabetesatlas.org/ [Accessed: 2016-02-15].

[5]   Funnell MM, Anderson RM. MSJAMA: The problem with compliance in diabetes. *JAMA*. 2000;284(13):1709. DOI: 10.1001/jama.284.13.1709-JMS1004-6-1.

[6]   American Diabetes Association. Diagnosis and classification of diabetes mellitus. *Diabetes Care*. 2014;37(Suppl. 1):S81–S90. DOI: 10.2337/dc14-S081.

[7]   Kulshrestha M, Seth S, Tripathi A, Seth A, Kumar A. Prevalence of complications and clinical audit of management of type 2 diabetes mellitus: A prospective hospital based study. *J Clin Diagnostic Res*. 2015;9(11):OC25–OC28. DOI: 10.7860/JCDR/2015/15369.6848.

[8]   Stratton IM, Adler AI, Neil AHW, et al. Association of glycaemia with macrovascular and microvascular complications of type 2 diabetes (UKPDS 35): prospective observational study. *BMJ*. 2000;321(7258):405–412. DOI: 10.1136/bmj.321.7258.405.

[9]   De Geest S, Sabaté E. Adherence to long-term therapies: evidence for action. *Eur J Cardiovasc Nurs*. 2003;2(4):323. DOI: 10.1016/S1474-5151(03)00091-4.

[10] Bailey CJ, Kodack M. Patient adherence to medication requirements for therapy of type 2 diabetes. *Int J Clin Pr*. 2011;65(3):314–322. DOI: 10.1111/j.1742-1241.2010.02544.x.

[11] Delamater AM. Improving patient adherence. *Clin Diabetes*. 2006;24(2):71–77. DOI: 10.2337/diaclin.24.2.71.

[12] Karter AJ, Ackerson LM, Darbinian JA, et al. Self-monitoring of blood glucose levels and glycemic control: the Northern California Kaiser Permanente Diabetes registry. *Am J Med*. 2001;111(1):1–9. DOI: 10.1016/S0002-9343(01)00742-2.

[13] Harris MI, National Health and Nutrition Examination Survey (NHANES). Frequency of blood glucose monitoring in relation to glycemic control in patients with type 2 diabetes. *Diabetes Care*. 2001;24(6):979–982. DOI: 10.2337/diacare.24.6.979.

[14] Wild H. The economic rationale for adherence in the treatment of type 2 diabetes mellitus. *Am J Manag Care*. 2012;18(Suppl. 3):S43–S48 [Internet]. Available from: http://www.ajmc.com/journals/supplement/2012/A405_12Apr_Diabetes/The-Economic-Rationale-for-Adherence-in-the-Treatment-of-Type-2-Diabetes-Mellitus/ [Accessed: 2016-02-15].

[15] Salas M, Hughes D, Zuluaga A, Vardeva K, Lebmeier M. Costs of medication nonadherence in patients with diabetes mellitus: a systematic review and critical analysis of the literature. *Value Heal*. 2009;12(6):915–922. DOI: 10.1111/j.1524-4733.2009.00539.x.

[16] Koenigsberg MR, Bartlett D, Cramer JS. Facilitating treatment adherence with lifestyle changes in diabetes. *Am Fam Physician*. 2004;69(2):309–316+319 [Internet]. Available from: http://www.aafp.org/afp/2004/0115/p309.html [Accessed: 2016-02-15].

[17] Chou AF, Brown AF, Jensen RE, Shih S, Pawlson G, Scholle SH. Gender and racial disparities in the management of diabetes mellitus among Medicare patients. *Women Heal Issues*. 2007;17(3):150–161.

[18] Delamater AM, Jacobson AM, Anderson B, et al. Psychosocial therapies in diabetes report of the psychosocial therapies working group. *Diabetes Care*. 2001;24(7):1286–1292. DOI: 10.2337/diacare.24.7.1286.

[19] Funnell MM, Anderson RM. Empowerment and self-management of diabetes. *Clin Diabetes*. 2004;22(3):123–127. DOI: 10.2337/diaclin.22.3.123.

[20] Stanford Patient Education Research Center. Chronic Disease Self-Management Program (Better Choices, Better Health® Workshop). Stanford Medicine [Internet]. Available from: http://patienteducation.stanford.edu/programs/diabeteseng.html [Accessed: 2016-02-15].

[21] Health Consumer Powerhouse AB. The Empowerment of the European Patient 2009 – options and implications. 2009:1–56 [Internet]. Available from: http://www.healthpowerhouse.com/files/EPEI-2009/european-patient-empowerment-2009-report.pdf [Accessed: 2016-02-15].

[22] Aikens JE, Zivin K, Trivedi R, Piette JD. Diabetes self-management support using mHealth and enhanced informal caregiving. *J Diabetes Complicat*. 2014;28(2):171–176. DOI: 10.1016/j.jdiacomp.2013.11.008.

[23] Krichbaum K, Aarestad V, Buethe M. Exploring the connection between self-efficacy and effective diabetes self-management. *Diabetes Educ*. 2003;29(4):653–662. DOI: 10.1177/014572170302900411.

[24] Norris SL, Lau J, Smith SJ, Schmid CH, Engelgau MM. Self-management education for adults with type 2 diabetes: a meta-analysis of the effect on glycemic control. *Diabetes Care*. 2002;25(7):1159–1171. DOI: 10.2337/diacare.25.7.1159.

[25] Chodosh J, Morton SC, Mojica W, et al. Meta-analysis: chronic disease self-management programs for older adults. *Ann Intern Med*. 2005;143(6):427–438. DOI: 10.7326/0003-4819-143-6-200509200-00007.

[26] Norris SL, Engelgau MM, Narayan KM. Effectiveness of self-management training in type 2 diabetes: a systematic review of randomized controlled trials. *Diabetes Care*. 2001;24(3):561–587. DOI: 10.2337/diacare.24.3.561.

[27] Weingarten SR, Henning JM, Badamgarav E, et al. Interventions used in disease management programmes for patients with chronic illness-which ones work? Meta-analysis of published reports. *BMJ*. 2002;325(7370):925. DOI: 10.1136/bmj.325.7370.925.

[28] McAllister M, Dunn G, Payne K, Davies L, Todd C. Patient empowerment: the need to consider it as a measurable patient-reported outcome for chronic conditions. *BMC Heal Serv Res*. 2012;12(1):1. DOI: 10.1186/1472-6963-12-157.

[29] Aujoulat I, Marcolongo R, Bonadiman L, Deccache A. Reconsidering patient empowerment in chronic illness: a critique of models of self-efficacy and bodily control. *Soc Sci Med*. 2008;66(5):1228–1239. DOI: 10.1016/j.socscimed.2007.11.034.

[30] Hernandez-Tejada MA, Campbell JA, Walker RJ, Smalls BL, Davis KS, Egede LE. Diabetes empowerment, medication adherence and self-care behaviors in adults with type 2 diabetes. *Diabetes Technol Ther*. 2012;14(7):630–634. DOI: 10.1089/dia.2011.0287.

[31] Fitbit [Internet]. Available from: http://www.fitbit.com/uk/home# [Accessed: 2016-02-15].

[32] BitBite Mindful Eating Habits [Internet]. Available from: http://www.thebitbite.com/ [Accessed: 2016-02-15].

[33] iHealth Innovative Mobile Healthcare Products [Internet]. Available from: https://ihealthlabs.com/ [Accessed: 2016-02-15].

[34] Medisana. VitaDock+ [Internet]. Available from: https://cloud.vitadock.com/ [Accessed: 2016-02-15].

[35] VPD [Internet]. Available from: http://www.vpd.si/ [Accessed: 2016-02-15].

[36] Abbott [Internet]. Available from: http://www.abbott.com/ [Accessed: 2016-02-15].

[37] Najafi B. SmartSox: a smart textile to prevent diabetic foot amputation. *Qatar Found Annu Res Forum Proc*. 2013:BIOP 013. DOI: 10.5339/qfarf.2013.BIOP-013.

[38] Stanford School of Medicine. Smartphones become "eye-phones" with low-cost devices developed by ophthalmologists. [Internet]. 2014. Available from: https://med.stanford.edu/news/all-news/2014/03/smartphones-become-eye-phones-with-low-cost-devices-developed-by-ophthalmologists.html [Accessed: 2016-02-15].

[39] Preventice Solutions. BodyGuardian [Internet]. Available from: http://www.preventicesolutions.com/healthcare-professionals.html [Accessed: 2016-02-15].

[40] Google. Google Fit [Internet]. Available from: https://fit.google.com/ [Accessed: 2016-02-15].

[41] Moves. Activity Diary of your Life [Internet]. Available from: https://www.moves-app.com/ [Accessed: 2016-02-15].

[42] Case MA, Burwick HA, Volpp KG, Patel MS. Accuracy of smartphone applications and wearable devices for tracking physical activity data. *JAMA*. 2015;313(6):625. DOI: 10.1001/jama.2014.17841.

[43] 24alife [Internet]. Available from: https://www.24alife.com/home [Accessed: 2016-02-15].

[44] Dacadoo. What's your Health Score? [Internet]. Available from: https://www.dacadoo.com/ [Accessed: 2016-02-15].

[45] LTFE. DeStress Assistant [Internet]. Available from: http://desa.ltfe.org/ [Accessed: 2016-02-15].

[46] SkyHealth LLC. Diabetes and Blood Sugar Management Software [Internet]. Available from: http://www.glucosebuddy.com/ [Accessed: 2016-02-15].

[47] Sieverdes JC, Treiber F, Jenkins C. Improving diabetes management with mobile health technology. *Am J Med Sci*. 2013;345(4):289–295. DOI: 10.1097/MAJ.0b013e3182896cee.

[48] Patel MS, Asch DA, Volpp KG. Wearable devices as facilitators, not drivers, of health behavior change. *JAMA*. 2015;3(313):459–460. DOI: 10.1001/jama.2014.14781.

[49] Polisena J, Tran K, Cimon K, Hutton B, McGill S, Palmer K. Home telehealth for diabetes management: a systematic review and meta-analysis. *Diabetes Obes Metab*. 2009;11(10): 913–930. DOI: 10.1111/j.1463-1326.2009.01057.x.

[50] Jackson CL, Bolen S, Brancati FL, Batts-Turner ML, Gary TL. A systematic review of interactive computer-assisted technology in diabetes care. *J Gen Intern Med*. 2006;21(2): 105–110.

[51] Vrbnjak D, Pajnkihar M, Stožer A, Dinevski D. M-health and diabetes mellitus. In: Proceedings of the 2014 Congress Better Information for More Health (MI'2014); 6-7 November 2014; Zreče. Ljubljana: SDMI. 2014. p. 28'33.

[52] Klonoff DC. The current status of mHealth for diabetes: will it be the next big thing? *J Diabetes Sci Technol*. 2013;77(33):749–758. DOI: 10.1177/193229681300700321.

[53] Anderson M. Technology Device Ownership: 2015. Pew Research Center. 2015 [Internet]. Available from: http://www.pewinternet.org/2015/10/29/technology-device-ownership-2015 [Accessed: 2016-02-15].

[54] Pew Research Center. Emerging Nations Embrace Internet, Mobile Technology. [Internet]. 2014. Available from: http://www.pewglobal.org/files/2014/02/Pew-Re-search-Center-Global-Attitudes-Project-Technology-Report-FINAL-Febru-ary-13-20147.pdf [Accessed: 2016-02-15].

[55] Vital Wave Consulting. mHealth for Development: The Opportunity of Mobile Technology for Healthcare in the Developing World. Washington, D.C. and Berkshire, UK: UN Foundation-Vodafone Foundation Partnership; 2009 [Internet]. Available from: http://www.globalproblems-globalsolutions-files.org/unf_website/assets/publications/technology/mhealth/mHealth_for_Development_full.pdf [Accessed: 2016-02-15].

[56] El-Gayar O, Timsina P, Nawar N, Eid W. Mobile applications for diabetes self-management: status and potential. *J Diabetes Sci Technol*. 2013;7(1):247–262. DOI: 10.1177/193229681300700130.

[57] Fiordelli M, Diviani N, Schulz PJ. Mapping mHealth research: a decade of evolution. *J Med Internet Res*. 2013;15(5):e95. DOI: 10.2196/jmir.2430.

[58] Arnhold M, Quade M, Kirch W. Mobile applications for diabetics: a systematic review and expert-based usability evaluation considering the special requirements of diabetes patients age 50 years or older. *J Med Internet Res*. 2014;16(4):e104. DOI: 10.2196/jmir. 2968.

[59] Chomutare T, Fernandez-Luque L, Arsand E, Hartvigsen G. Features of mobile diabetes applications: review of the literature and analysis of current applications compared against evidence-based guidelines. *J Med Internet Res*. 2011;13(3):e65. DOI: 10.2196/jmir. 1874.

[60] Årsand E, Frøisland DH, Skrøvseth SO, et al. Mobile health applications to assist patients with diabetes: lessons learned and design implications. *J Diabetes Sci Technol*. 2012;6(5):1197–1206. DOI: 10.1177/193229681200600525.

[61] Georga EI, Protopappas VC, Bellos C V, Fotiadis DI. Wearable systems and mobile applications for diabetes disease management. *Heal Technol*. 2014;4(2):101–112. DOI: 10.1007/s12553-014-0082-y.

[62] Parkin CG, Buskirk A, Hinnen DA, Axel-Schweitzer M. Results that matter: structured vs. unstructured self-monitoring of blood glucose in type 2 diabetes. *Diabetes Res Clin Pr*. 2012;97(1):6–15. DOI: 10.1016/j.diabres.2012.03.002.

[63] Polonsky WH, Fisher L, Schikman CH, et al. Structured self-monitoring of blood glucose significantly reduces A1C levels in poorly controlled, noninsulin-treated type 2 diabetes: results from the Structured Testing Program study. *Diabetes Care*. 2011;34(2): 262–267. DOI: 10.2337/dc10-1732.

[64] Goyal S, Morita P, Lewis GF, Yu C, Seto E, Cafazzo JA. The systematic design of a behavioural mobile health application for the self-management of type 2 diabetes. *Can J Diabetes*. 2016;40(1):95–104. DOI: 10.1016/j.jcjd.2015.06.007.

[65] Pal K, Eastwood S V, Michie S, et al. Computer-based interventions to improve self-management in adults with type 2 diabetes: a systematic review and meta-analysis. *Diabetes Care*. 2014;37(6):1759–1766. DOI: 10.2337/dc13-1386.

[66] Baron J, McBain H, Newman S. The impact of mobile monitoring technologies on glycosylated hemoglobin in diabetes: a systematic review. *J Diabetes Sci Technol*. 2012;6(5):1185–1196.

[67] Granado-Font E, Flores-Mateo G, Sorlí-Aguilar M, et al. Effectiveness of a smartphone application and wearable device for weight loss in overweight or obese primary care patients: protocol for a randomised controlled trial. *BMC Public Health*. 2015;15(1):531. DOI: 10.1186/s12889-015-1845-8.

[68] Yu Z, Sealey-Potts C, Rodriguez J. Dietary self-monitoring in weight management: current evidence on efficacy and adherence. *J Acad Nutr Diet*. 2015;115(12):1931–1938. DOI: 10.1016/j.jand.2015.04.005.

[69] Nelson KM, Reiber G, Boyko EJ, NHANES III. Diet and exercise among adults with type 2 diabetes: findings from the third national health and nutrition examination

survey (NHANES III). *Diabetes Care*. 2002;25(10):1722–1728. DOI: 10.2337/diacare. 25.10.1722.

[70] American Diabetes Association. Foundations of care: education, nutrition, physical activity, smoking cessation, psychosocial care, and immunization. Sec. 4. In Standards of Medical Care in Diabetes – 2015. *Diabetes Care*. 2015;38(Suppl. 1):S20–S30. DOI: 10.2337/dc15-S007.

[71] Wu W, Dasgupta S, Ramirez EE, Peterson C, Norman GJ. Classification accuracies of physical activities using smartphone motion sensors. *J Med Internet Res*. 2012;14(5):e130. DOI: 10.2196/jmir.2208.

[72] Hurling R, Catt M, Boni MD, et al. Using internet and mobile phone technology to deliver an automated physical activity program: randomized controlled trial. *J Med Internet Res*. 2007;9(2):e7. DOI: 10.2196/jmir.9.2.e7.

[73] Glynn LG, Hayes PS, Casey M, et al. Effectiveness of a smartphone application to promote physical activity in primary care: the SMART MOVE randomised controlled trial. *Br J Gen Pr*. 2014;64(624):e384–e391. DOI: 10.3399/bjgp14X680461.

[74] Direito A, Dale LP, Shields E, Dobson R, Whittaker R, Maddison R. Do physical activity and dietary smartphone applications incorporate evidence-based behaviour change techniques? *BMC Public Health*. 2014;14:646. DOI: 10.1186/1471-2458-14-646.

[75] Handelsman Y, Bloomgarden ZT, Grunberger G, et al. American association of clinical endocrinologists and American college of endocrinology – clinical practice guidelines for developing a diabetes mellitus comprehensive care plan – 2015. *Endocr Pr*. 2015;21(Suppl. 1):1–87. DOI: 10.4158/EP15672.GL.

[76] American Diabetes Association. Standards of medical care in diabetes – 2016. *Diabetes Care*. 2016;39(Suppl. 1):S1–S112. DOI: 10.2337/dc14-S014.

[77] Bays HE, Chapman RH, Grandy S, Group the SI. The relationship of body mass index to diabetes mellitus, hypertension and dyslipidaemia: comparison of data from two national surveys. *Int J Clin Pr*. 2007;61(5):737–747. DOI: 10.1111/j. 1742-1241.2007.01336.x.

[78] Bae JP, Lage MJ, Mo D, Nelson DR, Hoogwerf BJ. Obesity and glycemic control in patients with diabetes mellitus: analysis of physician electronic health records in the US from 2009–2011. *J Diabetes Complicat*. 2015. DOI: 10.1016/j.jdiacomp.2015.11.016.

[79] Wing RR, Lang W, Wadden TA, et al. Benefits of modest weight loss in improving cardiovascular risk factors in overweight and obese individuals with type 2 diabetes. *Diabetes Care*. 2011;34(7):1481–1486. DOI: 10.2337/dc10-2415.

[80] Carter MC, Burley VJ, Nykjaer C, Cade JE. Adherence to a smartphone application for weight loss compared to website and paper diary: pilot randomized controlled trial. *J Med Internet Res*. 2013;15(4):e32. DOI: 10.2196/jmir.2283.

[81] Burke LE, Conroy MB, Sereika SM, et al. The effect of electronic self-monitoring on weight loss and dietary intake: a randomized behavioral weight loss trial. *Obes (Silver Spring)*. 2011;19(2):338–344. DOI: 10.1038/oby.2010.208.

[82] Turner-McGrievy G, Tate D. Tweets, Apps, and Pods: results of the 6-month mobile pounds off digitally (mobile POD) randomized weight-loss intervention among adults. *J Med Internet Res*. 2011;13(4):e120. DOI: 10.2196/jmir.1841.

[83] American Diabetes Association. Cardiovascular disease and risk management. Sec. 8. In Standards of Medical Care in Diabetes – 2015. *Diabetes Care*. 2015;38(Suppl. 1):S49–S57. DOI: 10.2337/dc15-S011.

[84] Logan AG, Irvine MJ, McIsaac WJ, et al. Effect of home blood pressure telemonitoring with self-care support on uncontrolled systolic hypertension in diabetics. *Hypertension*. 2012;60(1):51–57. DOI: 10.1161/HYPERTENSIONAHA.111.188409.

[85] Madsen LB, Kirkegaard P, Pedersen EB. Blood pressure control during telemonitoring of home blood pressure. A randomized controlled trial during 6 months. *Blood Press*. 2008;17(2):78–86. DOI: 10.1080/08037050801915468.

[86] Vervloet M, Linn AJ, van Weert JC, de Bakker DH, Bouvy ML, van Dijk L. The effectiveness of interventions using electronic reminders to improve adherence to chronic medication: a systematic review of the literature. *J Am Med Informatics Assoc*. 2012;19(5): 696–704. DOI: 10.1136/amiajnl-2011-000748.

[87] Vervloet M, van Dijk L, de Bakker DH, et al. Short- and long-term effects of real-time medication monitoring with short message service (SMS) reminders for missed doses on the refill adherence of people with type 2 diabetes: evidence from a randomized controlled trial. *Diabet Med*. 2014;31(7):821–828. DOI: 10.1111/dme.12439.

[88] Vervloet M, van Dijk L, Santen-Reestman J, et al. SMS reminders improve adherence to oral medication in type 2 diabetes patients who are real time electronically monitored. *Int J Med Inf*. 2012;81(9):594–604. DOI: 10.1016/j.ijmedinf.2012.05.005.

[89] Brath H, Morak J, Kästenbauer T, et al. Mobile health (mHealth) based medication adherence measurement – a pilot trial using electronic blisters in diabetes patients. *Br J Clin Pharmacol*. 2013;76(Suppl. 1):47–55. DOI: 10.1111/bcp.12184.

[90] Haas L, Maryniuk M, Beck J, et al. National standards for diabetes self-management education and support. *Diabetes Care*. 2014;37(Suppl. 1):S144–S153. DOI: 10.2337/dc12-1707.

[91] Azar KMJ, Sukyung Chung M, Wang EJ, et al. Impact of education on weight in newly diagnosed type 2 diabetes: every little bit helps. *PLoS One*. 2015;10(6):e0129348. DOI: 10.1371/journal.pone.0129348.

[92] Izquierdo RE, Knudson PE, Meyer S, Kearns J, Ploutz-Snyder R, Weinstock RS. A comparison of diabetes education administered through telemedicine versus in person. *Diabetes Care*. 2003;26(4):1002–1007. DOI: 10.2337/diacare.26.4.1002.

[93] Saffari M, Ghanizadeh G, Koenig HG. Health education via mobile text messaging for glycemic control in adults with type 2 diabetes: a systematic review and meta-analysis. *Prim Care Diabetes*. 2014;8(4):275–285. DOI: 10.1016/j.pcd.2014.03.004.

[94] Han Y, Faulkner MS, Fritz H, et al. A pilot randomized trial of text-messaging for symptom awareness and diabetes knowledge in adolescents with type 1 diabetes. *J Pediat Nurs*. 2015;30(6):850–861. DOI: 10.1016/j.pedn.2015.02.002.

[95] Fijacko N, Brzan PP, Stiglic G. Mobile applications for type 2 diabetes risk estimation: a systematic review. *J Med Syst*. 2015;39(10):124. DOI: 10.1007/s10916-015-0319-y.

[96] Lee R, Wong TY, Sabanayagam C. Epidemiology of diabetic retinopathy, diabetic macular edema and related vision loss. *Eye Vis*. 2015;2:17. DOI: 10.1186/s40662-015-0026-2.

[97] American Diabetes Association. Microvascular complications and foot care. Sec. 9. In Standards of Medical Care in Diabetes—2015. *Diabetes Care*. 2015;38(Suppl. 1):S58–S66. DOI: 10.2337/dc15-S012.

[98] Bourouis A, Feham M, Hossain MA, Zhang L. An intelligent mobile based decision support system for retinal disease diagnosis. *Decis Support Syst*. 2014;59(1):341–350. DOI: 10.1016/j.dss.2014.01.005.

[99] Shojaiefard A, Khorgami Z, Larijani B. Independent risk factors for amputation in diabetic foot. *Int J Diabetes Dev Ctries*. 2008;28(2):32–37. DOI: 10.4103/0973-3930.43096.

[100] Hazenberg CE, van Baal JG, Manning E, Bril A, Bus SA. The validity and reliability of diagnosing foot ulcers and pre-ulcerative lesions in diabetes using advanced digital photography. *Diabetes Technol Ther*. 2010;12(12):1011–1017. DOI: 10.1089/dia.2010.0088.

[101] Foltynski P, Ladyzynski P, Wojcicki JM. A new smartphone-based method for wound area measurement. *Artif Organs*. 2014;38(4):346–352. DOI: 10.1111/aor.12169.

[102] Trief P, Morin P, Izquierdo R, et al. Depression and glycemic control in elderly ethnically diverse patients with diabetes. *Diabetes Care*. 2006;29(4):830–835.

[103] Baasterlar KMP, Pouwer F, Cuijpers P, Riper H, Snoek FJ. Web-based depression treatment for type 1 and type 2 diabetic patients. *Diabetes Care*. 2011;34:320–325. DOI: 10.2337/dc10-1248.

[104] Kwan RYC, Lai CKY. Can smartphones enhance telephone-based cognitive assessment (TBCA)? *Int J Environ Res Public Health*. 2013;10:7110–7125. DOI: 10.3390/ijerph10127110.

[105] Markle Foundation. Connecting for health. A public-private collaborative. The Personal Health Working Group Final Report. [Internet]. 2003. Available from: http://www.providersedge.com/ehdocs/ehr_articles/The_Personal_Health_Working_Group_Final_Report.pdf [Accessed: 2016-02-15].

[106] Shortliffe EH, Cimino JJ. Biomedical Informatics: Computer Applications in Health Care and Biomedicine. 4th ed. London: Springer-Verlag; 2014. DOI: 10.1007/978-1-4471-4474-8.

[107] Sevick MA, Zickmund S, Korytkowski M, et al. Design, feasibility, and acceptability of an intervention using personal digital assistant-based self-monitoring in managing type 2 diabetes. *Contemp Clin Trials*. 2008;29(3):396–409. DOI: 10.1016/j.cct.2007.09.004.

[108] Vuong A V, Huber JC, Brolin JN, et al. Factors affecting acceptability and usability of technological approaches to diabetes self-management: a case study. *Diabetes Technol Ther*. 2012;14(12):1178–1182. DOI: 10.1089/dia.2012.0139.

[109] Scheibe M, Reichelt J, Bellmann M, Kirch W. Acceptance factors of mobile apps for diabetes by patients aged 50 or older: a qualitative study. *Med 2 0*. 2015;4(1):e1. DOI: 10.2196/med20.3912.

[110] Rabbi M, Pfammatter A, Zhang M, Spring B, Choudhury T. Automated personalized feedback for physical activity and dietary behavior change with mobile phones: a randomized controlled trial on adults. *JMIR mHealth uHealth*. 2015;3(2):e42. DOI: 10.2196/mhealth.4160.

[111] Pulman A, Taylor J, Galvin K, Masding M. Ideas and enhancements related to mobile applications to support type 1 diabetes. *J Med Internet Res*. 2013;15(7):e12. DOI: 10.2196/mhealth.2567.

[112] Peterson A. Improving type 1 diabetes management with mobile tools: a systematic review. *J Diabetes Sci Technol*. 2014;8(4):859–864. DOI: 10.1177/1932296814529885.

[113] Ashurst EJ, Jones RB, Abraham C, et al. The diabetes app challenge: user-led development and piloting of internet applications enabling young people with diabetes to set the focus for their diabetes consultations. *Med 2 0*. 2014;3(2):e5. DOI: 10.2196/med20.3032.

[114] Huckvale K, Adomaviciute S, Prieto JT, Leow MK-S, Car J. Smartphone apps for calculating insulin dose: a systematic assessment. *BMC Med*. 2015;13(1):106. DOI: 10.1186/s12916-015-0314-7.

[115] Okazaki S, Castañeda JA, Sanz S, Henseler J. Factors affecting mobile diabetes monitoring adoption among physicians: questionnaire study and path model. *J Med Internet Res*. 2012;14(6):e83. DOI: 10.2196/jmir.2159.

[116] Tiefengrabner M, Domhardt M, Oostingh GJ, et al. Can smartphone-based logging support diabetologists in solving glycemic control problems? *Stud Health Technol Inform*. 2014;198:188–195. DOI: 10.3233/978-1-61499-397-1-188.

[117] Klonoff DC. Using telemedicine to improve outcomes in diabetes—an emerging technology. *J Diabetes Sci Technol*. 2009;3(4):624–628 [Internet]. Available from: http://www.ncbi.nlm.nih.gov/pmc/articles/PMC2769943/ [Accessed: 2016-02-15].

[118] Li R, Zhang P, Barker LE, Chowdhury FM, Zhang X. Cost-effectiveness of interventions to prevent and control diabetes mellitus: a systematic review. *Diabetes Care*. 2010;33(8): 1872–1894. DOI: 10.2337/dc10-0843.

[119] Javitt JC, Reese CS, Derrick MK. Deployment of an mHealth patient monitoring solution for diabetes-improved glucose monitoring leads to reduction in medical expenditure. *US Endocrinol*. 2013;9(2):119–123.

[120] Levin K, Madsen JR, Petersen I, Wanscher CE, Hangaard J. Telemedicine diabetes consultations are cost-effective, and effects on essential diabetes treatment parameters are similar to conventional treatment: 7-year results from the Svendborg Telemedicine Diabetes Project. *J Diabetes Sci Technol*. 2013;7(3):587–595.

[121] Gordon LG, Bird D, Oldenburg B, Friedman RH, Russell AW, Scuffham PA. A cost-effectiveness analysis of a telephone-linked care intervention for individuals with type 2 diabetes. *Diabetes Res Clin Pr*. 2014;104(1):103–111. DOI: 10.1016/j.diabres.2013.12.032.

[122] Henderson C, Knapp M, Fernández JL, et al. Cost effectiveness of telehealth for patients with long term conditions (Whole Systems Demonstrator telehealth questionnaire study): nested economic evaluation in a pragmatic, cluster randomised controlled trial. *BMJ*. 2013;346:f1035. DOI: 10.1136/bmj.f1035.

[123] Zhai YK, Zhu WJ, Cai YL, Sun DX, Zhao J. Clinical- and cost-effectiveness of telemedicine in type 2 diabetes mellitus: a systematic review and meta-analysis. *Med*. 2014;93(28):e312. DOI: 10.1097/MD.0000000000000312.

[124] Graschew G, Rakowsky S. Telemedicine Techniques and Applications. Intech. [Internet]. 2011. Available from: http://www.intechopen.com/books/telemedicine-techniques-and-applications [Accessed: 2016-02-15]. DOI: 10.5772/724

[125] Keith-Hynes P, Guerlain S, Mize B, et al. DiAs user interface: a patient-centric interface for mobile artificial pancreas systems. *J Diabetes Sci Technol*. 2013;7(6):1416–1426. DOI: 10.1177/193229681300700602.

9

The Practice of Medicine in the Age of Information Technology

Mark Dominik Alscher and Nico Schmidt

Abstract

Regarding the practice of medicine, we have to face the chances and challenges of all aspects of e-Health; however, the term "digitalization" is broader and spanning all aspects. However, the digitalization of medicine offers solutions for pressing problem. We know the factors that lead to excellence in medicine. Without the right amount of experiences based on a solid ground of knowledge, no excellence is achievable. The problem, nowadays, is that due to restriction of working hours, to the goals of life ("life-work-balance") and the restrictions of Generation Y, almost no education in medicine is spanning the needed 10,000 h experiences in practical medicine for excellence. Therefore, we will see the fading of medical excellence, if we could not establish other systems. A solution can be searched in decision-support systems. However, a requirement before is the need of a digitalization of all health data. We surely do not have enough evidences for all aspects of the practice of medicine, the intuition is fading away and therefore, we have to look around for other solutions. Big data generated by the digitalization of all health data could be the problem solver. In combination, IT will help to improve the quality of care.

Keywords: quality, practice of medicine, digitalization, health care, intuition, big data, randomized controlled trial (RCT)

1. Introduction

Nowadays we found a lot of changes of the frame works for all professions. The terms "digitalization," "Internet of Things," "disruption," and "big data" cover some aspects of these changes on different hierarchical levels. Regarding the practice of medicine, we have to face the chances and challenges of all aspects of e-Health; however, the term "digitalization" is broader and spanning all aspects [1]. In the following chapter, I try to highlight some aspects especially in the face of practical medicine.

2. Excellence in the practice of medicine

We know the factors that lead to excellence in medicine. Without the right amount of experiences based on a solid ground of knowledge, no excellence is achievable. However, without knowledge and without the ability for processing the experiences, excellence cannot be found [2]. Therefore, experiences alone are not the key to excellence [3]. It is the combination of genius, knowledge base, and experiences. Simon and Chase have found for master chess player that 10 years of practice are necessary [4]. In that time period, around 50,000 different patterns are stored that are essential for the intuitive part of the game. Ericsson was able to extend these findings to musicians and physicians [2]. For excellence, you must be worked in practice for about 10,000 h.

However, let us have a closer look to excellence in the practice of medicine. Colleagues were asked what makes the difference regarding excellence in their colleagues [5]. They gave four factors:

1. Extensive practical experiences.

2. Master in taking the medical history from patients.

3. Precise and critical integration of all information into the process of diagnosis reasoning.

4. Continuous learning of clinical practice.

In internal medicine, the process of diagnostic reasoning is key to excellence [6]. This process can be divided into two parts:

System 1: Intuition

System 2: Analysis

Both have different properties (**Table 1**). For the doctor in the practice of health care, due to time pressure and the big number of patients and problems a typical doctor has to treat, handle, and solve in short time, the system 1 (intuition) is the only practical way, that is in most part confined to the amount of experiences made before. However, from time to time,

System 1: Intuition	System 2: Analysis
Experimental-induction	Hypothesis-deduction
Rational limitations	Rational unlimited
Heuristic	Normative
Pattern recognition	Robust decisions
Modular ("hard-wired") decisions	Critical-logical thinking
Guidance by pattern recognition	Decision trees
Gut feeling	Logical reasoning

Table 1. Medical decision-making after Croskerry [6].

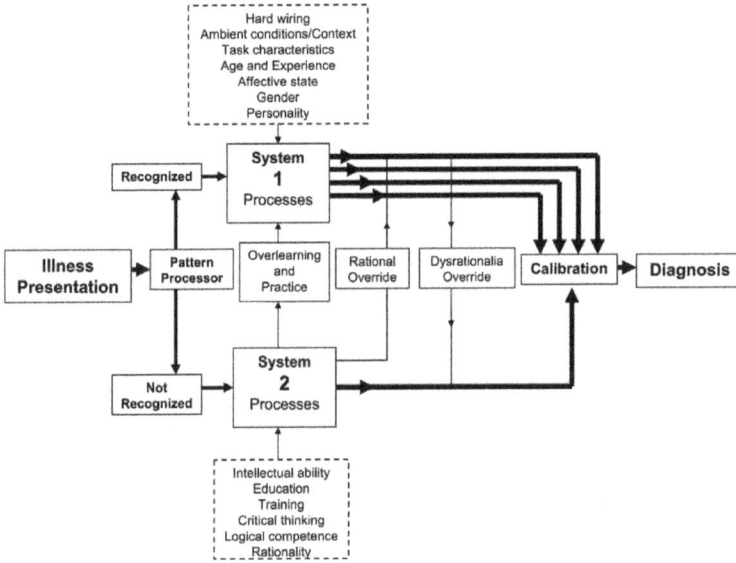

Figure 1. Combination of System 1 and System 2 in diagnostic reasoning [6].

the doctor will face a problem, he cannot solve by intuition, then he has to go to system 2 (analysis), that is time-consuming. Ideal would be an automatic adjustment of both systems in all decision-making during the process of diagnostic reasoning (**Figure 1**).

The problem nowadays is, that due to restriction of working hours, to the goals of life ("life-work-balance") and the restrictions of Generation Y, almost no education in medicine is spanning the mentioned 10,000 h experiences in practical medicine. Therefore, we will see the fading of medical excellence, if we could not establish other systems to replace system 1. The United States was leading in guarantee excellence in medicine by education since the days of Flexner [7]. The base of the excellence, however, was the precise and holistic learning of the medical knowledge base [8]. This is under pressure [9–11].

A solution can be searched in decision-support systems. However, before we need a digitalization of all health data. Electronic patient records are the key to accomplish that task [12]. Since we do not have the holistic solution, interfaces, and standards for that interfaces are highly needed [13, 14]. The analysis of data from the health system, often called "big data," is confined on a solution to those issues. Algorithms should give help in a world of overwhelming information load for the doctor and should release him from the pain of long working hours. This is the promise of big data from the viewpoint of the practitioner.

3. Big data versus randomized controlled trials (RCT)

Measurement of quality in diagnostic reasoning and decision-making is the evidence-based decision, based on precise evidences generated, at best, in randomized controlled trial (RCTs) [15]. RCTs revolutionized medicine and yearly we get the evidences from 40,000 trials [16]. However, we surely do not have enough evidences for all aspects of the practice of medicine,

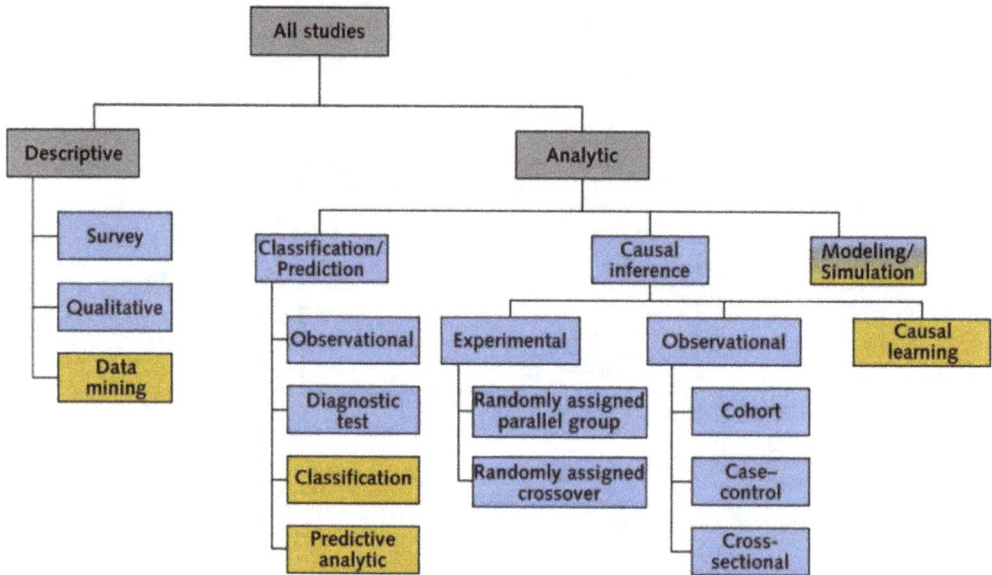

Figure 2. Big data (yellow) and randomized controlled trials (RCT = blue) [17].

the intuition is fading away and therefore, we have to look around for other solutions. Big data could be the problem solver [16]. The combination of RCTs and big data could be key to assure the quality and excellence in medicine in the future (**Figure 2**) [17].

4. Impact of modern machine learning in todays and future medicine practice

Machine learning (ML) technology already has a big impact on today's medical practice. From image classification in radiographs, over epidemic outbreak prediction to genome sequencing, computer algorithms become more and more prominent in modern medicine [18–21]. Projects of major companies like IBM Watson or Google's Deep Mind Health as well as numerous smaller privately and publicly funded research projects are pushing forward to close the gaps between medicine, mathematics, and computer science [22].

For narrow applications with clear regulations, ML algorithms already outperform human capabilities by far and even create new unseen strategies as recently shown by Google's Alpha Go Zero [22]. In this case, a self-trained algorithm mastered the game—more complex than chess—in less than 3 days. Although it has to be mentioned, that the reinforcement learning strategy used in this case might not be suitable in many medical applications, it is an indication of the potential of modern learning algorithms.

A closer look on the technology gives hope, that similar algorithms will not be limited to single and narrow applications, but rather can evolve in order to address the challenges of preserving the knowledge and intuition of experts and improve the quality of RCTs.

The reason for the great potential of machine learning lies in the nature of most of these new algorithms. Regardless whether Random Forests, Support Vector Machine or—most popular today—Deep Neural Networks are applied, they generate their functionality by converting the information contained in thousands and even millions or billions of examples into a highly nonlinear mathematical model [23–25]. In some ways, this is similar to the human learning process and hence may be the appropriate tool for conserving human experience in such models.

With medical data becoming increasingly available in a digitalized form, not only by clinical trials but rather from every day medical practice, the databases grow in size and in depth [26]. This provides the possibility for algorithms not only to become more precise in their predictions but also to become more general in a sense that they can include a huge variety of factors in their decision process. Some aspects of a fading in intuition may so be replaceable by recommendation systems not based on thousands of hours of experience but of millions of decisions already made by experts in the past. Of course, so far, humans are still more efficient in their learning capabilities, but the pure scale of data contained in the algorithmic models may overcome this lack in efficiency. Nevertheless, recommendation systems driven by machine learning algorithms are more likely to complement a physician's intuition in the very near future, than to completely surrogate it.

In a similar manner, classical RCTs can benefit from big data. In semi-supervised learning, for example, datasets of known and unknown outcomes are considered. Here one task is to identify corner cases in the data in order to increase the model accuracy most efficiently [27]. Such methods could help to identify suitable candidates for clinical trials to make their results more robust. Another opportunity in this direction is the analysis of already trained models by feature extraction methods, which may generate promising hypotheses for further investigation in RCT. Finally it is to mention, that although RCTs form the scientific backbone of medicine, factors like publication bias and poor reproducibility rates show, that permanent monitoring of standard clinical practice is necessary [28, 29]. The ability of machine learning algorithms to constantly adapt to new situations, they seem to be predestined for such a controlling task.

5. Conclusion

The excellence in the practice of medicine was bonded to long working hours and a relative small knowledge base. Nowadays, the framework for the practice of medicine is protecting the rights of the individual regarding long working hours, however, in combination with the fast growing of the knowledge base, the practice of medicine is under pressure regarding quality and excellence. The big data approach could help find a solution; however, the digitalization of all data used in the practice of medicine before are warranted. In combination, IT will help to improve the quality of care.

Conflict of interest

There is no "conflict of interest" declaration necessary.

Author details

Mark Dominik Alscher[1*] and Nico Schmidt[2]

*Address all correspondence to: dominik.alscher@rbk.de

1 Robert-Bosch-Hospital, Stuttgart, Germany

2 Bosch - Healthcare Solution GmbH, Waiblingen, Germany

References

[1] Alscher MD. Medicine in the digital age: Let's take the opportunities! Deutsche Medizinische Wochenschrift. 2017;**142**(5):313

[2] Ericsson KA. Deliberate practice and the acquisition and maintenance of expert performance in medicine and related domains. Academic Medicine. 2004;**79**:S70-S81

[3] Galton F. Hereditary Genius: An Inquiry into Its Laws and Consequences. London: Originally published in 1869: Julian Friedman Publishers; 1979. p. 1869

[4] Simon HA, Chase WG. Skill in chess. American Scientist. 1973;**61**:394-403

[5] Mylopoulos M, Lohfeld L, Norman GR, Dhaliwal G, Eva KW. Renowned physicians' perceptions of expert diagnostic practice. Academic Medicine. 2012;**87**(10):1413-1417

[6] Croskerry P. A universal model of diagnostic reasoning. Academic Medicine. 2009;**84**: 1022-1028

[7] Flexner A. Medical education in the United States and Canada. Carnegie Foundation for the Advancement of Teaching. 1910; Bulletin No. 4

[8] Stern DT, Papadakis M. The developing physician—Becoming a professional. New England Journal of Medicine. 2006;**355**:1794-1799

[9] Greenberg A, Verbalis JG, Amin AN, Burst VR, Chiodo 3rd JA, Chiong JR, et al. Current treatment practice and outcomes. Report of the hyponatremia registry. Kidney International. 2015;**88**(1):167-177

[10] Bickel J, Brown AJ. Generation X: Implications for faculty recruitment and development in academic health centers. Academic Medicine. 2005;**80**:205-210

[11] Eckleberry-Hunt J, Tucciarone J. The challenges and opportunities of teaching "generation y". Journal of Graduate Medical Education. 2011;**3**(4):458-461

[12] Kühn S, Haas P. Elektronische Patientenakte: Von der Dokumentenakte zur feingranularen Akte. Dtsch Arztebl International. 2008;**105**(18):20

[13] Henderson ML, Dayhoff RE, Titton CP, Casertano A. Using IHE and HL7 conformance to specify consistent PACS interoperability for a large multi-center enterprise. Journal of Healthcare Information Management. 2006;**20**(3):47-53

[14] Heinze O, Birkle M, Koster L, Bergh B. Architecture of a consent management suite and integration into IHE-based regional health information networks. BMC Medical Informatics and Decision Making. 2011;**11**:58

[15] Windeler J, Antes G, Behrens J, Donner-Banzhoff N, Lelgemann M. Randomised controlled trials (RCTs). Zeitschrift für Evidenz, Fortbildung und Qualität im Gesundheitswesen. 2008;**102**(5):321-325

[16] Angus DC. Fusing randomized trials with big data: The key to self-learning health care systems? Journal of the American Medical Association. 2015;**314**(8):767-768

[17] Sim I. Two ways of knowing: Big data and evidence based medicine. Annals of Internal Medicine. 2016;**164**:262-263

[18] DePristo MA, Banks E, Poplin R, Garimella KV, Maguire JR, Hartl C, et al. A framework for variation discovery and genotyping using next-generation DNA sequencing data. Nature Genetics. 2011;**43**(5):491-498

[19] Akgul CB, Rubin DL, Napel S, Beaulieu CF, Greenspan H, Acar B. Content-based image retrieval in radiology: Current status and future directions. Journal of Digital Imaging. 2011;**24**(2):208-222

[20] Kircher M, Stenzel U, Kelso J. Improved base calling for the Illumina Genome Analyzer using machine learning strategies. Genome Biology. 2009;**10**(8):R83

[21] Penedo MG, Carreira MJ, Mosquera A, Cabello D. Computer-aided diagnosis: A neural-network-based approach to lung nodule detection. IEEE Transactions on Medical Imaging. 1998;**17**(6):872-880

[22] Gibney E. What Google's winning Go algorithm will do next. Nature. 2016;**531**(7594): 284-285

[23] Basu S, Kumbier K, Brown JB, Yu B. Iterative random forests to discover predictive and stable high-order interactions. Proceedings of the National Academy of Sciences of the United States of America. January 19, 2018;**2017**:11236. (published ahead of print)

[24] Goodfellow I, Yoshua B, Courville A. Deep Learning. Cambridge: MIT press; Springer-Verlag New York. 2016. http://www.springer.com/978-0-387-77241-7

[25] Steinwart I, Andreas C. Support Vector Machines. New York: Springer-Verlag, Springer Science & Business Media; 2008

[26] Bellazzi R, Blaz Z. Predictive data mining in clinical medicine: Current issues and guidelines. International Journal of Medical Informatics. 2008;**77**(2):81-97

[27] Cohn D, Rich C, McCallum A. Semi-supervised clustering with user feedback. Constrained Clustering: Advances in Algorithms, Theory, and Applications. 2003;**4**(1):17-32

[28] Mobley A, Linder SK, Braeuer R, Ellis LM, Zwelling L. A survey on data reproducibility in cancer research provides insights into our limited ability to translate findings from the laboratory to the clinic. PLoS One. 2013;**8**(5):e63221

[29] Easterbrook PJ, Berlin JA, Gopalan R, Matthews DR. Publication bias in clinical research. Lancet. 1991;**337**(8746):867-872

10

Mobile Health Monitoring

Niloofar Mohammadzadeh and Reza Safdari

Abstract

Chronic diseases impose heavy burden and costs on the health industry in many countries. Suitable health procedures, management, and prevention of disease by continuous monitoring through modern technologies can lead to a decrease in health costs and improve people empowerment. Applying remote medical diagnosis and monitoring system based on mobile health systems can help significantly reduce health care costs and correct performance management particularly in chronic disease management. In this chapter, mHealth opportunities in patient monitoring with the introduction of various systems specifically in chronic disease are expressed. Also mHealth challenges in patient monitoring in general and specific aspects are identified. Some of the general challenges include threats to confidentiality and privacy, and lack of information communication technology (ICT), and mobile infrastructure. In specific aspect, some difficulties include lack of system interoperability with electronic health records and other IT tools, decrease in face-to-face communication between doctor and patient, ill-functioning of system that leads to medical errors and negative effects on care outcomes, patients, and personnel, and factors related to the telecommunication industry include reliability and sudden interruptions of telecommunication networks.

Keywords: monitor, challenge, advantage, mobile health, chronic disease

1. Introduction

Information technology, as a powerful tool, is the most important factor in increasing the efficiency and effectiveness of organizations. Various industries in order to maintain their existence in the current competitive environment and promotion of their outcomes have taken effective steps toward the use of these technologies. The health care industry is no exception from this rule. Different countries consider the information technology to promote the devel-

opment of health information and health system outcomes with regard to the importance of care industry, direct and indirect impacts on various aspects of community development [1].

Advent of mobile devices with capabilities of caring handy and easy is one of the modern effects of IT that application of them is growing especially in the industrial sector. Some of the mobile devices include cell phones, smart phones (mobile phones processing capabilities, storage, and intelligence communications), and personal digital assistants (PDA). These devices are equipped with communication capabilities such as the ability to connect through GSM/GPRS, Wireless LAN, and Bluetooth networks; hence their utilization will provide comfort for their users.

Using mobile devices seems inevitable because the health industry is facing challenges such as resource constraints like focusing resources on specific areas, for example, in large cities [2], rising health care costs, the need for immediate access to various health care data types such as audio, video, text for early detection and treatment of patients, especially in emergency situations, and difficult in rural areas, and increasing remote aid in telemedicine and home care [3].

A study in Denmark on the necessity of using mobile devices in hospital wards showed hospital staffs want to use mobile devices because of the need to participate in different physical locations, have instant access to information, and immediately contact specific individuals while serving the patients [4].

Easy to carry and quick access to information on mobile devices make them perfect tools for health care providers. Mobile devices provide opportunities and play an important role in consulting, diagnosis, treatment [5], medical education and research [6], conducting quick access to information during shift change sectors [7], chronic disease management [8], patient empowerment [9], rapid establishment of communication regardless of distance restraints [10], and lead to increase efficiency, effective management measures, and promotion of health achievements [11].

In a similar investigation at a cancer treatment center in Spain, it was found that short telephone calls for 3–5 min between medical staff and patients decreased emergency department visits and patients' visit to the center by 24–42% [12].

Wakadha et al. in Kenya showed in rural western Kenya mobile phone-based strategies and short message services (SMSs) are potentially useful to deliver reminders, cash transfers, and achieve high, timely, and sustainable immunization coverage [13].

Today, the use of health information systems which are fixed terminals just does not seem sufficient. Because these systems do not provide necessary information for health care providers in real time, the continuous rapid delivery of services to patients is interrupted [7]. Studies indicate that lack of timely access to patient information [14], discontinuity of the communication, and lack of coordination between service provider and health care team members [15] are the main causes of medical errors. The use of mobile devices in terms of emergency situation and telemedicine is crucial for instant access to patient information, entry and data processing of medical records on time, and when the shift health care services changes for providers of health services [16, 17].

The use of mobile health programs is very interesting due to numerous benefits; however using these tools is still has many challenges. One of the approaches that significantly helps to reduce barriers is survey of advantages and obstacles of mobile devices usage. Studies of opportunities and strengthening them and identifying problems help to design proper planning and a roadmap for promoting the achievements of mobile health systems.

We begin the following section by discussing about the necessity of mHealth in chronic disease management especially in diabetes. In next part, the advantages of mobile health in patient monitoring at two groups of agent and nonagent based system are explained. After that, we describe the challenges of patient monitoring based on mobile health systems in general and specific aspects. Finally, we explain one project as a case study about developing framework for agent-based diabetes disease management system in national level based on user's perspective.

2. Chronic disease management: necessity of mHealth approach

In most countries, chronic diseases lead to high health care costs and reduced productivity of people in society [18]. Diabetes is a common chronic disease in nearly all countries [19] and one of the most common metabolic diseases with an increasing incidence. More than 15% of national health budget is dedicated to diabetic care [20]. Diabetes as a hidden disease causes many complications such as various types of heart disease, nephropathy, retinopathy, and so on, thus imposing direct and indirect high costs to society. In Iran, diabetes complications contributed to 53% of the aggregate excess direct costs of diabetes [21].

The quality of diabetic care improves, on one hand, if patient monitoring is done according to the nutrition program and physician orders that are placed with high quality [22]. On the other hand, fast and accurate diagnosis due to continuous monitoring through information communication technology (ICT) devices leads to prevent the death of diabetic patients [23]. Telemedicine as a main tool to remote health care delivery and home care has advantages such as real-time access to health information [3, 24], reducing medical errors [25], and increasing coordination and cooperation among health care teams [1], reducing travel of patients and their families in remote area [26], and useful education tool for patients, their families, and health care providers [27]. Therefore, this technology has a very important role in decreasing costs and taking appropriate management actions especially in diabetes management and other chronic disease [28, 29]. The use of innovative technologies such as mobiles to enjoy the most advantages of telemedicine is necessary. Mobile health systems can be a good option for health care industry because of reducing delay and error in patient treatment, avoiding test duplication, providing remote and timely access of health care professionals to organizational database and patient information especially in the emergency situations [26, 30].

3. mHealth opportunities in patient monitoring

In this study, electronic chronic disease management systems based on mobile technology were divided into two types: agent-based systems and nonagent-based systems. Some electronic health system based on agent that studied in this research are:

- Integrated mobile information system (IMIS) in Sweden through mobile network communication platform provides the possibility of self-treatment and home care supervision for the diabetic patient. This system has six databases: (1) database for patients including all necessary information about diabetic health care centers, medical journals, dietary, food habits, etc.; (2) database for care providers containing whole information about physicians, home care services; (3) tools or instrument base including all aiding functions for implementation health care such as visit reserve, alarms, monitor; (4) community network include all relevant actors like diabetes centers, consultation, and so on links to each other; (5) database for laws, rules, and norms applied in health care including all legal and cultural documents about health care therefore can help with privacy, security, and quality of services; and (6) database for labor division in health care that determines who (health care provider) and what to do, this ensures to provide all the different patient needs [31–34].

- M2DM Telemedicine Service system in European Commission with the aim of presenting correct knowledge to correct people at correct time. Two types of agents are used in the M2DM: (1) communication server that is responsible for communication between different user terminals and (2) application server that is responsible for data analysis and processing. The architecture of this system includes multiaccess server, common database management system (DBMS), multiaccess organizer, communication server agent, and application server agent. The overall goal of M2DM is increasing quality of care through improving communication between patient and health care providers [35, 36].

Also other nonagent and useful e-health system survey in this section are:

- Personal Health Monitor (PHM), University of Sydney, Australia, uses PHM with focus on e-health services based on mobile devices at local level for monitoring patient in various situations therapeutic. Architecture of PHM comprises BAN devices, sensor front end, mobile base unit, back end [37, 38].

- Mobi Health and Body Area Network [BAN], most of the European countries use this system for remote patient monitoring and provide appropriate care to patients. A consortium of 14 European countries was set up to implement the health system project [39]. This project has been implemented in four countries: Spain, the Netherlands, Sweden, and Germany for different groups of patients, including home care and trauma, where the patient is located in an outdoor center. It aims to improve patients' quality of life and freedom in their daily activities and complete mobility. BAN devices, sensor front end, mobile base unit, and back end are the architecture elements [37, 40–42].

- In 2009, the first virtual diabetes clinic in Iran was inaugurated at Tehran University of Medical Sciences with common database, multiaccess server architecture, and organizer server is discussed in this chapter [43–45].

Some benefits of nonagent-based system in **Table 1** include disease prevention improvement, better self-care, increased life style quality, reduce unnecessary [re]hospitalizations, possibility of teleconsultation, and provide patients mobility to perform their daily works. Diabetes virtual clinic is used for monitoring system and as a proper tool that provides up-to-date, useful, relevant, and accurate information used to suitable self-care and remote health care. Access of all users to useful and necessary information about prevention, treatment, side effects, and ways to control diabetes and providing teleconsultation are most important advantages of a virtual clinic.

In PHM, data processing is done locally, and in Mobi health BAN processing can be done at server side. Some of the studied system implemented on PDA and mobile phone platforms,

System	Multi-agent	Development method	Usage	Access to data technology	Devices	Type of communication	Some of the capabilities
Integrated mobile information system (IMIS) [31–34]	Yes	User centered	Diabetic home-care, chronic, elderly care	Internet, SMS	Mobile computers, Nokia communicator, PDA, stationary computers home	Wired/wireless communications	(1) Integrate and co-ordinate various healthcare activities under the same fundamental activity system, (2) self-treatment, (3) preparation before face-to-face diagnoses, (4) access and share the same and right information on right time for a seamless co-operative work among organizations and among persons
M2DM Telemedicine service [35, 36]	Yes	Merging of telemedicine with knowledge management	Diabetes	Internet, WebTV, SMS, WAP, GPRS	Mobile computers, PDA, palmtops,	Wired/wireless communications	(1) Telecare, (2) visit management, (3) management of HER, (4) automatic generation of reports, (5) intelligent alarms, (6) tele-education, (7) intelligent knowledge management
PHM: Personal health monitor [37, 38]	No	Local, personal mHealth services	Cardiology, general well-being, chronic disease management, rehabilitation, monitoring: cardiac rhythm monitoring, cardiac rehabilitation, primary prevention	GPS, GSM, SMS, 3G, Internet	Mobile phone	Wired/wireless communications (Bluetooth)	(1) Triage of life data which can be personalized to the application domain, (2) data processing Viewing and reporting for physician, (3) physician can update sensor thresholds, (4) remote management of PHM equipment and patients, (5) password protected viewing by the patient [limited view], (6) synchronization between MBU and Back End
Mobihealth BAN [37, 40–42]	No	Telemonitoring or teletreatment services	Cardiology, obstetrics, trauma care, rheumatology, psychiatry, pulmonary medicine, gerontology, neurology, telemonitoring, teletreatment	SMS, WIFI, GPRS, Internet, GPS	Mobile phones, PDA, UMTS, Any mobile platform capable of running Java VM and RMI	Wired/wireless communications (Bluetooth)	(1) Application functionality specific to each individual clinical application and patient and HP user requirements, (2) BAN devices have alarm button, (3) viewing, streaming and management services for BANs and BAN data, analysis and interpretation algorithms, alarms, geospatial and location-based services, (4) various security and access control mechanism
Diabetes virtual clinic [43–45]	NO	User center	Diabetes	SMS, WIFI, Internet	Computers, mobile, PDA	Wired/wireless communications	(1) Self-care, (2) e-learning, (3) tele consultation, (4) integrate and co-ordinate various health care activities under the same fundamental activity system

Table 1. Electronic health system characteristics in chronic disease management.

and others implemented on mobile phone. Sending alarm to patients and health care providers and identify place of patients with GPS are possible in some of the studied systems. Wired and wireless communication in all system studied can be useful especially when mobility is desired.

Recently, health care systems shift toward fast achieving to right decision to solve problems with spending least costs. So to reach this goal, find suitable information from useful and reliable resources in the fastest time and the least possible effort for information searching, analyzing, and filtering is very important.

This requires high interoperability among different professionals and systems in various places. In fact for providing effective health care and shared information, all actions need to be coordinated. Facilitated decision making requires interoperability and effective communications between professionals. Finding standard software as a suitable solution for complex health challenges is not easy. Electronic health systems must be proactive in anticipating the health information needs and supporting communications.

Because of potential capabilities of agent technology like mobility [44], autonomy, interoperability, scalability and re-configurability, integrating disparate systems, improving distributed data and resources management, handling the complexity of solutions, modeling and organizing the interrelationships between components [31–36, 46–51], is very valuable tool for telemedicine and telecare.

Agent-based systems in this table increase quality of care management. For example in IMIS system, tasks were delegated and all users in each level can communicate with one another and share the relevant data. In M2DM system, various analytic ways through knowledge agent were combined and used for the identification of abnormal situations. Also sending alarms, analysis results and real-time feedbacks to users are some benefits of this system [31–36]. Agents can be implemented on portable and mobile devices like PDA and use web services to interact with other systems.

The IMIS platforM is based on the Internet and will be accessible by PC or wireless network PDA. Accessibility should be regulated by groups of users. Each step in this system by the user is followed with instant feedback. M2DM can be activated in three ways: based on user needs, with receiving data, and by system. This system uses inexpensive and widely accepted technologies. This system applies technologies such as WEB, WEB TV, and SMS that are supported with computers or mobile terminals. Also it combines innovative and advanced technologies like PDA, WAP, GPRS, and PALMTOPS. The use of such technologies is limited in small groups of users because of costs, accessibilities, and user skills required.

Overall, according to multiagent health systems advantages in comparison to other type of systems and challenges in health care systems especially in diabetics care management, it can be said that the use of agent technology as a new and modern technology to reach full advantages of telemedicine and telehealth is essential, and health systems in the world must move toward agent-based applications.

4. mHealth challenges in patient monitoring

Although mHealth technology has a key role in health care systems, yet its uptake has faced with general and specific challenges. Some problems in general dimension include organizational challenges like organizational culture, support of high-level management; technological barriers such as lack of ICT and mobile infrastructure [52]; human challenges, for example, lack of trained and skilled personnel at health care centers in this field [28], user attitudes, technology acceptance [53, 54], user characteristics like age, economic, social, and educational status [55]; and threats to confidentiality and privacy, legal, ethical, and administrative barriers, costs of system implementation and maintenance [28], dependence on IT [56], the cost of updating, costly modern systems [57], sufficient investment, delays in implementation and providing electronic devices and software [58]. Some barriers from specific aspects also include problems in interoperability between other health systems and information technology tools, poor and inappropriate design and implementation [59], effect on face-to-face communication between health care providers and patient [60], causes omission of human relationship and the negative effects of technology on relationships between individuals and social processes [56], designing of mHealth services content [55], failure to meet targets [58], virtual information control [61], medical errors due to malfunctioning of system [62], fault documentation [59] like data manipulation and rewriting, misrepresentation, and violation of patients' legal rights. Difficulties related to telecommunication industry such as reliability, sustainability of connections, sudden interruptions of telecommunication networks [63], device and sensor type that can be used, type of data and language presentation [56], scalability in terms of data rate, power and energy consumption; antenna design, quality of service, energy efficiency [64, 65] wearable devices weight, type of devices that used for patient monitoring that sometimes lead to problem in data processing, accuracy of gathering information depends on where data were collected, and user training to use wearable system [66].

As aforementioned, one of the items that can help mHealth infrastructure development is application of agent-based systems in patient monitoring. We perform research in Iran about diabetes as one of the most challenging chronic diseases. The aim of this research is developing framework for agent-based diabetes disease management system through mHealth according to user's perspective. Some of the most important results are as follows:

5. Case study

Endocrinology and metabolism research institute of Tehran University of Medical Sciences in collaboration with Health Information Management Research center in this University conducted a research in 2012–2013. The goal of this research was to provide a model based on mobile health and agent technology in national level for diabetes management information. This framework must have capabilities of agent and support decision-making, create alerts and remote monitoring of patient status, and provide appropriate treatment and preventive recommendations for diabetes.

A questionnaire was designed with a study of library resources and operation of major organizations in and out of the country and interviews with relevant medical experts.

To determine the validity of a questionnaire distributed among experts in three areas after analyzing the results, the reliability was evaluated. Questionnaire includes three parts. First section covers personal identification. Second section questions about the general features of agent-based systems for the management of diabetes. Finally, third section examines the specific features of the systems in hospitals. At the end of questionnaire, an open question captured the opinions of experts concerning diabetes management system structure based on agent technology. Results of the questionnaires were analyzed with SPSS17 and were plotted with FREEPLANE mind map software. Finally, essential agents according to tasks of diabetes management system were determined. Some of the results obtained from this study are explained below.

Most diabetics must monitor and measure their blood glucose levels during the day. Like measuring glucose after every insulin injection and record it, along with the amount of daily insulin injections and diet and information about their lifestyle. Using information technology tools and a telemedicine system helps process management of health service, allows real-time monitoring, and provides early treatment for diabetes. To achieve these goals are possible through multi agent systems can be performed with using different agents. Based on this study, a diabetes management system has necessary business process including:

1. Information processing

2. Monitor patient status

3. Consultation

4. Diagnosis

5. Archiving relevant documents and patient records

6. Decision support system

7. Appropriate interface for communication between patients and health electronic systems

8. Monitoring operations and service delivery and allocate tasks to perform

Important services and processes through the implementation of software systems in the field of diabetes management from the experts, perspectives are plotted (see **Figure 1**).

From the experts' point of view in this research, proposed framework must be used in priority order for home care, outpatient, and inpatient. Best development method to such system in priority order is telemonitoring or teletreatment services, user centered, merging of telemedicine with knowledge management, local and personal health services. Access to data technology in this system in priority order is mobile, SMS, Email, Internet in devices including web, phone, WIFI, and PDA. Also according to studies, to provide better health services, the communication should be used through wired or wireless connection tools.

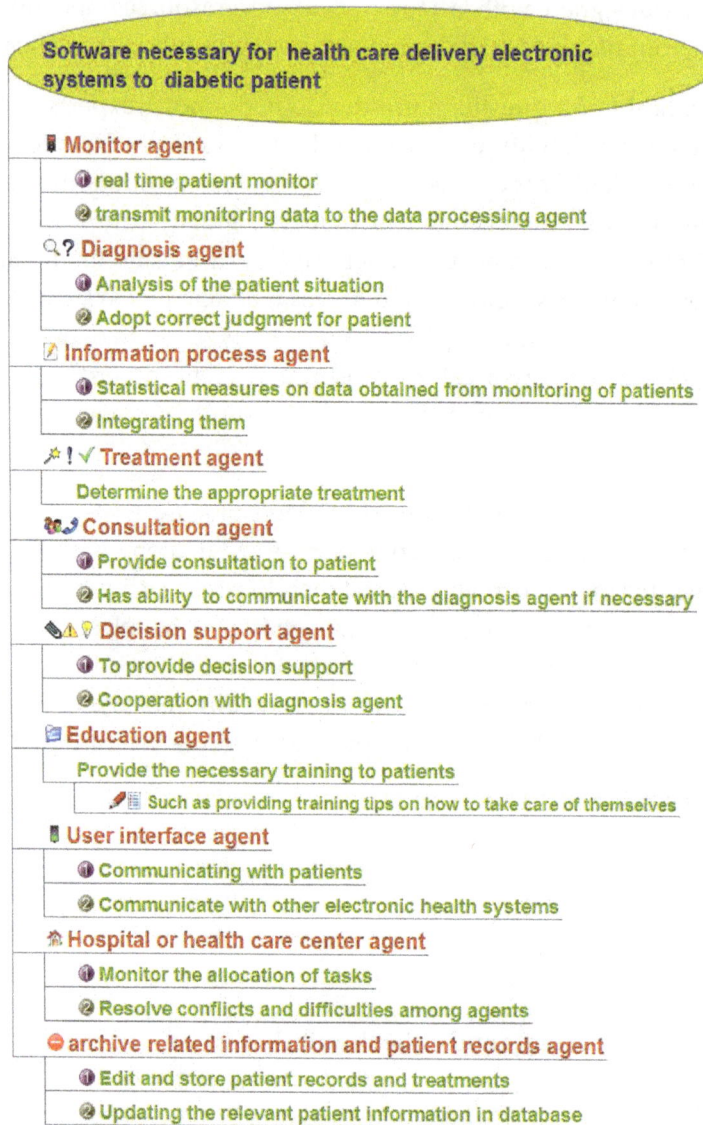

Figure 1. Software necessary for health care delivery electronic systems for diabetic patients.

Capabilities for diabetes management system based on agent technology in medical centers and hospitals section based on research findings with FREE PLANE software are depicted in **Figure 2**.

Also capabilities for diabetes management system based on agent technology for health care personnel based on research findings are: (1) remote education, (2) knowledge management, (3) intelligent alarms, and (4) electronic health records management. From the experts' point of view, diabetes management system based on agent technology must have these abilities for patients in the following order: (1) remote education, (2) intelligent alarms and reminders, (3) patient monitoring, (4) self-management, and (5) determining the exact location of medical centers and hospitals.

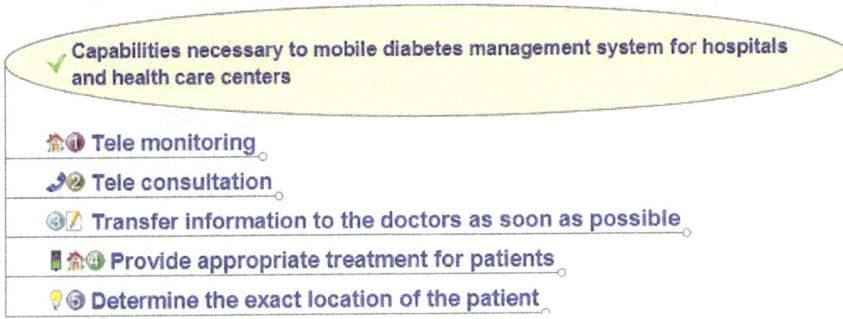

Figure 2. Capabilities necessary for mobile diabetes management system for hospitals and health care centers.

Experts in this research believed that proposed framework must be delivered through remote education to diabetes patients. Suitable remote education formats recommended in order of priority include imaging, audio, model questions and answers, and text tutorials. Patients on remote education should be able to search based on their needs, choice of content, and personalization and have the possibility to download the contents.

The weakness of this project is that benefits of experts surveyed only from health information management, software and physician in diabetic research center fields. To design and implement more appropriate conceptual models, involved experts should be from various fields such as telecommunication and addressing various aspects are very helpful, and the gained result is a more practical.

6. Discussion

Nowadays real-time access to reliable and proper information in order to deliver continuous health care and increase quality of care is very much in demand. So in order to achieve this goal, interoperability and coordination among providers involved in patient treatment for exchange of health information is a critical need. Chronic disease management especially diabetes based on IT tools has impressive benefits and some challenges. In this chapter, diabetic management system is classified into two groups: agent-based system and nonagent-based system.

Better self-care, improved prevention, increased quality life style, and teleconsultation are most important benefits of nonagent-based systems. Also these systems confront some challenges. The use of agent systems as a modern technology to decrease these barriers and take full advantages of telemedicine is essential and health systems must move using agent-based applications. In the second group, some of the benefits of agent technology in telemedicine services delivery include providing immediate feedback to patients, promoting interaction of the patient with organization that provides remote health care, reinforcing their motivation for the use of telemedicine systems and patients, and clinicians focusing on abnormal data that will prevent future occurrence of dangerous situations.

Agent-based systems improve interoperability, maintain the autonomy of the collaborating participants, communicate between themselves for exchanging health information, provide expert knowledge management, and improve e-learning. Multiagent systems are inherently compatible with mobile devices. Architecture of these systems allows high interoperability and quality information management and appropriate sharing data. Diabetes virtual clinic in Iran is one of the nonagent systems that provides some important health services to the people and assist them to improve knowledge about diabetes care. This system needs to move toward the use of artificial intelligence tools and expert systems like agents for further development and increased capabilities. Our finding in 2013 research showed that to accelerate the development of diabetes management systems based on artificial intelligence tools, we must consider these items: (1) promote organizational cultural, (2) note to suitable technical infrastructure, (3) provide appropriate security and privacy, (4) adequate investment, (5) user participation, and (6) involvement of private sections. Also note to structure, proper system, and database design that can support different kinds of training formats and tasks, and provide backup are very important. Ease of use and user friendliness of system should be considered especially for elderly people. Also design of drug and injection reminders for patients in addition to the built-in alarm system is a key factor.

It should be noted that the use of agent systems only with technical view does not lead to elimination of obstacles. In delivering health care to diabetic patients or other chronic disease patients, paying attention to human aspect and social dimension is very important. Some users dislike computers and do not trust them. So these challenges in designing diabetes system based on mobile devices must be considered. In other words, note to all dimensions for implementation of mobile health systems especially agent system like user satisfaction, user acceptance, costs, motivation, structural and organizational factors, and standards, individual's affordability, identification challenges and opportunity, and so on are necessary. Also accelerating the application and implementation of multiagent diabetes management systems and use of mobile devices need to development of strategies to encourage health care providers for make greater use of mobile devices in deliver health care services to patients and providing the necessitate infrastructure and appropriate readiness. Stakeholders' support to apply of agent technology is essential.

7. Conclusion

Application of electronic health systems for patient monitoring has significant advantages. The use of these tools in health care organizations needs to study about these technologies, compare their benefits and limitations, note to organizational resources including human, technical, financial; suitable planning, and affordability of these facilities. Determining and decreasing challenges and identifying opportunities that affect on successful implementation of these technologies have critical roles in proper application of each of these systems.

Health care systems based on mobile technology are faced with important limitations such as user attitude and acceptance, budget, technical standard, equipment, and tools required for mobile communication, security and good infrastructure, increasing the accuracy of critical signals, interoperability between different systems, bandwidth limitations, quality of health services, battery life limited tools, and so on.

User acceptance is improved through the provision of advisable training and cultural awareness. It also provides an environment in which innovations in organizations are appreciated. Key factors to increase user acceptance include staff participation and involvement in all stages of the process from planning to implementation, clear and effective communication between managers and all staff members involved in the project, describing the advantages of technology and change management.

Note to important factors such as adequate bandwidth, preparation of standard tools that provide maximum mobility and flexibility for users, decreasing obstacles which interrupt network communications, insurance coverage, and supporting patients who use remote monitoring devices, data encryption while transferring, paying attention to legal and ethical aspects are all necessary in the success of these systems in health care organizations.

8. Future trends

For future work, we suggest that try to provide inexpensive mHealth services, so that more people can use these services. Insurance companies especially in developing countries consider situations and are motivated to cover these types of health care services. Decreased dependence of communication protocols with mobile device types can help generalize and extend the use of mobile health devices.

Acknowledgements

The authors would like to thank the anonymous reviewers for their valuable comments and suggestions, which improved this chapter.

Author details

Niloofar Mohammadzadeh and Reza Safdari*

*Address all correspondence to: rsafdari@tums.ac.ir

Department of Health Information Management, Tehran University of Medical Sciences, Tehran, Iran

References

[1] Safdari R, Mohammadzadeh N. Multi-agent systems and health information management. In 2nd eHospital and Telemedicine Conference. Tehran University of Medical
Sciences. Tehran. Iran. 2011.

[2] Kahn GJ, Yang SJ, Kahn SJ. 'Mobile' health needs and opportunities in developing
countries. Health Affairs 2010.29(2):252–258. doi:10.1377/hlthaff.2009.0965.

[3] Tan J. Medical Informatics: Concepts, Methodologies, Tools, and Applications, Volume
1, Chapter 7.5. Securing Mobile Data Computing in Healthcare, Hershey, New York.
2009. p: 1930.

[4] Bøne E, Hasvold P, Henriksen E, Strandenæs T. Risk analysis of information security
in a mobile instant messaging and presence system for healthcare. International Journal
of Medical Informatics 2007.76:677–687. doi: http://dx.doi.org/10.1016/j.ijmedinf.
2006.06.002

[5] World Health Organization. mHealth New horizons for health through mobile
technologies. 2011. ISBN 978 92 4 156425 0. Available from: http://www.who.int/goe/
publications/goe_mhealth_web.pdf [Accessed: 5 June 2013]

[6] Pawar P, Jones V, van Beijnum BJ, Hermens H. A framework for the comparison of
mobile patient monitoring systems. Journal of Biomedical Informatics 2012.45(3):544–
556. doi: 10.1016/j.jbi.2012.02.007.

[7] Prgomet M, Georgiou A, Westbrook JI. The impact of mobile handheld technology on
hospital physicians' work practices and patient care: a systematic review. Journal of
the American Medical Informatics Association 2009.16:792–801. doi: 10.1197/
jamia.M3215.

[8] Strandbygaard U, Thomsen SF, Backer V. A daily SMS reminder increases adherence
to asthma treatment: a three-month follow-up study. Respiratory Medicine 2010.104(2):
166–171. doi: 10.1016/j.rmed.2009.10.003.

[9] Suter P, Suter WN, Johnston D. Theory-based telehealth and patient empowerment.
Population Health Management 2011.14(2):87–92. doi:10.1089/pop.2010.0013.

[10] Warren I, Weerasinghe T, Maddison R, Wang Y. Odin telehealth: a mobile service
platform for telehealth. Procedia Computer Science 2011.5:681–688. doi:10.1016/j.procs.
2011.07.089.

[11] Bellini P, Boncinelli S, Grossi F, Mangini M, Nesi P, Sequi L. Mobile emergency, an
emergency support system for hospitals in mobile devices: pilot study. JMIR Research
Protocols 2013.2(1):e19. doi:10.2196/resprot.2293.

[12] Ferrer-Roca O, Subirana R. A four-year study of telephone support for oncology patients using a non-supervised call centre. Journal of Telemedicine and Telecare 2002.8(6):331. doi:10.1258/135763302320939211.

[13] Wakadha H, Chandir S, Were Elijah V, Rubin A, Obor D, Levine OS, Gibson DG, Odhiambo F, Laserson KF, Feikin DR. The feasibility of using mobile-phone based SMS reminders and conditional cash transfers to improve timely immunization in rural Kenya. Vaccine 2013.31:987–993. doi:10.1016/j.vaccine.2012.11.093.

[14] Martins M, Henrique G. Mobilizing Health Information to Support Healthcare-related Knowledge Work. INSTICC Press: Portugal. 2009. p. 69

[15] Khairat S, Gong Y. Understanding effective clinical communication in medical errors. Studies in Health Technology Informatics 2010.160(Pt 1):704–708. doi: 10.3233/978-1-60750-588-4-704.

[16] Goldbach H, Chang AY, Kyer A, Ketshogileng D, Taylor L, Chandra A, Dacso M, Kung SJ, Rijken T, Fontelo P, Littman-Quinn R, Seymour AK, Kovarik CL. Evaluation of generic medical information accessed via mobile phones at the point of care in resource-limited settings. Journal of the American Medical Informatics Association 2014.21(1): 37–42. doi:10.1136/amiajnl-2012-001276.

[17] Tubaro M. An organized system of emergency care for patients with myocardial infarction: a reality? Future Cardiology 2010.6(4):483–489. doi:10.2217/fca.10.25.

[18] Engelgau M, Rosenhouse S, El-Saharty S, Mahal A. The economic effect of noncommunicable diseases on households and nations: a review of existing evidence. Journal of Health Communication: International Perspectives 2011.16(2):75–81. doi: 10.1080/10810730.2011.601394.

[19] Zhang P, Zhang X, Brown J, Vistisen D, Sicree R, Shaw J, Nichols G. Global healthcare expenditure on diabetes for 2010 and 2030. Diabetes Research and Clinical Practice 2010.87(3):293–301. doi:10.1016/j.diabres.2010.01.026.

[20] World Health Organization. Global status report on non communicable diseases 2010. World Health Organization 2011 Reprinted 2011. ISBN 978 92 4 156422 9. ISBN 978 92 4 068645 8 (PDF). Available from: http://www.who.int/nmh/publications/ncd_report_full_en.pdf [Accessed 30 June 2013].

[21] Esteghamati A, Khalilzadeh O, Anvari M, Meysamie A, Abbasi M, Forouzanfar M, Alaeddini F. The economic costs of diabetes: a population-based study in Tehran, Iran. Diabetologia 2009.52:1520–1527. doi:10.1007/s00125-009-1398-4.

[22] McAndrew LM, Napolitano MA, Pogach LM, Quigley KS, Shantz K, Vander Veur SS, Foster GD. The impact of self-monitoring of blood glucose on a behavioral weight loss intervention for patients with Type 2 diabetes. The Diabetes Educator 2013.39(3):397–405. doi:10.1177/0145721712449434.

[23] Paré G, Moqadem K, Pineau G, St-Hilaire C. Clinical effects of home tele monitoring in the context of diabetes, asthma, heart failure and hypertension: a systematic review. Journal of Medical Internet Research 2010.12(2):e21. doi:10.2196/jmir.1357.

[24] Barjis J, Kolfschoten G, Maritz J. A sustainable and affordable support system for rural healthcare delivery. Decision Support Systems 2013.56:223–233. doi:10.1016/j.dss. 2013.06.005. Available from: http://dx.doi.org/10.1016/j.dss.2013.06.005 [Accessed 24 June 2013].

[25] Skolnik NS. Electronic Medical Records: A Practical Guide for Primary Care. New York: Springer Humana Press; 2011. p: 1.

[26] Finn N, Bria W. Digital Communication in Medical Practice. London: Springer-Verlag; 2009. p: 70–73.

[27] Toledo FG, Triola A, Ruppert K, Siminerio LM. Telemedicine Consultations: an alternative model to increase access to diabetes specialist care in underserved rural communities. JMIR Research Protocols 2012.1(2):e14. doi:10.2196/resprot.2235.

[28] Khoumbati K, Dwivedi Y, Srivastava A, Lal B. Handbook of Research on Advances in Health Informatics and Electronic Healthcare Applications: Global Adoption and Impact of Information Communication Technologies. Hershey. New York: Medical Information Science Reference; 2010. p: 91, 10, 156.

[29] Safdari R, Mohammadzadeh N. Patient Health Monitoring Through Mobile Health Systems. Lecture in International Conference on 2012 Electronic Health (ICEH 2012). Medical Council of Islamic Republic of Iran. Tehran. Iran.

[30] McDaniel J. Advances in Information Technology and Communication in Health. Amsterdam: IOS Press; 2009. p: 467–471.

[31] Integrated Mobile Information Research. 2010. Available from: http://www.bth.se/research/imis/ [Accessed 4 July 2013]

[32] Shaheen A, Ahmad Khan W. Intelligent Decision Support System in Diabetic eHealth Care From the perspective of Elders. [Master Thesis]. Computer Science. Blekinge Institute of Technology. Sweden. 2009. Available from: http://www.bth.se/fou/cuppsats.nsf/all/89449be91369ee27c12575d60071c747/$file/Master_thesis_asma.pdf [Accessed 4 July 2013]

[33] Zhang P. Multi-agent Systems in Diabetic Health Care. Blekinge Institute of Technology Licentiate Series. Issue 5. Karlskrona: Blekinge Institute of Technology. ISBN: 91-7295-060-9. 2005. Available from: http://www.bth.se/fou/forskinfo.nsf/all/07625d65f3f89ee6c1256fef00220c36?OpenDocument [Accessed 4 July 2013].

[34] Bellazzi R, Carson ER, Cobelli C, Hernando E, Gomez EJ, Nabih-Kamel-Boulos M, Rendschmidt T, Roudsari V, et al. Merging Telemedicine With Knowledge Management: The M2DM Project. Published in: Engineering in Medicine and Biology Society.

Proceedings of the 23rd Annual International Conference of the IEEE, Volume 4, 2001. p: 4117–4120. doi:10.1109/IEMBS.2001.1019762.

[35] Hernando M E, Garsia A, Javiar Perdices F, Torralba V, Gomez E J. del Pozo F. Multi agent architecture for the provision of intelligent telemedicine services in diabetes management. Available from: http://cyber.felk.cvut.cz/EUNITE03-BIO/pdf/EHernando.pdf [Accessed 4 July 2013]

[36] Jones V, Gay V, Leijdekkers P. Body Sensor Networks for Mobile Health Monitoring: Experience in Europe and Australia. Accepted for 4th International Conference on Digital Society, ICDS 2010, February 10–16, 2010, ICDS '10. Fourth International Conference on. Netherlands: Digital Society; 2010.

[37] Leijdekkers P, Gay V. A Self-Test to Detect a Heart Attack Using a Mobile Phone and Wearable Sensors. 21st IEEE International Symposium on Computer-Based Medical Systems; 2008. p: 93-98. ISBN: 978-0-7695-3165-6.

[38] Jones M, Bults G, Konstantas D, Vierhout P. Healthcare PANs: Personal Area Networks for trauma care and home care, Proceedings Fourth International Symposium on Wireless Personal Multimedia Communications. [WPMC], Sept. 9–12, 2001, Aalborg, Denmark. 2001. Available from: http://wpmc01.org/, ISBN 87-988568-0-4.

[39] Otto C, Milenkovic A, Sanders C, Jovanov E.System Architecture of a wireless body area sensor network for ubiquitous health monitoring. Journal of Mobile Multimedia 2006.1(4):307–326.

[40] Halteren Aart V, Bults R, Wac K, Konstantas D, Widya I, Dokovsky N, Koprinkov G, Jones V, Herzog R. Mobile patient monitoring: the MobiHealth system. Journal on Information Technology in Healthcare 2004.2(5):365–373. ISSN 1479-649X.

[41] MobiHealth—Shaping the Future of Healthcare. Available from: http://www.ltu.se/cms_fs/1.90345!/file/Mobihealth%20brochure.pdf [Accessed 4 July 2013].

[42] Inaugurate first diabetes virtual clinic in Iran at Tehran university of medical sciences (in Persian). Available from: http://publicrelations.tums.ac.ir/news/detail.asp?newsID=13114 [Accessed 4 July 2013].

[43] For the first time in Iran, virtual clinic for diabetes opening in Shariati hospital. (in Persian). Available from: http://www.pezeshkan.ir/view.asp?id=99119 [Accessed 4 July 2013].

[44] Diabetes Virtual Clinic. Available from: http://emri.tums.ac.ir/pages/mainpage.asp?I=S54M5P2C1 [Accessed 4 July 2013].

[45] Annicchiarico R, Cortés U, Urdiales C. Agent Technology and e-Health. Switzerland: Birkhäuser Verlag; 2008. p: 141–148.

[46] Isabelle B, Sachin V, Ashlesha J, Lakhmi J.Computational Intelligence in Healthcare 4. Berlin: Springer-Verlag; 2010. p: 25–48.

[47] Sánchez D, Isern D, Rodríguez Á, Moreno A. General purpose agent-based parallel computing. In: Omatu S, Rocha MP, Bravo J, Fernández F, Corchado E, Bustillo A, Corchado JM. [eds.] IWANN. LNCS, Heidelberg: Springer; 2009. vol. 5518, p: 231–238.

[48] Mohammadzadeh N, Safdari R. Artificial intelligence tools in health information management. International Journal of Hospital Research 2012.1(1):65–70.

[49] Isern D, Sánchez D, Moreno A. Agents applied in health care: a review. International Journal of Medical Informatics 2010.79:145–166. doi:10.1016/j.ijmedinf.2010.01.003.

[50] Safdari R, Mohammadzadeh N. Electronic Health Information Systems. Tehran: Mirmah; 2011. p: 152–156 (in Persian).

[51] Cripps H, Standing C. The implementation of electronic health records: a case study of bush computing the Ngaanyatjarra Lands. International Journal of Medical Informatics 2011.80(12):841–848. doi:10.1016/j.ijmedinf.2011.09.007.

[52] Cresswell K, Sheikh A. Organizational issues in the implementation and adoption of health information technology innovations: an interpretative review. International journal of medical informatics 2013.82(5):e73–e86. doi:10.1016/j.ijmedinf.2012.10.007.

[53] Venkatesh V, Thong J Y L, Xu X. Consumer acceptance and use of information technology: extending the unified theory of acceptance and use of technology. Forthcoming in MIS Quarterly 2012.36(1):157–178.

[54] Hardiker NR, Grant MJ. Factors that influence public engagement with eHealth: a literature review. International Journal of Medical Informatics 2011.80(1):1–12. doi: 10.1016/j.ijmedinf.2010.10.017.

[55] Taniar D. Mobile Computing: Concepts, Methodologies, Tools, and Applications. New York: Information Science reference; 2009. p: 791–792, 432–433. ISBN 978-1-60566-054-7 (hardcover) — ISBN 978-1-60566-055-4 (ebook).

[56] Blumenthal D. Stimulating the adoption of health information technology. The New England Journal of Medicine 2009.360:1477–1479. doi:10.1056/NEJMp0901592.

[57] Lucas H. Information and communications technology for future health systems in developing countries. Social Science & Medicine 2008.66:2122–2132. doi:10.1016/ j.socscimed.2008.01.033.

[58] Lawler EK, Hedge A, Pavlovic-Veselinovic S. Cognitive ergonomics, socio-technical systems, and the impact of healthcare information technologies. International Journal of Industrial Ergonomics 2011.41:336–344. doi:10.1016/j.ergon.2011.02.006.

[59] Viitanen J, Hyppönen H, Lääveri T, Vänskä J, Reponen J, Winblad I. National questionnaire study on clinical ICT systems proofs: physicians suffer from poor usability. International Journal of Medical Informatics 2011.80(10):708–25. doi:10.1016/j.ijmedinf. 2011.06.010.

[60] Lluch M. Healthcare professionals' organizational barriers to health information technologies: a literature review. International Journal of Medical Informatics 2011.80(12):849–862. doi:10.1016/j.ijmedinf.2011.09.005.

[61] While A, Dewsbury G. Nursing and information and communication technology (ICT): a discussion of trends and future directions. International Journal of Nursing Studies 2011.48:1302–1310. doi:10.1016/j.ijnurstu.2011.02.020.

[62] Nykänen P, Brender J, Talmon J, de Keizer N, Rigby M, Beuscart-Zephir M, Ammen-werth E. Guideline for good evaluation practice in health informatics (GEP-HI). International Journal of Medical Informatics 2011.80:815–827. doi:10.1016/j.ijmedinf.2011.08.004.

[63] Aggarwal NK. Applying mobile technologies to mental health service delivery in South Asia. Asian Journal of Psychiatry 2012.5:225–230. doi:10.1016/j.ajp.2011.12.009.

[64] Patel M, Jianfeng W. Applications, challenges, and prospective in emerging body area networking technologies. IEEE Wireless Communications. 2010.17(1):80–88. doi:10.1109/MWC.2010.5416354.

[65] Klingeberg T, Schilling M. Mobile wearable device for long term monitoring of vital signs. Computer Methods and Programs in Biomedicine 2012.106:89–96. doi:10.1016/j.cmpb.2011.12.009.

[66] Chan M, Estève D, Fourniols J, Escriba C, Campo E. Smart wearable systems: current status and future challenges. Artificial Intelligence in Medicine 2012.56:137–156. doi:10.1016/j.artmed.2012.09.003

11

Using Patient Registries to Identify Triggers of Rare Diseases

Feras M. Ghazawi, Steven J. Glassman,
Denis Sasseville and Ivan V. Litvinov

Abstract

Mapping the distribution of patients and analyzing disease clusters is an effective method in epidemiology, where the non-random aggregation of patients is carefully investigated. This can aid in the search for clues to the etiology of diseases, particularly the rare ones. Indeed, with the increased incidence of rare diseases in certain populations and/or geographic areas and with proper analysis of common exposures, it is possible to identify the likely promoters/triggers of these diseases at a given time. In this chapter, we will highlight the appropriate methodology and demonstrate several examples of cluster analyses that lead to the recognition of environmental, occupational and communicable preventable triggers of several rare diseases.

Keywords: cluster investigation, epidemiology, rare diseases, exposures, disease triggers, patient registries

1. Introduction

Many diseases are preventable with lifestyle modifications and by minimizing exposures to harmful substances. In fact, it was recently reported that nearly half of all cancer-related deaths in the United States were attributable to modifiable and preventable risk factors [1]. Through epidemiological studies and careful examination of public health data such as disease registries, and by studying disease distribution, incidence, prevalence and mortality trends, the occurrence of diseases in defined populations can be estimated and can be related to different external factors. Disease clusters are aggregates of patients with a particular disease in a specified time period and at a defined geographical level, occurring at a rate markedly higher than expected. Analyzing and mapping the incidence rates of diseases indeed can help identify non-random distributions of patient clusters, while a proper assessment of the population demographics as well as the surrounding environment can implicate occupational, communicable and environmental exposures as potential causes for a given disease. For instance, in the 1800's, despite limited knowledge on the etiology of many diseases such as cholera, clustering analysis was the method that enabled physicians and scientists to establish a definite link between the disease outbreaks and causative or potentiating agents from the surrounding environment. In the case of cholera, water from a contaminated pump infected with *Vibrio cholerae* bacterium was clearly identified as a disease source in London, England. As highlighted in the examples in Section 2.2, it will be evident to the reader that geographic clustering analyses of patient populations can shed light on the triggers of many rare diseases.

2. Cluster investigation analysis

2.1. Cluster investigations

In epidemiology, trends and causes of diseases and their progression and regression rates can be monitored over time and the occurrence of diseases within the defined populations can be estimated. There are several types of epidemiologic studies including cohort, case–control, cross-sectional, ecologic and cluster studies. Epidemiological studies have a significant impact on public health outcomes as they identify increased disease incidence/prevalence rates, which shape health policies including preventative measures and resource allocation planning, accordingly. Spatial epidemiology is the description and geographical analysis of health data, taking into account patients' demographics, and risk factors including socioeconomic, genetic, environmental, behavioral, infectious and noninfectious exposures [2]. Detection of disease clusters is an integral component of spatial epidemiology as it identifies disproportionately high rates of a disease in a given population, which ultimately generates hypotheses that can help elucidate disease triggers/promoters.

Clustering analyses can be characterized as either general (non-focused) or specific (focused). In a general clustering analysis, the precise location of disease clusters is not studied but rather the clustering tendency of the disease and the overall distribution of disease is examined [3, 4]. On the other hand, specific disease clustering analysis carefully describes unusual nonrandom accumulation of disease outbreaks and the precise location of clusters, in time or space, that are unlikely to be due to chance alone [3, 4]. These investigations can be applied to formulate hypotheses and elucidate potential causes of diseases. Further, clustering patterns of diseases have many applications beyond identifying disease triggers, including identification of areas with high disease prevalence in order to optimize medical management and resource allocation. This will be discussed in Section 2.2.

2.2. Applications of cluster investigations in identifying disease triggers

2.2.1. Cholera

Cholera is an acute infectious diarrheal disease that can be fatal within days if left untreated. This disease became a major health threat in the 1800s, with several outbreaks that had

devastating outcomes. The accepted explanation of cholera outbreaks at the time was attributed to the "Miasma theory", which suggested that poisonous vapor or mist filled with
substances from decomposed matter ("Miasmata") caused many diseases including cholera, chlamydia and plague [5]. In 1854, a severe outbreak of cholera occurred in London,
England, killing more than 600 people. Dr. John Snow, an English physician, investigated
the cause of this epidemic by analyzing the geographic distribution of cholera and plotting
cholera cases on a map, along with certain landmarks in the city including providers of
potable water (**Figure 1**). Notably, most of the cholera cases occurred within 250 yards of the
intersection of Broad and Cambridge streets and in close proximity to a public water pump
on Broad street. This observation prompted the local council to disable the water pump
which halted the spread of cholera. This analysis enabled the identification of the precise
source of the cholera outbreak in London as the public water pump, which was built near
an old open toilet. This work established for the first time that cholera can spread via contaminated water [6]. The breakthrough in fact paved the way for the field of epidemiology.

2.2.2. Mesothelioma

Mesothelioma is a rare but aggressive cancer that arises in the mesothelium, the lining of the
pleura, peritoneum, and pericardium. Studying the prevalence of mesotheliomas in asbestos
miners of South Africa established asbestos exposure as a critical factor responsible for this
deadly malignancy. In a study by Wagner and colleagues, it was noted that while mesothelioma is a very rare disease in the Northwest Cape province of South Africa, 33 cases were
described in the area, each having occupational exposure to crocidolite asbestos mining [8].
This finding was shortly followed by several population studies in Quebec Canada, United
Kingdom, The Netherlands, Germany, Scotland and Northern Ireland, demonstrating that

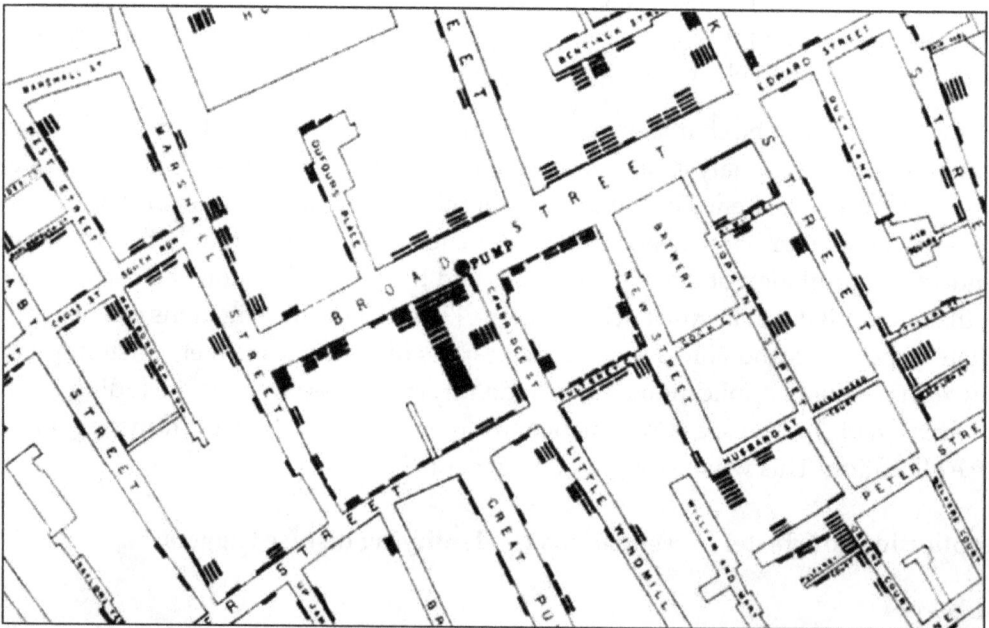

Figure 1. Original map by Dr. John Snow illustrating clustering of cholera cases in the London epidemic of 1854. Cholera
cases are highlighted as black lines [7].

most of the described mesothelioma patients clustered in several communities where occupational exposure to asbestos was routine. At that time asbestos was commonly used in insulation, construction, factory work as well as in shipyards. This analysis confirmed the causal link between asbestos and mesotheliomas and led to a legislative action to ban the use of this carcinogen in construction and other workplaces [9].

2.2.3. Squamous cell carcinoma

For many centuries, arsenic was used by the Egyptians, Greeks, Asians and Romans for many applications including the treatment of rheumatism and for facial hair removal. Little was known about the carcinogenic effects of arsenic at that time. In 1898, Geyer conducted a detailed population study in Reichenstein, Silesia (Prussia). In this small arsenic-mining town, chronic poisoning took place primarily through the use of drinking water contaminated by precipitating arsenical fumes in the rain. This work shed light on the carcinogenic effects of arsenic [10]. Affected individuals developed a constellation of symptoms including pigmentation changes and hyperkeratosis (wart-like lesions) on the palms and soles. The latter had a high risk of progression to cutaneous squamous cell carcinomas. This condition was referred to as "Reichenstein's disease" [11]. The significant increase of this disease in the residents of this town helped establish the link between arsenic and the occurrence of arsenical keratoses and squamous cell carcinomas of the skin. This example further demonstrates the importance of non-random clustering of rare diseases in identifying novel environmental or occupational disease triggers.

2.2.4. Cutaneous T-cell lymphoma

Cutaneous T-cell lymphoma (CTCL) is a rare group of non-Hodgkin lymphomas that primarily involves the skin. Patients with CTCL typically present with persistent, red itchy patches and thickened plaques that are located mostly on the trunk. As the malignancy progresses, patients can develop skin tumors with concomitant involvement of lymph nodes and visceral organs. In some stages, the disease involves the blood and patients can develop erythroderma (generalized redness and desquamation of the skin) and suffer intractable pruritus as well as B-symptoms of lymphoma. Many advanced disease patients succumb to this malignancy within 2–3 years. Unfortunately, the risk factors and promoters for this disease remained poorly understood for many years. It is recognized that disruption of molecular pathways in skin lymphocytes by bacterial, viral or environmental factors can lead to cutaneous lymphomas [12–14]. Although progress has been made in the past few decades, the precise pathogenesis by which CTCL develops remains poorly understood. Several reports from different parts of the world examined the distribution of CTCL patients illustrating non-random clustering of cases. This was shown in Sweden [15], Houston, Texas (**Figure 2**) [16, 17] and the Pittsburgh metropolitan area [18]. Furthermore, the unusually high incidence of CTCL in married couples [19], and in families [20] was also noted. These clustering patterns of CTCL patients strongly argue for the existence of external and potentially preventable risk factors for this rare skin cancer.

Several factors have been implicated in CTCL carcinogenesis, including immunosuppression, vitamin D deficiency, bacterial agents (*Staphylococcus aureus*, *Mycobacterium leprae* and *Chlamydophila pneumoniae*), medications (calcium channel blockers, angiotensin converting enzyme inhibitors, hydrochlorothiazide, and serotonin reuptake inhibitors), dermatophytes and viruses (EBV, HSV and HTLV-1) [21]. However, none of these agents have been definitively linked with this skin lymphoma.

In addition, recent studies in Canada further confirmed the existence of disease clusters and areas completely spared by this malignancy and implicated industrial exposure and living in a proximity to major transportation junctions as potential triggers for CTCL [22, 23]. Considering that the majority of skin cancers are caused by external and often preventable triggers (e.g. UV radiation, HPV, polyomaviruses, etc.) it is not surprising that skin lymphomas

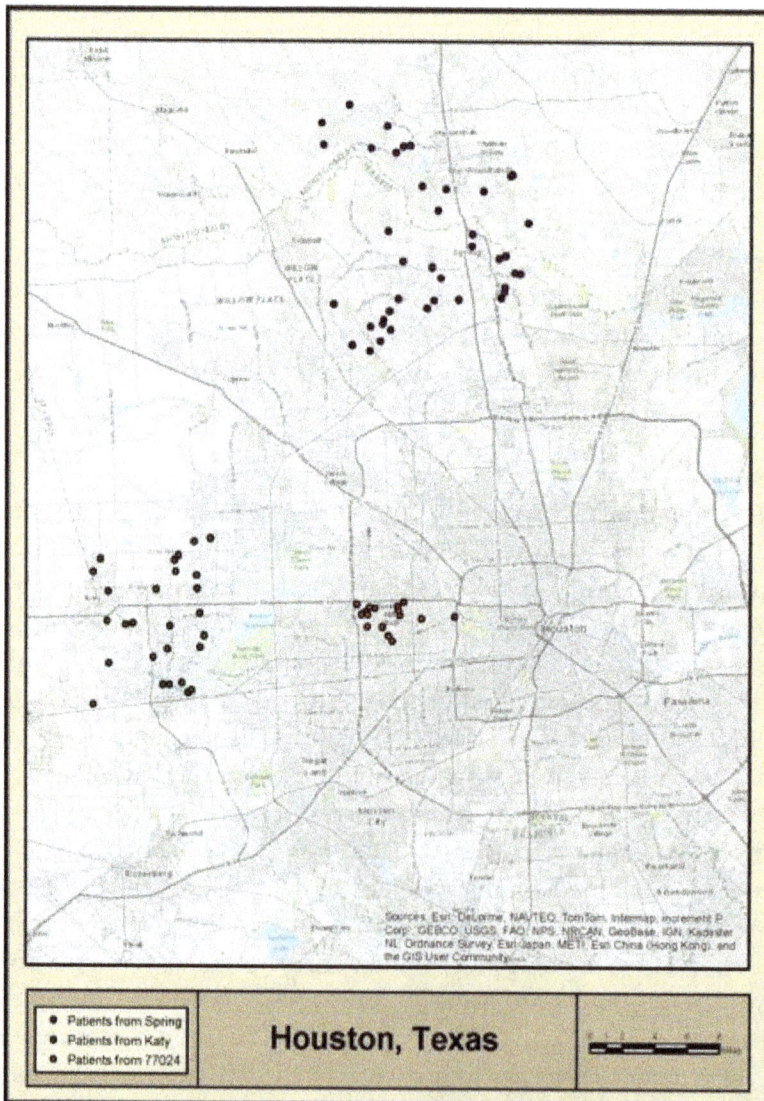

Figure 2. Geographic mapping of cutaneous T-cell lymphoma cases in Houston, Texas demonstrating clustering pattern of patients with this rare malignancy with incidence rates 5–20-fold higher than expected. Patients in 'Spring' community are indicated by violet, patients in 'Katy' community are indicated by green, and patients residing in the Houston memorial area are indicated by orange. Adapted from [17].

could also be caused by an external trigger. Currently, the search for such trigger(s) for this malignancy is ongoing.

2.2.5. Childhood leukemia

Another example revealing a cause of an important disease came from an observation in the early 1980s in Woburn, Massachusetts, where an elevated incidence rate of childhood leukemia was documented. An extensive investigation of the geographical distribution of these patients helped implicate chlorinated organic compounds contaminating two of eight municipal wells servicing Woburn as a cause of childhood leukemia. Specifically, it was shown that select dwellings where the patients with this cancer resided, were provided water from these contaminated wells [24].

2.2.6. Bladder cancer

Bladder cancer is a disease of significant morbidity and mortality [25]. Cluster investigation recently helped identify occupational and behavioral promoters for this cancer. These factors are potentially modifiable and thus rates of this malignancy could possibly be reduced with primary prevention. The astute observation in 1895 by Rehn, a German physician, showed that the incidence rates of bladder cancer were remarkably high in aniline dye industry workers. This was the first evidence that occupational risk factors can be directly implicated in this malignancy [26]. By carefully analyzing the incidence of bladder cancers in industrial workers, it was possible to identify aromatic amines, polycyclic aromatic hydrocarbons and chlorinated hydrocarbons that are now well recognized as causative agents for this disease [25].

2.2.7. Emerging trends

2.2.7.1. Multiple sclerosis

Multiple sclerosis (MS) is an autoimmune demyelinating disease, affecting the central nervous system and resulting in a spectrum of neurological symptoms including vision problems, fatigue, pains, spasms and cognitive decline. The precise triggers of this rare disease have not yet been described or identified. However, studying the epidemiology and geographic distribution of MS globally has yielded many interesting trends that allowed generation of a number of hypotheses addressing the cause of MS. Clusters of new MS cases have been reported in many communities around the world including the United States, Canada, Europe, Israel, New Zealand, Australia and Russia [27–30]. Many studies indicated significant variation in the global distribution of MS patients, where the incidence of this autoimmune disease is relatively uncommon in tropical climates, but is much more common in temperate zones and in the Western Hemisphere [31]. Furthermore, remarkably elevated incidence rates in northern latitudes were reported [32, 33]. Many theories have been postulated to implicate promoters of MS, such as diet, soil minerals and deficiency in vitamin D [32, 33]. The identity of a definite trigger for MS remains unknown, and extensive follow up of identified clusters may potentially provide some clues in the future.

2.2.7.2. Alzheimer's disease

Alzheimer's disease is a common, yet incompletely understood form of dementia. Differences in the geographical distribution of patients with Alzheimer's disease were reported, highlighting the possible contribution of nutritional or socio-environmental factors in the development and progression of the disease [34]. Indeed, levels of essential trace elements including selenium, magnesium, iron, copper and zinc were shown to be markedly reduced in Alzheimer's patients compared to same age healthy individuals [35]. This illustrates that further epidemiologic studies can be used to associate nutritional deficiencies with diseases.

2.3. Applications of cluster investigations in identifying nutritional deficiencies

2.3.1. Scurvy

Deficiency in micronutrients and vitamins can result in a variety of diseases. For instance, vitamin A deficiency is a known cause of keratomalacia, while vitamin D deficiency in childhood invariably causes rickets. One important use of clustering analysis in epidemiology is to identify nutritional deficiencies.

During the Age of Discovery in the fifteenth and sixteenth century, particularly during long transatlantic journeys, it was noted that the incidence of scurvy, a rare disease caused by a severe deficiency of vitamin C (ascorbic acid), was much higher in sailors, pirates and other sea explorers. Also, the disease later affected soldiers in world wars. Scurvy is characterized by general weakness, gingivitis and bleeding disorders. It was noted that eating citrus fruits prevented and cured this disease in sailors, which enabled later confirmation that vitamin C deficiency is the sole cause of scurvy. Thus, careful demographic and epidemiologic analyses of these individuals, who did not have access to fresh fruit and vegetables, established a link between nutritional deficiency and disease.

2.3.2. Goiter

Thyroid goiters, which represent enlargement of the thyroid gland, are caused by iodine deficiency. Fortification of table salt, medications and common foods like bread with iodine has largely eliminated the once pandemic goiter, but the condition persists in some regions of the developing world. The first hypothesis linking iodine with the treatment of goiter was made in the mid-1800s by a French chemist, Adolphe Chatin [36]. However, fortification of table salt with iodine was not implemented in the United States until the early 1920s [37], and this was, at least in part, driven by epidemiological research.

It was noted that the prevalence of goiter was very high (in approximately 26–70% of children) in the upper Midwest and Great Lakes regions of the United States. In fact, this endemic region was known at the time as the "Goiter Belt" [38]. The prevalence was also reported as high as 64.4% in some areas of Michigan [39]. This highlighted the severity of the problem, sparking a major public health initiative to supplement table salt with iodine. The intervention was very successful, as the incidence of goiter in Michigan dropped by up to 90% within a decade of iodine supplementation [40]. Currently, several areas have remarkably high prevalence of goiter, such as parts of India and the Himalayan/sub-Himalayan belts [41]. In fact, despite efforts to implement iodine supplementation and table salt fortification with iodine, the goiter prevalence in these communities has not decreased significantly [42]. Thus, more work needs to be done to address logistic, cultural and other obstacles to eliminate suffering from goiter in these regions. In conclusion, recognizing the high prevalence of 'uncommon' diseases such as goiter has important clinical implications. These studies help detect regions with micronutrient deficiency, which can serve as surrogate markers for poor nutrition and encourage prioritizing resource allocation to the affected communities.

2.4. Conducting a proper cluster investigation analysis

2.4.1. Systematic approach to conducting a cluster analysis

The study of the incidence/prevalence of a disease and mapping its distribution requires a systematic approach when trying to implicate occupational and environmental exposures as disease triggers/promoters. Mapping and exposure investigations are critical to highlight the existence and significance of identified clusters. However, it is not enough to only learn about the geographical disease clusters (i.e., disease hot-spots). It is also important to identify regions that are significantly spared by the disease (i.e., disease cold-spots). Detailed epidemiological and statistical analysis of both can help rule-in or rule-out environmental contamination or exposures as disease triggers [43]. A point-by-point guide of a systematic approach to conducting a cluster investigation is provided below:

1. Define the disease and population(s) to be examined.

2. Obtain 'background' information about patient demographics to enable standardization of incidence and mortality rates (such as standardization by age, gender, race, socioeconomic status, etc.).

3. Obtain census or other population information to enable calculating incidence and mortality rates per country, territory/state/province, city and postal code. It is also helpful to learn about common exposures or diseases in that population to adjust for potential confounders. For instance, when studying the incidence of hepatitis C infection in a population, the rate of HIV prevalence would be an important confounder, since in many patients there is co-infection with both viruses due to shared risk factors for viral transmission. Population demographic parameters often vary and can be useful for subsequent analysis of collected data. The specific parameters of interest will differ for each disease, but often include population size, age ranges, race, gender distribution, socioeconomic status, data on lifestyle/behaviors, other environmental, occupational, or local rates of communicable diseases, etc.

4. Obtain public health data on patients with the disease of interest (e.g. local or national cancer registries and Centers for Disease Control, etc.). It is critical to obtain the data from population-based registries since it is often very difficult to draw conclusions from data based on a single medical center or a few select hospitals' experience. One must always seek to correlate single center evidence with population-based registries/databases.

Relevant collected information should include age at diagnosis, year of diagnosis (for incidence calculation), gender, ethnic background (to study disease ethnic predilection), patients' addresses (for geographical mapping), age at death, year of death (for mortality calculation), disease stage, etc.

5. Subsequent calculations of incidence can be easily performed using the obtained data (incidence rate per year = number of new patients per year/population at risk per year). A plot of incidence rates (y axis) *vs.* year (x axis) will enable calculating an average incidence rate and trending the change of rate over time. Mortality calculations are done similarly, using number of deceased patients per year/population at risk.

6. Incidence rates in smaller geographical regions can be calculated similarly. For rare diseases, it is important to include only locations with at least >5000–10,000 residents per geographical area to reduce erroneous false-positive hits, in which a few cases of disease occurring within a scarcely populated area (e.g., <5000 residents) may artificially inflate the incidence/mortality rate.

7. The calculated incidence/mortality rates can be normalized to several variables (such as age, gender, ethnicity) or to a known distribution of relevant disease-specific variables (such as communicable diseases, geographical latitude, socioeconomic status, etc.) This is important to account for potential confounding variables and to highlight trends that can be 'masked' if rates are not normalized in subsequent analyses.

8. Conduct proper statistical analysis to determine statistically significant high and low incidence/mortality rates per geographical region at all levels. Two of the most commonly used methods of statistical analysis are the chi-square test (comparing observed number of cases to that expected under an assumed Poisson distribution) and the Knox test for time–space interaction, among more than 70 different methods, which have been used in previously published studies [43].

9. Plot the incidence rates in a specialized computer program such as ArcGIS or other geographic information system (GIS) software. Generate several maps, choosing appropriate color schemes representing standardized rates. It may also be advantageous to generate maps representing rates of statistical significance. Maps should serve as a clear, rapid and informative summary of complex geographical information and should help the reader identify interesting trends and generate relevant hypotheses.

10. Repeat the mapping analysis (step 9) using different normalized rates. Map the data in different formats and beware of "biased mapping" which was discussed elsewhere [44]. Ensure plotting maps that convey the message clearly and accurately.

11. Visualize and further analyze the plotted maps and note the presence of disease clusters ("disease hot-spots") as well as areas of significantly low incidence/mortality rates ("cold-spots"). Observe for interesting trends, particularly, if several of these clusters occur geographically side-by-side and are supported by hypotheses/current evidence of disease pathogenesis. It is often useful to compare generated disease maps with land-use maps that can be obtained from local authorities.

12. Perform sub-analysis of the identified "disease hot-spots" and correlate with the surrounding environment for any prevalent occupations, exposures, environmental factors, etc. If the patients within the area of high incidence (e.g. within a zip/postal code or a city) demonstrate an additional level of clustering (e.g., living on the same street or up and down the stream or river) it can further strengthen clustering findings and provide clues regarding possible triggers/exposures.

2.4.2. Limitations and bias

As illustrated in this chapter, studying the spatial patterns and geographical distribution of diseases has many benefits including the identification of disease clusters. This can be a powerful tool to help identify disease triggers and to better allocate financial and logistic resources for better management of these medical conditions. When the analysis is conducted properly, results are often specific. However, as in any type of analysis, one must be aware of potential limitations and intrinsic bias of the method. When analyzing clusters of patients in a given geographical region, one must be aware that there is a possibility that at least some of the observed clusters may be occurring by chance alone. Another important point, when studying the incidence of rare diseases in small regions: it is imperative to bracket the population analysis to at least 5000–10,000 residents per geographical area to reduce erroneous false-positive hits. Also, association does not always imply causality. Extensive additional field and experimental work must be performed to link identified associations causally with a given disease. Finally, one must be careful when directly comparing different geographic clustering studies as differences in the inclusion criteria, statistical methods or intrinsic differences of the populations at risk can produce divergent results.

3. Conclusions

The applications of cluster studies in medicine have developed rather rapidly in recent decades. These will enable us to focus on studying risk factors and possible etiologic triggers of rare cancers and other conditions. Furthermore, this work can help make informed decisions regarding resource allocation and promote the development of primary prevention programs.

Acknowledgements

The authors would like to sincerely thank both Dr. Linda Moreau and Dr. Elham Rahme for their generous support and valuable advice.

Conflict of interest

The authors declare no potential conflicts of interest with respect to the research, authorship, and/or publication of this book chapter.

Author details

Feras M. Ghazawi[1], Steven J. Glassman[1], Denis Sasseville[2] and Ivan V. Litvinov[2*]

*Address all correspondence to: ivan.litvinov@mcgill.ca

1 Division of Dermatology, University of Ottawa, Ottawa, Ontario, Canada

2 Division of Dermatology, McGill University Health Centre, Montréal, Québec, Canada

References

[1] Islami F, Goding Sauer A, Miller KD, Siegel RL, Fedewa SA, Jacobs EJ, et al. Proportion and number of cancer cases and deaths attributable to potentially modifiable risk factors in the United States. CA: A Cancer Journal for Clinicians. 2017;**68**(1):31-54. Epub 2017/11/22

[2] Elliott P, Wartenberg D. Spatial epidemiology: Current approaches and future challenges. Environmental Health Perspectives. 2004;**112**(9):998-1006 Epub 2004/06/17

[3] Rezaeian M, Dunn G, St Leger S, Appleby L. Geographical epidemiology, spatial analysis and geographical information systems: A multidisciplinary glossary. Journal of Epidemiology and Community Health. 2007;**61**(2):98-102 Epub 2007/01/20

[4] Torabi M, Rosychuk RJ. An examination of five spatial disease clustering methodologies for the identification of childhood cancer clusters in Alberta, Canada. Spatial and Spatio-Temporal Epidemiology. 2011;**2**(4):321-330 Epub 2012/07/04

[5] Halliday S. Death and miasma in Victorian London: An obstinate belief. BMJ. 2001;**323**(7327):1469-1471 Epub 2001/12/26

[6] Snow SJ. John snow: The making of a hero? Lancet. 2008;**372**(9632):22-23 Epub 2008/07/10

[7] Snow J. On the Mode of Communication of Cholera. 2nd ed. London,: J. Churchill. 1855;**vii**(1):162

[8] Wagner JC, Sleggs CA, Marchand P. Diffuse pleural mesothelioma and asbestos exposure in the north western Cape Province. British Journal of Industrial Medicine. 1960;**17**:260-271 Epub 1960/10/01

[9] McDonald JC. Epidemiology of malignant mesothelioma—An outline. The Annals of Occupational Hygiene. 2010;**54**(8):851-857 Epub 2010/11/10

[10] Geyer L. Über die chronischen Hautveränderungen beim Arsenicismus und Betrachtungen über die Massenerkrankungen in Reichenstein in Schlesien. Archiv für Dermatologie und Syphilis. 1898;**43**(1):221-280

[11] Schwartz RA. Reichenstein disease. International Journal of Dermatology. 1991;**30**(4):304-305 Epub 1991/04/01

[12] Bogle MA, Riddle CC, Triana EM, Jones D, Duvic M. Primary cutaneous B-cell lymphoma. Journal of the American Academy of Dermatology. 2005;**53**(3):479-484

[13] Suzuki R. Pathogenesis and treatment of extranodal natural killer/T-cell lymphoma. Seminars in Hematology. 2014;**51**(1):42-51

[14] Tsukasaki K, Tobinai K. Human T-cell lymphotropic virus type I-associated adult T-cell leukemia-lymphoma: New directions in clinical research. Clinical Cancer Research: An Official Journal of the American Association for Cancer Research. 2014;**20**(20):5217-5225

[15] Gip L, Nilsson E. Ansamling av mycosis fungoides i Vasternorrlands lan [Clustering of mycosis fungoides in the county of Vasternorrland]. Lakartidningen. 1977;**74**(12):1174-1176 Epub 1977/03/23

[16] Litvinov IV, Tetzlaff MT, Rahme E, Jennings MA, Risser DR, Gangar P, et al. Demographic patterns of cutaneous T-cell lymphoma incidence in Texas based on two different cancer registries. Cancer Medicine. 2015;**4**(9):1440-1447 Epub 2015/07/03

[17] Litvinov IV, Tetzlaff MT, Rahme E, Habel Y, Risser DR, Gangar P, et al. Identification of geographic clustering and regions spared by cutaneous T-cell lymphoma in Texas using 2 distinct cancer registries. Cancer. 2015;**121**(12):1993-2003 Epub 2015/03/03

[18] Moreau JF, Buchanich JM, Geskin JZ, Akilov OE, Geskin LJ. Non-random geographic distribution of patients with cutaneous T-cell lymphoma in the greater Pittsburgh area. Dermatology Online Journal. 2014;**20**(7):pii: 13030/qt4nw7592w. Epub 2014/07/22

[19] Hazen PG, Michel B. Hodgkin's disease and mycosis fungoides in a married couple. Dermatologica. 1977;**154**(5):257-260 Epub 1977/01/01

[20] Hodak E, Klein T, Gabay B, Ben-Amitai D, Bergman R, Gdalevich M, et al. Familial mycosis fungoides: Report of 6 kindreds and a study of the HLA system. Journal of the American Academy of Dermatology. 2005;**52**(3 Pt 1):393-402 Epub 2005/03/12

[21] Litvinov IV, Shtreis A, Kobayashi K, Glassman S, Tsang M, Woetmann A, et al. Investigating potential exogenous tumor initiating and promoting factors for cutaneous T-cell lymphomas (CTCL), a rare skin malignancy. Oncoimmunology. 2016;**5**(7):e1175799 Epub 2016/09/14

[22] Ghazawi FM, Netchiporouk E, Rahme E, Tsang M, Moreau L, Glassman S, et al. Comprehensive analysis of cutaneous T-cell lymphoma (CTCL) incidence and mortality in Canada reveals changing trends and geographic clustering for this malignancy. Cancer. 2017;**123**(18):3550-3567 Epub 2017/05/12

[23] Ghazawi FM, Netchiporouk E, Rahme E, Tsang M, Moreau L, Glassman S, et al. Distribution and clustering of cutaneous T-cell lymphoma (CTCL) cases in Canada during 1992 to 2010. Journal of Cutaneous Medicine and Surgery. 2018 Mar/Apr;**22**(2): 154-165. DOI: 10.1177/1203475417745825. Epub 2017/12/16

[24] Zelen SWLBJWM. An analysis of contaminated well water and health effects in Woburn, Massachusetts. Journal of the American Statistical Society. 1986;**81**:583-596

[25] Burger M, Catto JW, Dalbagni G, Grossman HB, Herr H, Karakiewicz P, et al. Epidemiology and risk factors of urothelial bladder cancer. European Urology. 2013;**63**(2):234-241 Epub 2012/08/11

[26] Frumin E, Velez H, Bingham E, Gillen M, Brathwaite M, LaBarck R. Occupational bladder cancer in textile dyeing and printing workers: Six cases and their significance for screening programs. Journal of Occupational Medicine. 1990;**32**(9):887-890 Epub 1990/09/01

[27] Kurtzke JF. Multiple sclerosis in time and space—Geographic clues to cause. Journal of Neurovirology. 2000;**6**(Suppl 2):S134-S140 Epub 2000/06/29

[28] Bezzini D, Pepe P, Profili F, Meucci G, Ulivelli M, Bartalini S, et al. Multiple sclerosis spatial cluster in Tuscany. Neurological Sciences. 2017;**38**(12):2183-2187. Epub 2017/10/12

[29] Sheremata WA, Poskanzer DC, Withum DG, MacLeod CL, Whiteside ME. Unusual occurrence on a tropical island of multiple sclerosis. Lancet. 1985;**2**(8455):618 Epub 1985/09/14

[30] Schiffer RB, McDermott MP, Copley C. A multiple sclerosis cluster associated with a small, north-central Illinois community. Archives of Environmental Health. 2001;**56**(5):389-395 Epub 2002/01/05

[31] Jin Y, de Pedro-Cuesta J, Soderstrom M, Stawiarz L, Link H. Seasonal patterns in optic neuritis and multiple sclerosis: A meta-analysis. Journal of the Neurological Sciences. 2000;**181**(1-2):56-64 Epub 2000/12/02

[32] Simpson S Jr, Blizzard L, Otahal P, Van der Mei I, Taylor B. Latitude is significantly associated with the prevalence of multiple sclerosis: A meta-analysis. Journal of Neurology, Neurosurgery, and Psychiatry. 2011;**82**(10):1132-1141 Epub 2011/04/12

[33] Koch-Henriksen N, Sorensen PS. The changing demographic pattern of multiple sclerosis epidemiology. The Lancet Neurology. 2010;**9**(5):520-532 Epub 2010/04/20

[34] Russ TC, Batty GD, Hearnshaw GF, Fenton C, Starr JM. Geographical variation in dementia: Systematic review with meta-analysis. International Journal of Epidemiology. 2012;**41**(4):1012-1032 Epub 2012/07/17

[35] Vural H, Demirin H, Kara Y, Eren I, Delibas N. Alterations of plasma magnesium, copper, zinc, iron and selenium concentrations and some related erythrocyte antioxidant enzyme activities in patients with Alzheimer's disease. Journal of Trace Elements in Medicine and Biology. 2010;**24**(3):169-173 Epub 2010/06/24

[36] Chatin A. Recherches sur l'iode des eaux douces; de la presence de ce xorps sand les plantes at les animaux terrestes. Comptes Rendus de l'Académie des Sciences. 1852;**35**:505-517

[37] Leung AM, Braverman LE, Pearce EN. History of U.S. iodine fortification and supplementation. Nutrients. 2012;**4**(11):1740-1746 Epub 2012/12/04

[38] Pearce EN. National trends in iodine nutrition: Is everyone getting enough? Thyroid: Official Journal of the American Thyroid Association. 2007;**17**(9):823-827 Epub 2007/10/25

[39] Markel H. "When it rains it pours": Endemic goiter, iodized salt, and David Murray Cowie, MD. American Journal of Public Health. 1987;**77**(2):219-229 Epub 1987/02/01

[40] Markel H. A grain of salt. The Milbank Quarterly. 2014;**92**(3):407-412 Epub 2014/09/10

[41] Manjunath B, Suman G, Hemanth T, Shivaraj NS, Murthy NS. Prevalence and factors associated with goitre among 6-12-year-old children in a rural area of Karnataka in South India. Biological Trace Element Research. 2016;**169**(1):22-26 Epub 2015/06/13

[42] Gupta RK, Langer B, Raina SK, Kumari R, Jan R, Rani R. Goiter prevalence in school-going children: A cross-sectional study in two border districts of sub-Himalayan Jammu and Kashmir. Journal of Family Medicine and Primary Care. 2016;**5**(4):825-828 Epub 2017/03/30

[43] Wartenberg D. Using disease-cluster and small-area analyses to study environmental justice. In: Toward Environmental Justice: Research, Education, and Health Policy Needs. USA: National Academies Press; 1999:23-35

[44] Monmonier MS. How to Lie with Maps, Vol. xiii. 2nd ed. Chicago: University of Chicago Press; 1996. p. 207

12

Telemedicine Programs in Respiratory Diseases

Gonzalo Segrelles-Calvo and Daniel López-Padilla

Abstract

Telemedicine programs are widely used in respiratory diseases, more often in patients with chronic obstructive pulmonary diseases (COPD). Telemedicine platforms use several devices to measure vital signs such as heart rate, respiratory rate, pulsioximetry or blood pressure between others. It is not unusual that patients could do questionnaires about clinical situation or communicate with their nurses via telephone, videocalling and/or Skype. The majority of results has been positive, with reduction in the number of emergency visits, hospitalizations and noninvasive ventilations. Despite their promising results, telemedicine programs/platforms are slow to implement. In this chapter, we reviewed some of the factors related to telemedicine implementation such as patients' adherence, impact of telemedicine design and professionals' resistance to change between others.

Keywords: COPD, eHealth, home telemonitoring, telemedicine, telemedicine platforms

1. Introduction

Chronic obstructive pulmonary diseases (COPD), asthma and lung transplantation have been, by far, the respiratory diseases or conditions more studied, in terms of telemedicine. However, the interest of telehealth providers in new areas also related to neurologic conditions, such as neuromuscular diseases in need of home noninvasive ventilation (NIV) due to chronic respiratory failure, or sleep-related breathing disorders, has arisen in recent years.

Existing evidence reveals promising results regarding reliability and validity of measures across all pulmonary conditions, and patients usually show a positive attitude toward telecare technologies. Other positive effects, for instance, detection of complications, better disease control, immediate feedback, and adequate medication use, have also been addressed [1]. Yet, there is still somewhat decreased adherence within time, possibly secondary to poor health status, time conflicts, device problems, and lack of ability to operate the system [2]. Furthermore, there is no solid evidence about the utilization of healthcare resources, as well as cost-effectiveness, paramount scenarios to advocate in favor of this new way of approaching chronic respiratory patients.

In the following section, current evidence apropos specific respiratory diseases (COPD, asthma, lung transplantation, neuromuscular diseases, and SRBD) will be disclosed, focusing on the positive results, along with the pitfalls found so far.

1.1. Telemedicine

Telemedicine (TM) has several definitions and all of them emphasize the role of telemedicine to enable the completion of the medical act at distance (**Table 1**) [3–5]. Norrit et al. define TM as a scientific area that uses information and communication technologies (ICT) to share medical information [6]. Thanks to ICT development, TM clinical opportunities are increasing. The information provided by TM programs can be useful for diagnosis and treatment of several diseases, as well as for enhancing their follow-up.

	Ref	Definition
WHO	[3]	The delivery of health care services, where distance is a critical factor, by all health care professionals using information and communication technologies for the exchange of valid information for diagnosis, treatment and prevention of disease and injuries, research and evaluation, and for the continuing education of health care providers, all in the interests of advancing the health of individuals and their communities.
ATA	[4]	Telemedicine is the use of medical information exchanged from one site to another via electronic communications to improve a patient's clinical health status. Telemedicine includes a growing variety of applications and services using two-way video, email, smart phones, wireless tools, and other forms of telecommunications technology.
Bashur R	[5]	Telemedicine is conceived of as an integrated system of health-care delivery that employs telecommunications and computer technology as a substitute for face-to-face contact between provider and client.

WHO: World Health Organization; ATA: American Telemedicine Association, Ref: Reference.

Table 1. Telemedicine's definitions.

Historically, Dr. Graham Bell performed the first TM experience, when he used the telephone calling for help when he was sick. Also, in 1923, Sahlgrenska University (Gothenburg) used the Morse code to provide medical advice. TM programs were funded by the privacy industries in 1990 for the first time, and in 1993, the first telemedicine symposium was celebrated. Over 50 years, TM has been used for different programs such as: monitored surgeries, remote assistance in rural zones of Arizona, or vital signs monitoring of astronauts in space, just like

Bashur et al. demonstrated [7]. In fact, aerospace technology development has been one of the most important factors in TM evolution. In 1976, the Hermes satellite was put into orbit with the main objective of improving communications in remote areas of Canada. Since then, the Western Ontario University has been using it for telemonitoring of vital signs, sharing medical information between hospitals and, finally, sharing radiographies [8]. Moreover, the National Aeronautics and Space Administration (NASA) also has used TM to give medical assistance if a disaster takes place.

Generally speaking, TM applications could be classified into three groups: (a) normal clinical activity (teleconsult, telediagnosis, teletreatment, etc.), (b) remote assistance, and (c) administration labors and patient management.

1.1.1. Clinical activity

Almost all studies are aimed for telemonitoring patients or sharing medical data, where this medical act at distance needs a TM platform and a clinical response. We could classify the clinical response into two groups: synchronic or asynchronic response (**Figure 1**). The main difference is the time to response [9]. While in the first group, the clinical response is immediate and allows performing a live medical act, the second group clinical response is deferred (minutes or few hours). Asynchronic response is useful in telepatologhy or teleradiology, or in other telediagnosis programs.

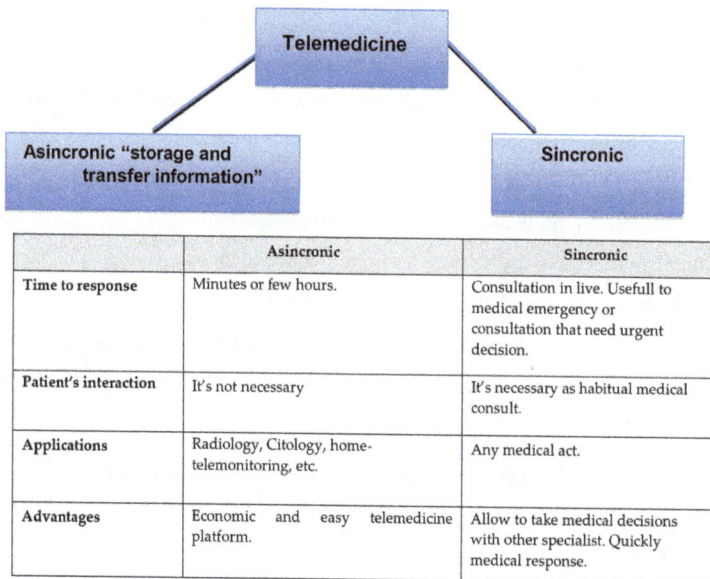

	Asincronic	Sincronic
Time to response	Minutes or few hours.	Consultation in live. Usefull to medical emergency or consultation that need urgent decision.
Patient's interaction	It's not necessary	It's necessary as habitual medical consult.
Applications	Radiology, Citology, home-telemonitoring, etc.	Any medical act.
Advantages	Economic and easy telemedicine platform.	Allow to take medical decisions with other specialist. Quickly medical response.

Figure 1. Telemedicine classification.

1.1.2. Remote assistance

In this group, several medical actions are included such as online records for consulting previous medical charts, establishing a direct communication between patients and physicians, or teleconference between primary and specialized care doctors, useful for discussing difficult cases and take decisions for complex patients (terminal disease, multiple comorbidities, social exclusion, impossibility to attend the hospital, etc.).

1.1.3. Patients' management

Nowadays, patients manage their medical events via Internet more often, and their doctors can use the same way to give medical recommendations (rehabilitation, nutritional care, tobacco information, or health life recommendations). Obviously, TM is a helpful tool for health care personnel as well. In this case, TM is used to access scientific information or as a type of communication for multicentric and international clinical trials.

1.2. Telemedicine: barriers and benefits

According to the Europe Institute of Technologies findings, only 14.2% of citizens had used the Internet to solve their health related doubts. The more frequent searches regarding these issues were: disease description, clinical trials, medical literature, or patients' disease associations (**Table 2**).

	Information related to	EEUU (% total)	EU-15 (% total)
Patients	Disease description	68,49	55,78
	Clinical Trials	33,14	21,93
	Medical literature	81,51	58,74
	Disease associations	27,81	30,11
Professionals	Disease description	65,91	57,23
	Clinical Trials	39,94	50,21
	Medical literature	90,58	89,36
	Disease associations	18,18	16,17

Table 2. Search topics by patients and healthcare professionals.

There are several studies that have showed important barriers for applying TM programs. Segrelles-Calvo et al. suggested that healthcare policy, lacking studies about economic burden and cost-effectiveness of TM, no laws regarding the handling of information in TM programs and the resistance to change "usual medicine conception," are some causes that explain slow TM implantation [10]. According to the concept of "resistant to change usual care," Mira-Solves et al. presented the results of the ValCrònic program [11], in which authors discussed the causes to leave a TM program. The main reasons were: (1) difficulty to use the devices, (2) complex measures, (3) nonadherence with TM program, (4) technical problems, and (5) caregivers preferences.

Another important barrier not well studied is the opinion of health professionals toward TM programs. Telemedicine collects a lot of information and their belief is that TM increases workload. However, this belief is not displayed in scientific studies. Jódar-Sánchez et al. [12] showed indeed that a specialized nurse could solve most of the clinical urgencies detected, where only 8 of 40 cases needed a pneumologist intervention. Similar results were published by Vitacca et al. [13] reporting that in 63% of alerts, these could be resolved only by a nurse, and in the rest of them both physician and nurse gave the clinical response. As conclusion, it seems that there are external factors acting as barriers in the TM implantation, and further works are required to establish them. Motulsky et al. [14] and Cresswell et al. [15] pooled those external factors in three groups: (1) healthcare institutions policy, (2) the urge of guidelines about TM, and (3) the need of specific formation and educational resources.

Telemedicine offers four fundamental benefits [4]:

a. *Improved access:* Telemedicine has been used to bring healthcare services to patients in distant locations.

b. *Cost efficiencies*: Telemedicine reduces the number of hospitalizations and the cost related to these events. Telemedicine program reduce patient displacement to Hospital and reduced travel times.

c. *Improved quality*: Studies have consistently shown that the quality of healthcare services delivered via telemedicine is as good as those given in traditional in-person consultations.

d. *Patient demand:* The greatest impact of telemedicine is on the patient, their family and their community. Telemedicine could reduce travel time and related stresses for the patient. Almost all studies have shown that patient and caregiver's satisfaction is very high.

1.3. Telemedicine platforms

In general, there is a common objective in telemedicine programs; however, there are several platforms in which TM could be offered. Telemedicine platforms are related to ICT. The most common scheme in telemedicine (**Figure 2**) is the one that includes devices to measure different vital signs or questionnaires, in order to perform a teleconsultation or to send educational resources to patients. Those measures could be made by the patients, anywhere and anytime. Clinical information is sent to a call center or a health professional by different means (telephone, Internet, etc.), and the clinical response is made according to all information regarding.

Some of the ICT used in telemedicine platform are as follows:

Videoconference. Possibly this ICT was one of the most important technological advances as a telemedicine platform. Mahmud et al. [16] made a follow-up platform of patients with chronic diseases (heart failure, COPD, cerebrovascular disease). In seven cases, the number of emergency department visits and hospitalizations were reduced, and the authors did not found complications in the use of the videoconference platform. These results were confirmed in 2000 by Johnston et al. [17] and by Nakamura et al. [18]. Johnston determined a reduction of 17% of home visits as well as a 27% reduction of costs in the telemedicine group. Moreover, Nakamura reported an improvement of daily activities in the telemedicine group. Recent studies have used videoconference to improve adherence to a telerehabilitation program [19], to follow-up patients with bipolar disorder [20] or to monitoring tuberculosis therapy compliance [21], among other topics. According to these studies, in our view the videoconference is a remarkable technology, facilitating the follow-up of patients to improve their adherence to treatment.

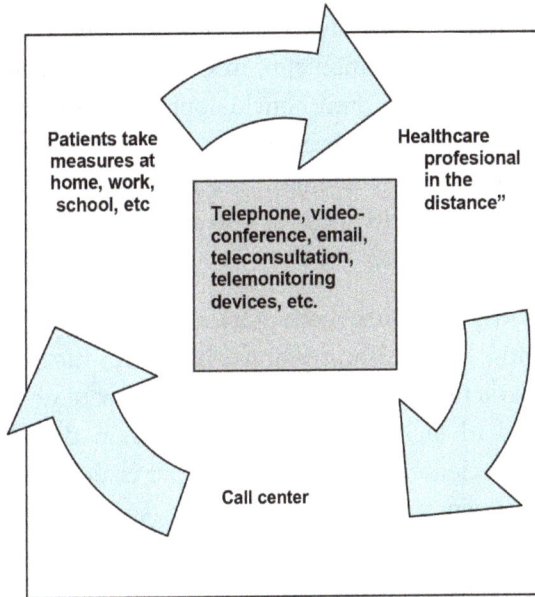

Figure 2. Telemedicine platform.

Telephone. Mainly, studies have focused in the telephone as a device to follow-up of patients but Balas et al. [22] described five possible actions that we could also do via telephone: (1) follow-up, (2) videoconsultation due to interactive telephone, (3) telephonic reminders of taking a medicine or doing an exercise, (4) calling health professionals if case of clinical deterioration, and (5) clinical investigation.

E-mail. Email is a rather quick tool for the patients to communicate with health professionals, making it easier for the latter to perform questionnaires so any given doubt of the patient or caregiver could be cleared up.

2. Chronic obstructive pulmonary diseases

It is now consensually agreed that an estimated number of 328 million people have COPD worldwide, that is, 168 million men and 160 million women. Moreover, COPD causes the death of 2.9 million people annually and it is projected to be the third cause of mortality by 2020 [23].

Whereas the three most important factors in individual patients that determine the economic and social costs of COPD are disease severity, presence of frequent exacerbations of disease and the presence of comorbidities, which are common (30–57%) in COPD patients [24], the current short-term and long-term strategies to reduce the burden of COPD comprise the triad of smoking cessation, minimizing acute exacerbations and management and prevention of comorbidities [25].

Hence, a high priority should be given to interventions aimed at delaying the progression of disease, preventing exacerbations and reducing the risk of comorbidities in order to alleviate the clinical and economic burden of COPD in Western countries [26]. Among these interventions, telemedicine has shown some promising results although no conclusive evidence has been accomplished. The effects of telemedicine in COPD have been addressed in previous systematic reviews [27, 28]; however, their conclusions are not consistent since the types of tested interventions have been rather heterogeneous. These interventions range from simple telephone or video interviews to daily telemonitoring of physiological parameters or symptoms data, and that is why comparativeness of one study to the other does not come along easily.

So far, there is moderate evidence of the benefit of telemedicine in COPD, in terms of increasing quality of life and reducing hospital admissions. Basically, the problem has been that in previous years the studies included in systematic reviews were underpowered, had heterogeneous populations and had lack of detailed intervention descriptions and of the care processes that accompanied telemonitoring [29]. Another issue is the clinical scenario where patients are usually recruited. For instance, telemedicine can be offered to those patients prone to exacerbations that are in stable condition [30], or right after admission regardless of the number of previous exacerbations or FEV_1 obstruction severity [31].

Regarding telemonitoring (understood as retrieving periodically clinical data such as oxygen saturation, heart rate, symptoms, etc.), recent data including randomized clinical trials of good quality are now available; however, some of them are still underpowered. In terms of hospital admissions, one of the latest systematic reviews on the matter, which included eight studies with 486 patients randomized to home telemonitoring or usual care, determined a significant lower risk of hospitalizations in the telemonitoring group. However, healthcare utilization in general was similar in both groups, since it was not clear whether the utilization was due to respiratory events specifically, and the lower range of compliance to telemonitoring reported by some studies may have influenced the ability of detecting clinical deterioration [32]. Moreover, even between this data retrieved on a daily basis there were different clinical features measured, which end up inevitability in being quite difficult to integrate quantitative variables because of missing or noncomparative data. Thus, the extrapolation of these results to the general population should be carried out with absolute caution. The usual problem with these systematic reviews is that, due to the heterogeneity of outcomes and the way the studies have assessed them, it is troublesome to determine the true effect of telemonitoring on COPD patients. For instance, adding a closer approach to patients with videoconsultations to the usual telemonitoring, which would be ideal in order to obtain higher rates of compliance or reduction of the use of healthcare resources in general, failed to demonstrate differences in hospital admissions or time to first admission or all-cause hospital admissions [33].

Detection and management of COPD exacerbations in early stages is an important step in order to reduce hospital admissions and the consequent increase of quality of life and reduction of health costs in general. So far, telemedicine has proven to be a useful tool to achieve this.

Physical activity, one of the strong mortality predictors in COPD patients, if not the strongest, has not been properly issued. Although no conclusive evidence of telemedicine benefit exists on this regard, the use of telehealthcare may lead to increased physical activity level [34]. A recent study that evaluated the feasibility of a telerehabilitation program compared to a regular outpatient program, showed an increase of physical activity measured by steps/day in the telerehabilitation group, with acceptable rates of satisfaction with the service, although no differences were found when the 6-minute walking test, dyspnea measured by the Medical Research Council or quality of life measured by the St. George's Respiratory Questionnaire were compared [35].

The cost-effectiveness of telemedicine in COPD is yet to be determined. In fact, a recent study carried out in the United Kingdom, which recruited 3230 patients where both at baseline and follow-up participants with COPD made up the largest telehealth intervention group, showed that costs of self-reported service use, combined with telehealth intervention costs, were greater for the group randomized to telehealth in addition to standard care than for the group randomized to usual care alone [36]. However, the validity of this conclusion may be biased for two reasons. First, the trial recruiters had foreknowledge of the allocation groups in many cases [37], and second, its transferability to other healthcare systems was not taken in consideration since the trial did not include all community and healthcare resources. Thus, a recent Danish trial (TeleCare North) will determine the real benefit of telemedicine in COPD in terms of health-related quality of life and the incremental cost-effectiveness ratio through a large-scale, pragmatic, cluster-randomized trial with nested economic evaluation [38].

Quality of life, a paramount feature in COPD and a strong predictor of mortality, has been analyzed irregularly. Once again, the instruments used to determine the health related quality of life vary greatly among the telemedicine studies (i.e., Chronic Respiratory Disease Questionnaire, Chronic Respiratory Questionnaire, St. George's Respiratory Questionnaire (SGRQ), Clinical COPD Questionnaire, EURO-QOL-5D Questionnaire, Medical Outcome Study Short-Form 36 Questionnaire), so comparative data is deficient. Overall, no significant differences have been found between a home telemonitoring group and the usual care group [32].

The aim of telemedicine toward COPD patients should be to keep this population outside the hospital or the emergency rooms. Although there is evidence that this aim has been achieved in some studies, we are still in need of larger clinical trials which include a rigorous cost-effectiveness analysis in terms of use of healthcare resources separated by respiratory diseases or not, quality of life, and mortality. Furthermore, a 6- or 12-month follow-up is insufficient to determine conclusive differences in favor of telemedicine.

3. Asthma

Asthma is a worldwide disease affecting 300 million of people, and its economic and social costs are mostly related to emergency visits and hospital admissions. Self-monitoring of symptoms and peak flow, following a written action plan and attending regular visits to their physician, have demonstrated to improve asthma control [39], and that is why approaches through telemedicine have been done to increase its control and follow-up. It has been hypothesized that providing self-monitoring tools such as easy-to-use handheld electronic monitoring devices or symptom questionnaires, patients can gain insight into their level of asthma control which gives them suggestions for subsequent treatment adjustment [40]. This is why telemedicine for asthma appears to be a promising tool to achieve this so wished for self-control and management of the disease.

However, there are some pitfalls regarding telemedicine for asthma. If noncomparative data due to the different sort of interventions is a main issue for COPD, the problem is probably more serious for asthma. One of the most relevant systematic reviews in the matter included 21 studies, of which nine consisted in telephone calls, two in videoconferences, two in using the Internet, one in short text messaging, one in a combination of short text and Internet, and six more using other networked communications. This study demonstrated no improvement of quality of life and even a nonsignificant increase of emergency room visits in the telemedicine group, although a significant reduction of hospitalizations was observed [41]. However, some authors have stated some concerns about these meta-analysis conclusions. First of all, there were only few examples of a comprehensive telemanagement approach in asthma (defined as a treatment plan, self-monitoring of lung function by FEV_1 and asthma control with feedback and e-communication with a professional to support this self-management), and second, patients in the control strategies often received an enhanced form of usual care, which makes it difficult to draw final conclusions on the effectiveness of telemanagement in asthma [40]. A more recent meta-analysis of 20 trials involving 10,406 asthmatic patients where common outcomes employed were healthcare utilization, quality of life and symptoms, concluded that the median effect of telemedicine was weakly positive, and that there were not differences between the types of interventions (telemonitoring, routine voice contact or videoconferencing). But the problem with this positive effect is that a publication bias exists due to the tendency of more positive results reported in earlier studies, which contained heterogeneous outcomes measurement and assessment [42].

Regarding cost-effectiveness we are still in need of studies addressing the topic specifically, situation that withholds the use of telemedicine for asthma unquestionably. Probably the only evidence of cost-effectiveness of Internet-based self-management compared with usual care, showed no significant differences during a follow-up of one year. However, this study had several limitations, acknowledge by the authors. First, the quality adjusted life year estimates were calculated out of only two measurements throughout one year. Second, patients were inevitable conscious of the allocated group, which may have influenced their utility ratings. And third, the economic evaluation was limited to one year only [43]. Regarding a specific feature of telemedicine, another study showed that telephone consultations led by experienced nurses enabled a greater proportion of asthma patients to be reviewed at no additional cost to the health service, although these findings should not be extrapolated as a thorough cost-effectiveness analysis, compared to the comprehensive telemanagement as explained before [44, 45].

Despite the similar moderate evidence either for asthma or COPD, there are some differences when telehealthcare main purposes are compared between the two diseases. While in COPD telemedicine aims to reduce exacerbations or their early detection in order to avoid emergency rooms visits or hospital admissions, in asthma these objectives are usually directed at assuring a better symptoms self-control and adherence to treatment, considering that undertreatment is the most common problem in European asthmatic subjects [46], and its usual presentation at early stages of life. A fitter control of asthma has been reported possibly secondary to the opportunity of register symptoms continually, thus, the patient obtained a more accurate picture of his disease severity and complied to treatment with a closer and efficient self-monitoring. However, this severity awareness led to an increased number of unscheduled visits and a harmful consumption of inhaled corticosteroids, which increased their adverse effects [47]. In a similar fashion, another study revealed that 43 patients under a mobile telephone interactive self-control system and compared with a control group, presented significantly higher mean daily dosage of either inhaled or systemic corticosteroids during the study period. Nonetheless, this system also demonstrated fewer unscheduled visits to the emergency department; higher peak expiratory flows at 4, 5, and 6 moths; higher FEV_1 at 6 months; and better quality of life at 3 months after inclusion [48].

Compliance to new technologies is a relevant feature of telemedicine since not all of public health systems can afford them, and there are still underprivileged groups who are not familiar to these sorts of interventions. It seems that telemedicine for asthma is feasible, although when compared to a web based self-management, patients presented higher rates of adherence to the classic paper based strategies of self-control of symptoms and action plans, though other critical feature such as lung function data was not reliable when the patient wrote it down on his own [49].

In the pediatric population there is also lacking evidence of telemedicine benefit. Telemonitoring of lung function on daily home spirometry in 44 children with professional feedback did not reduce the frequency of exacerbations significantly when compared to conventional treatment, nor the number of unscheduled visits, FEV_1, quality of life or use of inhaled corticosteroids [50]. This finding could be explained by the fact that a highly variable peak expiratory flow and FEV_1 values at time of symptoms and a complete overlap in distributions between symptoms-free days and at times of symptoms [51], and also by the underpowered nature of the study.

In conclusion, even though telemedicine for asthma seems to be a useful and promising tool for empowering the asthmatic patients in order to guarantee the self-control of the disease, the evidence of its benefit is still unclear. The short follow-ups, the heterogeneity of subjects and the insufficient evidence of its cost-effectiveness, are paramount aspects that restrain the use of telemedicine for asthmatic patients. We advocate for the tailoring treatment to the individual needs as the cornerstone of telehealthcare, although more studies are called for so the real effect of this new technologies can be elucidated.]

4. Sleep-related breathing disorders and obstructive sleep apnea

Speaking of sleep-related breathing disorders, obstructive sleep apnea (OSA) is a prevalent disease that affects approximately 6–7% of global population, although these figures probably underestimate the real OSA prevalence. OSA is a sleep disorder in wich breathing repeatedly stops and starts, which lead to hypoxemia, subsequent arousals, sleep fragmentation, thus, a poor sleep quality in general. The main symptom is excessive daytime sleepiness, and is now acknowledge as an independent cardiovascular risk factor, increasing the probability of presenting hypertension, coronary artery disease, congestive cardiac failure, and stroke [52]. Attended full in-lab polysomnography (PSG) is the gold standard for OSA diagnosis, an expensive test that demands plenty of time as well as fully trained technicians, and that is why simplified sleep data recollection systems have been approved by the scientific societies for patients with high or low pretest probability of OSA, in order to reduce the waiting list for PSG [53]. Despite the increase of accredited sleep units, the demand of sleep studies has also increased over the years considering the prevalence of the disease. Therefore, waiting lists remain long [54]. Finally, continuous positive airway pressure (CPAP) is by far the recommended treatment for symptomatic or severe OSA, and it is known to reduce cardiovascular death and non-fatal cardiovascular events [55], however, adherence to treatment has been a troublesome factor in such a way that the first year of long-term treatment usually between 25 and 30% of patients drop out the device [56]. Having said this, there have been some efforts to reduce the long waiting lists and increase the rates of CPAP adherence through telemedicine.

Regarding OSA diagnosis, the evidence of telemedicine usefulness is limited. So far, the American Academy of Sleep Medicine has classified the sleep recording devices into four categories. Full-attended in-lab PSG would be type 1; comprehensive portable unattended PSG with a minimum of seven channels (including electroencephalogram, electrooculogram, chin electromyogram, electrocardiogram or heart rate, airflow, respiratory effort, and oxygen saturation) corresponds to type 2; type 3 comprises modified portable systems with a minimum of four channels monitored, including ventilation or airflow (at least two channels or respiratory movement, or respiratory movement and airflow), heart rate or electrocardiogram, and oxygen saturation comprise; and finally type 4 includes continuous single or dual bioparameters with one or two channels, typically including oxygen saturation or airflow [57]. Despite the limitations of sensor losses that lead to technically inadequate recordings, the inability to assess sleep time duration or the distinction of apneas (central or obstructive), and the vast heterogeneity of sensors and recorders, the studies have confirmed the overall usefulness of type 3 devices, especially if they focus on the outcome which results in earlier access to treatment for the patient, specially those at high-risk of OSA. An alternative to type 3 devices is the home-polysomnography (H-PSG), which enables the home centered care for patients and a complete sleep evaluation allowing the possibility of diagnosing a large panel of sleep disorders. Thus, this H-PSG intends to perform as well as a full-attended PSG though in an unattended surrounding, without continuous supervision. A technician hooks-up the device, and this factor limits the wide us of this technique [58]. Since the loss of data is still a big issue with type 2 or 3 devices, potential future developments include the use of assistive technology and telemedicine to allow real-time remote monitoring.

To enhance the quality of H-PSG signal, real-time telematics data transmission has been tested generating successful and high-fidelity recordings through a cell phone for an easily deployed home monitor device [59], and a failure rate of 11% of telemonitored in-hospital unattended PSG compared to a 23% failure for unattended H-PSG was observed in another study [60]. Moreover, a pilot study, where 90% of recordings were of excellent quality, consisted in a wireless device to obtain real-time remote supervision of H-PSG from the sleep lab [61]. With this amount of evidence, it seems telemedicine for sleep studies recordings is feasible and may be an important step to reduce the failure rates of home devices; however, there are important barriers for implementing telemedicine for sleep studies regularly. Telemonitoring devices are complex as well as their software; hence, incompatibility problems with other computer programs should be expected. Furthermore, the cost-effectiveness of these systems is yet to be determined considering the fact that the home must be equipped with a computer and Internet connection, along with high specifications for computer programs. However, investigations using integrated circuits available on the market (mobile telephony) have been conducted to simplify access to these technologies [62]. Last but not least, there are also problems related to privacy protection and security of medical data transmission [58]. An ongoing telehealth out-of-laboratory "Fast Track for Sleep Apnea" program for veterans has been reported, that has helped to relieve clinical load at the central sleep program, improved local access to sleep care, and improved patient satisfaction with health care for sleep-related breathing disorders. Nonetheless, the following challenges have been acknowledged so far: the programs needed to be properly integrated with other data management systems and data storage devices must be interfaced with computers attached to the VA server; data loss; and maintaining quality control using metrics [63]. Either way, further research is required to determine the role of telemedicine in sleep-related breathing disorders diagnosis, especially for OSA.

CPAP has shown to wipe out the adverse effect of severe OSA, especially those effects related to cardiovascular diseases. However, the rates of adherence to CPAP are still far of being acceptable. That is way any measure to achieve CPAP adherence is needed, and new approaches such as telemedicine seems to be feasible and cost-effective. Compliance to CPAP is a complex process that involves the participation of the device itself, family support, physicians, health care personal, sleep unit, and government politics [64]. So far, low-quality evidence justifies the use of supportive interventions added to the usual clinical practice to increase CPAP adherence [65] and, similar to previous items, more clinical trials are called for to clear up the role of these interventions, where telemedicine is included. Earlier works presented contradictory results. A statistically significant higher adherence was found in a telemedicine-guided naïve to CPAP patients recently diagnosed with OSA along with greater satisfaction, concluding that telehealth might be cost-effective for CPAP adherence management [66]; while no differences were found in hours of CPAP use, functional status or client satisfaction in another study [67]. It is worth to mention that these two studies followed the patients for a 12-week and 30 days period, respectively. More recent clinical trials have added some light to the subject. A 12-month telemedicine intervention resulted in a median CPAP usage that was 0.9 h/night higher than that of an attention control group after 6 months, and 2.0 h/night higher after 12 months in a clinical trial including 250 patients, although the median adherence of all patients was low, with 19% of patients refusing the use of CPAP at all [68]. Another clinical trial of 75 patients, showed higher rates of adherence to CPAP after 3 months of telemedicine intervention, which was determined as a significant predictor of adherence, apart from age and sleepiness symptoms measured by the Epworth Sleepiness Scale [69]. Finally, although no difference in hours of CPAP use was found in a study including 139 OSA patients, telemedicine showed to be more cost-effective than the usual face-to-face management, with travel costs and lost work time being the most important sources of savings [70].

Improvement in case detection and the resulting higher healthcare demand has not been accompanied by any real improvement in OSA management. In addition, health resources assigned to OSA and its treatment have been found to be inadequate [71]. Telemedicine is an appealing approach that needs to be explored and taken into consideration in order to obtain a diagnosis and follow-up of sleep-related breathing disorders in a more timely fashion, which would help to achieve the desirable management of these diseases.

5. Lung transplantation

[Lung transplantation is offered for a great variety on respiratory diseases that have reached their end-stage, where no other treatment would obtain a reasonable survival. They are complex patients who are in need of aggressive immunosuppressive treatment for a lifetime that exposes them to opportunistic infections; so numerous complications are often taking place. By far, the major problem for every lung transplant patient is the allograft dysfunction, either acute or chronic (basically in its form of bronchiolitis obstructive syndrome). Allograft dysfunction is characterized for a functional decline of the implant, which is usually measured by FEV_1 [72], and daily home spirometry has been shown to lead to earlier detection and staging of bronchiolitis obstructive syndrome when compared with standard pulmonary function testing [73]. Concerning the need of retrieving daily spirometric data, telemedicine has been studied as a feasible instrument, making some interesting progress conducive to a more efficient follow-up of patients and the prompt recognition of a possible complication.

Earlier works determined the telemonitored spirometry as feasible, valid, reliable, and repeatable, when compared to the regular in-clinic functional testing [74–76]. Although these studies were clearly underpowered due to the small samples included. While on earlier works the objective is to determine the technical aspects of collecting acceptable spirometries, recent works have carried out clinical trials to demonstrate that a computerized rule-based decision support algorithm for nursing triage of potential acute bronchopulmonary events is effective [72, 77], or the identification of these events taking decision rules developed using wavelet analysis of declines in spirometry and increases in respiratory symptoms [78]. In conclusion, the evidence of the increase of quality of life and reduction of hospital admissions seems fairly positive, though we are still in need of more studies [79] and the training process for both medical staff and patients needs to be thorough [80] A different approach was revised by another study where telemedicine was employed in a clinical trial for lung transplant candidates, and clinical outcome measures were monitoring adherence and level of communication (for monitor acceptability and utilization), hospital length of stay after transplantation and survival at 4 months. However, no significant differences in clinical outcomes between groups were determined [81].

Similar to the previous three respiratory conditions, telemedicine for lung transplant patients is feasible. Still and all, no cost-effectiveness has been demonstrated, thus, larger clinical trials are required to establish the position of these new techniques in lung transplantation.

6. Conclusions

Telemedicine is a helpful tool to improve chronic respiratory patient management. Almost all results shows reduction in Emergency visits and the number of hospitalizations but despite of these results its implementation is troublesome and with different kind of factors relationship with this slowly development. Most users report that the difficult to use the devices or technology platform is the most important factor related to refuse telemedicine by users. We need to work to improve its implementation through educational programs to healthcare professionals and patients.

Author details

Gonzalo Segrelles-Calvo[1*] and Daniel López-Padilla[2]

*Address all correspondence to: gsegrelles@hotmail.com

1 Pneumology Department, University Hospital Rey Juan Carlos, Mostoles, Spain

2 Pneumology Department, University Hospital Gregorio Maranon, Madrid, Spain

References

[1] Jaana M, Paré G, Sicotte C. Home telemonitoring for respiratory conditions: a systematic review. Am J Manag Care. 2009;15:313–20.

[2] Sabati N, Snyder M, Edin-Stibbe C, Lindgren B, Finkelstein S. Facilitators and barriers to adherence with home monitoring using electronic spirometry. AACN Clin Issues. 2001;12:178–85.

[3]   World Health Organization. http://www.who.it. Last up to date 21st December 2015.

[4]   American Telemedicine Association (ATA). http://atmedad.org. Last up to date 21st December 2015.

[5]   Bashur RL. On the definition and evaluation of telemedicine. J Telemed Telecare. 1995;1:19–30.

[6]   Norris TG. Telemedicine and teleradiology. Radiol Technol. 1997;71:139–64.

[7]   Bashur R, Lovett J. Assessment of telemedicine: results of initial experience. Aviat Space Environ Med. 1997;48:65–70.

[8]   House AM, Roberts JM. Telemedicine in Canada. Can Med Assoc J. 1997;117:386–8.

[9]   Kopec A, Salazar AJ. Generalities about telemedicine. In: Bustamante MA, Rodríguez G, editors. Uses of telecommunication in Health in Andean region. Telemedicina. Perú: ORAS-CONHU; 2006.

[10] Segrelles-Calvo G, Chiner E, Fernández-Fabrellas E. Acceptance of telemedicine among healthcare professionals. Arch Bronconeumol. 2015;51:611–2.

[11] Mira-Solves JJ, Orozco-Beltrán D, Sánchez-Molla M, Sánchez-García J. Chronic patients satisfaction about telemedicine devices and the care received. ValCrònic Program. Aten Primaria. 2014;46:16-23.

[12] Jódar-Sánchez F, Ortega F, Parra C, Gómez-Suárez C, Jordán A, Pérez P, et al. Implementation of a telehealth programme for patients with severe chronic obstructive pulmonary disease treated with long-term oxygen therapy. J Telemed Telecare. 2013;19:11–7.

[13] Vitacca M, Bianchi L, Guerra A, Fracchia C, Spanavello A, Balbi B, et al. Tele-assistance in chronic respiratory failure patients: a randomised clinical trial. Eur Respir J. 2009;33:411–8.

[14] Motulsky A, Sicotte C, Lamothe L, Winslade N, Tamblyn R. Electronic prescriptions and disruptions to the jurisdiction of community pharmacists. Soc Sci Med. 2011;73:121–8.

[15] Cresswell K, Coleman J, Slee A, Williams R, Sheikh A; ePrescribing Programme Team. Investigating and learning lessons from early experiences of implementing ePrescribing systems into NHS hospitals: a questionnaire study. PLoS One. 2013;8:e71238–49.

[16] Mahmud K, LeSage K. Telemedicine—a new idea for home care. Caring. 1995;14:48–50.

[17] Johnston B, Wheeler L, Deuser J, Sousa KH. Outcomes of the Kaiser Permanente Tele-Home Health Research Project. Arch Fam Med. 2000;9:40–5.

[18] Nakamura K, Takano T, Akao C. The effectiveness of videophones in home healthcare for the elderly. Med Care. 1999;37:117–25.

[19] Hoaas H, Andreassen HK, Lien LA, Hjalmarsen A, Zanaboni P. Adherence and factors affecting satisfaction in long-term telerehabilitation for patients with chronic obstructive pulmonary disease: a mixed methods study. BMC Med Inform Decis Mak. 2016;16:26.

[20] Bauer MS, Krawczyk L, Miller CJ, Abel E, Osser DN, Franz A, et al. Team-based telecare for bipolar disorder. Telemed J E Health. 2016 (in press).

[21] Story A, Garfein RS, Hayward A, Rusovich V, Dadu A, Soltan V, et al. Monitoring therapy compliance of tuberculosis patients by using video-enabled electronic devices. Emerg Infect Dis. 2016;22:538-40

[22] Balas EA, Jaffrey F, Kuperman GJ, Boren SA, Brown GD, Pinciroli F, et al. Electronic communication with patients. Evaluation of distance medicine technology. JAMA. 1997;278:152–9.

[23] Vos T, Flaxman AD, Naghavi M, Lozano R, Michaud C, Ezzati M, Shibuya K, Salomon JA, Abdalla S, Aboyans V, et al. Years lived with disability (YLDs) for 1160 sequelae of 289 diseases and injuries 1990–2010: a systematic analysis for the Global Burden of Disease study 2010. Lancet. 2012;380:2163–96.

[24] Mannino DM, Buist AS. Global burden of COPD: risk factors, prevalence, and future trends. Lancet. 2007;370:765–73.

[25] López-Campos JL, Tan W, Soriano JB. Global burden of COPD. Respirology. 2016;21:14–23. doi: 10.1111/resp.12660.

[26] Mannino DM, Higuchi K, Yu TC, Zhou H, Li Y, Tian H, Suh K. Economic burden of chronic obstructive pulmonary disease by presence of comorbidities. Chest. 2015;148:138–50.

[27] Polisena J, Tran K, Cimon K, Hutton B, McGill S, Palmer K, Scott RE. Home telehealth for chronic obstructive pulmonary disease: a systematic review and meta-analysis. J Telemed Telecare. 2010;16:120–7. doi: 10.1258/jtt.2009.090812.

[28] McLean S, Nurmatov U, Liu JL, Pagliari C, Car J, Sheikh A. Telehealthcare for chronic obstructive pulmonary disease: Cochrane Review and meta-analysis. Br J Gen Pract. 2012;62:e739–49. doi: 10.3399/bjgp12X658269.

[29] Bolton CE, Waters CS, Peirce S, Elwyn G; EPSRC and MRC Grand Challenge Team. Insufficient evidence of benefit: a systematic review of home telemonitoring for COPD. J Eval Clin Pract. 2011;17:1216–22. doi: 10.1111/j.1365-2753.2010.01536.x.

[30] Segrelles Calvo G, Gómez-Suárez C, Soriano JB, Zamora E, Gónzalez-Gamarra A, González-Béjar M, Jordán A, Tadeo E, Sebastián A, Fernández G, Ancochea. A home telehealth program for patients with severe COPD: the PROMETE study. Respir Med. 2014;108:453–62. doi: 10.1016/j.rmed.2013.12.003.

[31]   Gottlieb M, Marsaa K, Andreassen H, Strømstad G, Godtfredsen N. Feasibility of a telecare solution for patients admitted with COPD exacerbation: screening data from a pulmonary ward in a university hospital. Eur Clin Respir J. 2014;1:24193

[32]   Cruz J, Brooks D, Marques A. Home telemonitoring effectiveness in COPD: a systematic review. Int J Clin Pract. 2014;68:369–78. doi: 10.1111/ijcp.12345.

[33]   Ringbæk T, Green A, Laursen LC, Frausing E, Brøndum E, Ulrik CS. Effect of tele health care on exacerbations and hospital admissions in patients with chronic obstructive pulmonary disease: a randomized clinical trial. Int J Chron Obstruct Pulmon Dis. 2015;10:1801–8. doi: 10.2147/COPD.S85596.

[34]   Lundell S, Holmner Å, Rehn B, Nyberg A, Wadell K. Telehealthcare in COPD: a systematic review and meta-analysis on physical outcomes and dyspnea. Respir Med. 2015;109:11–26. doi: 10.1016/j.rmed.2014.10.008.

[35]   Paneroni M, Colombo F, Papalia A, Colitta A, Borghi G, Saleri M, Cabiaglia A, Azzalini E, Vitacca M. Is telerehabilitation a safe and viable option for patients with COPD? A feasibility study. COPD. 2015;12:217–25. doi: 10.3109/15412555.2014.933794.

[36]   Henderson C, Knapp M, Fernández JL, Beecham J, Hirani SP, Cartwright M, Rixon L, Beynon M, Rogers A, Bower P, Doll H, Fitzpatrick R, Steventon A, Bardsley M, Hendy J, Newman SP; Whole System Demonstrator evaluation team. Cost effectiveness of telehealth for patients with long term conditions (Whole Systems Demonstrator telehealth questionnaire study): nested economic evaluation in a pragmatic, cluster randomised controlled trial. BMJ. 2013;346:f1035. doi: 10.1136/bmj.f1035.

[37]   Steventon A, Bardsley M, Billings J, Dixon J, Doll H, Hirani S, Cartwright M, Rixon L, Knapp M, Henderson C, Rogers A, Fitzpatrick R, Hendy J, Newman S; Whole System Demonstrator Evaluation Team. Effect of telehealth on use of secondary care and mortality: findings from the Whole System Demonstrator cluster randomised trial. BMJ. 2012;344:e3874. doi: 10.1136/bmj.e3874.

[38]   Udsen FW, Lilholt PH, Hejlesen O, Ehlers LH. Effectiveness and cost-effectiveness of telehealthcare for chronic obstructive pulmonary disease: study protocol for a cluster randomized controlled trial. Trials. 2014;15:178. doi: 10.1186/1745-6215-15-178.

[39]   Gibson PG, Powell H, Coughlan J, Wilson AJ, Abramson M, Haywood P, et al. Self management education and regular practitioner review for adults with asthma (Cochrane review). In: The Cochrane Library, Issue 4. Chichester, UK: John Wiley and Sons, Ltd; 2003.

[40]   Van Gaalen JL, Hashimoto S, Sont JK. Telemanagement in asthma: an innovative and effective approach. Curr Opin Allergy Clin Immunol. 2012;12:235–40. doi: 10.1097/ACI. 0b013e3283533700.

[41]   McLean S, Chandler D, Nurmatov U, Liu J, Pagliari C, Car J, Sheikh A. Telehealthcare for asthma: a Cochrane review. CMAJ. 2011;183:E733–42. doi: 10.1503/cmaj.101146.

[42] Wootton R. Twenty years of telemedicine in chronic disease management—an evidence synthesis. J Telemed Telecare. 2012;18:211–20. doi: 10.1258/jtt.2012.12021.

[43] van der Meer V, van den Hout WB, Bakker MJ, Rabe KF, Sterk PJ, Assendelft WJ, Kievit J, Sont JK; SMASHING (Self-Management in Asthma Supported by Hospitals, ICT, Nurses and General Practitioners) Study Group. Cost-effectiveness of Internet-based self-management compared with usual care in asthma. PLoS One. 2011;6:e27108. doi: 10.1371/journal.pone.0027108.

[44] Pinnock H, McKenzie L, Price D, Sheikh A. Cost-effectiveness of telephone or surgery asthma reviews: economic analysis of a randomised controlled trial. Br J Gen Pract. 2005;55:119–24.

[45] Pinnock H, Adlem L, Gaskin S, Harris J, Snellgrove C, Sheikh A. Accessibility, clinical effectiveness, and practice costs of providing a telephone option for routine asthma reviews: phase IV controlled implementation study. Br J Gen Pract. 2007;57:714–22.

[46] Raben KF, Vermeire PA, Soriano JB, Maier WC. Clinical management of asthma in 1999: the Asthma Insights and Reality in Europe (AIRE) study. Eur Respir J. 2000;16:802–7.

[47] Rasmussen LM, Phanareth K, Nolte H, Backer V. Internet-based monitoring of asthma: a long-term, randomized clinical study of 300 asthmatic subjects. J Allergy Clin Immunol. 2005;115:1137–42.

[48] Liu WT, Huang CD, Wang CH, Lee KY, Lin SM, Kuo HP. A mobile telephone-based interactive self-care system improves asthma control. Eur Respir J. 2011;37:310–7. doi: 10.1183/09031936.00000810.

[49] Araújo L, Jacinto T, Moreira A, Castel-Branco MG, Delgado L, Costa-Pereira A, Fonseca J. Clinical efficacy of web-based versus standard asthma self-management. J Investig Allergol Clin Immunol. 2012;22:28–34.

[50] Deschildre A, Béghin L, Salleron J, Iliescu C, Thumerelle C, Santos C, Hoorelbeke A, Scalbert M, Pouessel G, Gnansounou M, Edmé JL, Matran R. Home telemonitoring (forced expiratory volume in 1 s) in children with severe asthma does not reduce exacerbations. Eur Respir J. 2012;39:290–6. doi: 10.1183/09031936.00185310.

[51] Brouwer AF, Brand PL, Roorda RJ, Duiverman EJ. Airway obstruction at time of symptoms prompting use of reliever therapy in children with asthma. Acta Paediatr. 2010;99:871–6. doi: 10.1111/j.1651-2227.2010.01715.x.

[52] Ge X, Han F, Huang Y, Zhang Y, Yang T, Bai C, Guo X. Is obstructive sleep apnea associated with cardiovascular and all-cause mortality? PLoS One. 2013;8:e69432. doi: 10.1371/journal.pone.0069432.

[53] Collop NA. Clinical guidelines for the use of unattended portable monitors in the diagnosis of obstructive sleep apnea in adult patients. J Clin Sleep Med. 2007;3:737e47.

[54] Masa Jimenez JF, Barbé Illa F, Capote Gil F, Chiner Vives E. Resources and delays in the diagnosis of sleep apnea-hypopnea syndrome. Arch Bronconeumol. 2007;43:188e98.

[55] Wang J, Yu W, Gao M, Zhang F, Li Q, Gu C, Yu Y, Wei Y. Continuous positive airway pressure treatment reduces cardiovascular death and non-fatal cardiovascular events in patients with obstructive sleep apnea: a meta-analysis of 11 studies. Int J Cardiol. 2015;191:128–31. doi: 10.1016/j.ijcard.2015.05.003.

[56] Meurice JC. Improving compliance to CPAP in sleep apnea syndrome: from coaching to telemedicine. Rev Mal Respir. 2012;29:7–10. doi: 10.1016/j.rmr.2011.12.007.

[57] Chesson AL Jr, Berry RB, Pack A; American Academy of Sleep Medicine; American Thoracic Society; American College of Chest Physicians. Practice parameters for the use of portable monitoring devices in the investigation of suspected obstructive sleep apnea in adults. Sleep. 2003;26:907–13.

[58] Bruyneel M, Ninane V. Unattended home-based polysomnography for sleep disordered breathing: current concepts and perspectives. Sleep Med Rev. 2014;18:341–7. doi: 10.1016/j.smrv.2013.12.002.

[59] Kayyali HA, Weimer S, Frederick C, Martin C, Basa D, Juguilon JA, Jugilioni F. Remotely attended home monitoring of sleep disorders. Telemed J E Health. 2008;14:371–4. doi: 10.1089/tmj.2007.0058.

[60] Gagnadoux F, Pelletier-Fleury N, Philippe C, Rakotonanahary D, Fleury B. Home unattended vs hospital telemonitored polysomnography in suspected obstructive sleep apnea syndrome: a randomized crossover trial. Chest. 2002;121:753e8.

[61] Bruyneel M, Van den Broecke S, Libert W, Ninane V. Real-time attended home-polysomnography with telematic data transmission. Int J Med Inform. 2013;82:696e701.

[62] Dellaca R, Montserrat JM, Govoni L, Pedotti A, Navajas D, Farré R. Telemetric CPAP titration at home in patients with sleep apnea-hypopnea syndrome. Sleep Med. 2011;12:153e7.

[63] Hirshkowitz M, Sharafkhaneh A. A telemedicine program for diagnosis and management of sleep-disordered breathing: the fast-track for sleep apnea tele-sleep program. Semin Respir Crit Care Med. 2014;35:560–70. doi: 10.1055/s-0034-1390069.

[64] Shapiro GK, Shapiro CM. Factors that influence CPAP adherence: an overview. Sleep Breath. 2010;14:323–35.

[65] Wozniak DR, Lasserson TJ, Smith I. Educational, supportive and behavioural interventions to improve usage of continuous positive airway pressure machines in adults with obstructive sleep apnoea. Cochrane Database Syst Rev. 2014;1:CD007736. doi: 10.1002/14651858.CD007736.pub2.

[66] Smith CE, Dauz ER, Clements F, Puno FN, Cook D, Doolittle G, Leeds W. Telehealth services to improve nonadherence: a placebo-controlled study. Telemed J E Health. 2006;12:289–96.

[67] Taylor Y, Eliasson A, Andrada T, Kristo D, Howard R. The role of telemedicine in CPAP compliance for patients with obstructive sleep apnea syndrome. Sleep Breath. 2006;10:132–8.

[68] Sparrow D, Aloia M, Demolles DA, Gottlieb DJ. A telemedicine intervention to improve adherence to continuous positive airway pressure: a randomised controlled trial. Thorax. 2010;65:1061–6. doi: 10.1136/thx.2009.133215.

[69] Fox N, Hirsch-Allen AJ, Goodfellow E, Wenner J, Fleetham J, Ryan CF, Kwiatkowska M, Ayas NT. The impact of a telemedicine monitoring system on positive airway pressure adherence in patients with obstructive sleep apnea: a randomized controlled trial. Sleep. 2012;35:477–81. doi: 10.5665/sleep.1728.

[70] Isetta V, Negrín MA, Monasterio C, Masa JF, Feu N, Álvarez A, Campos-Rodriguez F, Ruiz C, Abad J, Vázquez-Polo FJ, Farré R, Galdeano M, Lloberes P, Embid C, de la Peña M, Puertas J, Dalmases M, Salord N, Corral J, Jurado B, León C, Egea C, Muñoz A, Parra O, Cambrodi R, Martel-Escobar M, Arqué M, Montserrat JM; SPANISH SLEEP NETWORK. A Bayesian cost-effectiveness analysis of a telemedicine-based strategy for the management of sleep apnoea: a multicentre randomised controlled trial. Thorax. 2015;70:1054–61. doi: 10.1136/thoraxjnl-2015-207032.

[71] Rotenberg B, George C, Sullivan K, Wong E. Wait times for sleep apnea care in Ontario: a multidisciplinary assessment. Can Respir J. 2010;17:170–4.

[72] Finkelstein SM, Scudiero A, Lindgren B, Snyder M, Hertz MI. Decision support for the triage of lung transplant recipients on the basis of home-monitoring spirometry and symptom reporting. Heart Lung. 2005;34:201–8.

[73] Robson KS, West AJ. Improving survival outcomes in lung transplant recipients through early detection of bronchiolitis obliterans: daily home spirometry versus standard pulmonary function testing. Can J Respir Ther. 2014;50:17–22.

[74] Finkelstein SM, Snyder M, Edin-Stibbe C, Chlan L, Prasad B, Dutta P, Lindgren B, Wielinski C, Hertz MI. Monitoring progress after lung transplantation from home-patient adherence. J Med Eng Technol. 1996;20:203–10.

[75] Lindgren BR, Finkelstein SM, Prasad B, Dutta P, Killoren T, Scherber J, Stibbe CL, Snyder M, Hertz MI. Determination of reliability and validity in home monitoring data of pulmonary function tests following lung transplantation. Res Nurs Health. 1997;20:539–50.

[76] Wagner FM, Weber A, Park JW, Schiemanck S, Tugtekin SM, Gulielmos V, Schüler S. New telemetric system for daily pulmonary function surveillance of lung transplant recipients. Ann Thorac Surg. 1999;68:2033–8.

[77] Finkelstein SM, Lindgren BR, Robiner W, Lindquist R, Hertz M, Carlin BP, VanWormer A. A randomized controlled trial comparing health and quality of life of lung transplant recipients following nurse and computer-based triage utilizing home spirometry monitoring. Telemed J E Health. 2013;19:897–903. doi: 10.1089/tmj.2013.0049.

[78] Wang W, Finkelstein SM, Hertz MI. Automatic event detection in lung transplant recipients based on home monitoring of spirometry and symptoms. Telemed J E Health. 2013;19:658–63. doi: 10.1089/tmj.2012.0290.

[79] Fadaizadeh L, Najafizadeh K, Shafaghi S, Hosseini MS, Ghoroghi A. Using home spirometry for follow up of lung transplant recipients: "A Pilot Study". Tanaffos. 2013;12:64–9.

[80] Fadaizadeh L, Najafizadeh K, Shajareh E, Shafaghi S, Hosseini M, Heydari G. Home spirometry: assessment of patient compliance and satisfaction and its impact on early diagnosis of pulmonary symptoms in post-lung transplantation patients. J Telemed Telecare. 2016;22:127–31

[81] Mullan B, Snyder M, Lindgren B, Finkelstein SM, Hertz MI. Home monitoring for lung transplant candidates. Prog Transplant. 2003;13:176–82.

Permissions

List of Contributors

Sinchai Kamolphiwong, Thossapon Kamolphiwong and Soontorn Saechow
Department of Computer Engineering, Faculty of Engineering, Prince of Songkla University, Hatyai, Songkla, Thailand

Verapol Chandeeying
Faculty of Medicine, University of Phayao, Muang, Phayao, Thailand

Marcia R. Friesen, Bennet Gigliotti and Tik Wai (Kiral) Poon
Electrical & Computer Engineering, University of Manitoba, Winnipeg, Manitoba, Canada

Geletaw Sahle Tegenaw
Faculty of Computing, Jimma Institute of Technology, Jimma University (JU), Ethiopia

Fang Zhao and Meng Li
Brain and Behavior Discovery Institute and Department of Neurology, Medical College of Georgia, Augusta University, Augusta, Georgia, USA

Joe Z. Tsien
Brain and Behavior Discovery Institute and Department of Neurology, Medical College of Georgia, Augusta University, Augusta, Georgia, USA
Banna Biomedical Research Institute, Xi-Shuang-Ban-Na Prefecture, Yunnan Province, China

Sahr Wali and Catherine Demers
McMaster University, Hamilton, Canada

Karim Keshavjee
InfoClin Inc, Toronto, Canada

Chin-Feng Lin, Chung-Cheng Chang,Chao-Sheng Wang, Shiue-Li Cheng, Shiou-Yu Li and Lan-Yu Wu
Department of Electrical Engineering, National Taiwan Ocean University, Keelung, Taiwan

Shere-Er Wang
Department of Nursing, Ching Kuo Institute of Management and Health, Keelung, Taiwan

Yen-Chiao Lu
Department of Nursing, Chung Shan Medical University, Taichung, Taiwan

Chung-I Lin
Health Center of Gongliao, New Taipei City, Taiwan

Tim Yeh, Candice Lee and Jeffson Huang
Microlife, Taipei, Taiwan

Chic-Erh Weng and Sue-Hsien Chen
Department of Nursing Division, Chang Cung Memorial Hospital, Keelung Branch, Keelung, Taiwan

Bing-Leung Sun
Department of Applied Information and Multimedia, Ching Kuo Institute of Management and Health, Keelung, Taiwan

Sandeep Reddy
School of Medicine, Faculty of Health, Deakin University, Australia

Matjaž Krošel, Lana Švegl and Dejan Dinevski
Faculty of Medicine, University of Maribor, Maribor, Slovenia

Luka Vidmar
Telekom Slovenije d.d., Ljubljana, Slovenia

Mark Dominik Alscher
Robert-Bosch-Hospital, Stuttgart, Germany

Nico Schmidt
Bosch - Healthcare Solution GmbH, Waiblingen, Germany

Niloofar Mohammadzadeh and Reza Safdari
Department of Health Information Management, Tehran University of Medical Sciences, Tehran, Iran

Feras M. Ghazawi and Steven J. Glassman
Division of Dermatology, University of Ottawa, Ottawa, Ontario, Canada

Denis Sasseville and Ivan V. Litvinov
Division of Dermatology, McGill University Health Centre, Montréal, Québec, Canada

Gonzalo Segrelles-Calvo
Pneumology Department, University Hospital Rey Juan Carlos, Mostoles, Spain

Daniel López-Padilla
Pneumology Department, University Hospital Gregorio Maranon, Madrid, Spain

Index

www.ingramcontent.com/pod-product-compliance
Lightning Source LLC
Chambersburg PA
CBHW061947190326
41458CB00009B/2806